Blueprints **Notes & Cases**
Microbiology and Immunology

Blueprints **Notes & Cases**
Series Editor: Aaron B. Caughey MD, MPP, MPH

Blueprints *Notes & Cases—Microbiology and Immunology*
Monica Gandhi, Paul Baum, C. Bradley Hare, Aaron B. Caughey

Blueprints *Notes & Cases—Biochemistry, Genetics, and Embryology*
Juan E. Vargas, Aaron B. Caughey, Annie Tan, Jonathan Z. Li

Blueprints *Notes & Cases—Pharmacology*
Katherine Y. Yang, Larissa R. Graff, Aaron B. Caughey

Blueprints *Notes & Cases—Pathophysiology: Cardiovascular, Endocrine, and Reproduction*
Gordon Leung, Susan H. Tran, Tina O. Tan, Aaron B. Caughey

Blueprints *Notes & Cases—Pathophysiology: Pulmonary, Gastrointestinal, and Rheumatology*
Michael Filbin, Lisa M. Lee, Brian L. Shaffer, Aaron B. Caughey

Blueprints *Notes & Cases—Pathophysiology: Renal, Hematology, and Oncology*
Aaron B. Caughey, Christie del Castillo, Nancy Palmer, Karen Spizer, Dana N. Tuttle

Blueprints *Notes & Cases—Neuroscience*
Robert T. Wechsler, Alexander M. Morss, Courtney J. Wusthoff, Aaron B. Caughey

Blueprints *Notes & Cases—Behavioral Science and Epidemiology*
Judith Neugroschl, Jennifer Hoblyn, Christie del Castillo, Aaron B. Caughey

Blueprints **Notes & Cases**
Microbiology and Immunology

Monica Gandhi MD, MPH
Assistant Professor
Division of Infectious Diseases
Department of Medicine
University of California, San Francisco
San Francisco, California

Paul Baum, MD, PhD
Clinical Fellow
Division of Infectious Diseases
University of California at San Francisco
Postdoctoral Fellow
Gladstone Institute of Virology and Immunology
San Francisco General Hospital
San Francisco, California

C. Bradley Hare, MD
Assistant Professor
Division of Infectious Diseases
Department of Medicine
University of California, San Francisco
San Francisco, California

Aaron B. Caughey, MD, MPP, MPH
Clinical Instructor in Maternal-Fetal Medicine
Department of Obstetrics and Gynecology
University of California, San Francisco
San Francisco, California
Doctoral Candidate, Health Services and Policy Analysis
University of California, Berkeley
Berkeley, California

Series Editor: Aaron B. Caughey, MD, MPP, MPH

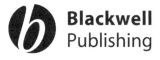
Blackwell
Publishing

© 2004 by Blackwell Publishing

Blackwell Publishing, Inc., 350 Main Street, Malden, Massachusetts 02148-5018, USA
Blackwell Publishing Ltd, 9600 Garsington Road, Oxford OX4 2DQ, UK
Blackwell Science Asia Pty Ltd, 550 Swanston Street, Carlton, Victoria 3053, Australia

03 04 05 06 5 4 3 2 1

ISBN: 1–4051-0347–7

Library of Congress Cataloging-in-Publication Data

Blueprints notes & cases : microbiology and immunology / Monica Gandhi .... [et al.].
    p. ; cm. — (Blueprints notes & cases)
  Includes index.
  ISBN 1-4051-0347-7 (pbk.)
  1. Medical microbiology—Case studies. 2. Immunology—Case studies.
  [DNLM: 1. Microbiology—Case Report. 2. Microbiology—Problems and Exercises. 3. Immunity—Case Report.
  4. Immunity—Problems and Exercises. QW 18.2 B658 2004] I. Title: Microbiology and immunology. II. Title: Blueprints notes
  and cases. III. Gandhi, Monica. IV. Series.
    QR46.B565 2004
    616'.01—dc21   2003010570

A catalogue record for this title is available from the British Library

Acquisitions: Beverly Copland
Development: Julia Casson
Production: Debra Lally
Cover design: Hannus Design Associates
Interior design: Janet Bollow Associates
Typesetter: Peirce Graphic Services in Stuart, Florida
Printed and bound by Courier Companies in Westford, MA

For further information on Blackwell Publishing, visit our website: www.blackwellpublishing.com

Notice: The indications and dosages of all drugs in this book have been recommended in the
medical literature and conform to the practices of the general community. The medications
described do not necessarily have specific approval by the Food and Drug Administration for
use in the diseases and dosages for which they are recommended. The package insert for each
drug should be consulted for use and dosage as approved by the FDA. Because standards for
usage change, it is advisable to keep abreast of revised recommendations, particularly those
concerning new drugs.

Contents

I. MICROBIOLOGY

II. IMMUNOLOGY

Contributor

Christie del Castillo
Class of 2003
University of California, San Francisco, School of Medicine
San Francisco, CA

Reviewers

Kelly Duckett
Class of 2004
Lake Erie College of Osteopathic Medicine
Erie, Pennsylvania

Puneet Gupta
Class of 2004
University of Texas Southwestern Medical School
Dallas, Texas

Amitha Harish
Class of 2004
Albany Medical College
Albany, New York

Jason Lane
Class of 2004
Tulane School of Medicine
New Orleans, Louisiana

Arne Olson
Class of 2004
Medical College of Wisconsin
Milwaukee, Wisconsin

Leigh Simmons
Class of 2004
Vanderbilt University School of Medicine
Nashville, Tennessee

Preface

The first two years of medical school are a demanding time for medical students. Whether the school follows a traditional curriculum or one that is case-based, every student is expected to learn and be able to apply basic science information in a clinical situation.

Medical schools are increasingly using clinical presentations as the background to teach the basic sciences. Case-based learning has become more common at many medical schools as it offers a way to catalogue the multitude of symptoms, syndromes, and diseases in medicine.

Blueprints **Notes & Cases is a new series by Blackwell Publishing designed to provide students a textbook to study the basic science topics combined with clinical data.** This method of learning is also the way to prepare for the clinical case format of USMLE questions. The eight books in this series will make the basic science topics not only more interesting, but also more meaningful and memorable. Students will be learning not only the why of a principle, but also how it might commonly be seen in practice.

The books in the *Blueprints* *Notes & Cases* series feature a comprehensive collection of cases that are designed to introduce one or more basic science topics. Through these cases, students gain an understanding of the coursework as they learn to:

- Think through the cases
- Look for classic presentations of most common diseases and syndromes
- Integrate the basic science content with clinical application
- Prepare for course exams and Step 1 USMLE
- Be prepared for clinical rotations

This series covers all the essential material needed in the basic science courses. Where possible, the books are organized in an organ-based system.

Clinical cases lead off and are the basis for discussion of the basic science content. A list of **"thought questions"** follows the case presentation. These questions are designed to challenge the reader to begin to think about how basic science topics apply to real-life clinical situations. The **answers to these questions** are integrated within the **basic science review and discussion** that follows. This offers a clinical framework from which to understand the basic content.

The discussion section is followed by a high-yield **Thumbnail table and Key Points box** which highlight and summarize the essential information presented in the discussion.

The cases also include two to four **multiple-choice questions** that allow readers to check their knowledge of that topic. Many of the answer explanations provide an opportunity for further discussion by delving into more depth in related areas. An **answer key** for these questions is at the end of the section for easy reference, and **full answer explanations** can be found at the end of the book.

This new series was designed to provide comprehensive content in a concise and templated format for ease in learning. A dedicated attempt was made to include sufficient art, tables, and clinical treatment, all while keeping the books from becoming too lengthy. We know you have much to read and that what you want is high-yield, vital facts.

The authors and series editor for these eight books, as well as everyone in editorial, production, sales and marketing at Blackwell Publishing, have worked long and hard to provide new textbooks to help you learn and be able to apply what you've learned. We engaged in multiple student email surveys and many focus groups to "hear what you needed" in new basic science level textbooks to meet the current curriculums, tests, and coursework. We know that you value this "student to student" approach, and sincerely hope you like what we have put together **just for you.**

Blackwell Publishing and the authors wish you success in your studies and your future medical career. Please feel free to offer us any comments or suggestions on these new books at blue@bos.blackwellpublishing.com.

Acknowledgments

I dedicate this book to Rajesh and Leena, as well as all the amazing Infectious Diseases doctors (especially Harry L., Ruth, and Dick) who've helped me love this field so much!
—Monica Gandhi

To Fran, Burt, Julie, Maurice, and the unsung Mrs. Ohara.
—Paul Baum

I would like to thank my parents, Charles and Donna, for their continued support and encouragement.
—C. Bradley Hare

We would like to thank all of the staff at Blackwell, in particular Julia and Jen who kept us organized and on track. I want to thank Monica, Brad, and Paul for doing a great job with this material. I would also like to acknowledge the support I receive from my mentors at UCSF and UC Berkeley, Gene Washington, Mary Norton, Miriam Kuppermann, Hal Luft, Jamie Robinson, Matthew Rabin, and Teh-Wei Hu. I also want to thank my parents, Bill and Carol, my siblings, Ethan and Samara, my closest friends, Jim and Wendy, and my wife, Susan, for all of the support over the years.
—Aaron B. Caughey

Abbreviations

AAC	antibiotic associated colitis		F	female
AaDO$_2$	alveolar arterial oxygen gradient		FDA	Food and Drug Administration
ACE	angiotensin converting enzyme		FTA-ABS	fluorescent treponemal antibody absorption
ADP	adenosine diphosphate		GABA	gamma aminobutyric acid
AFB	acid fast bacilli		GFR	glomerular filtration rate
AIDS	acquired immune deficiency syndrome		GI	gastrointestinal
ALT	alanine aminotransferase		GU	genito urinary
AMP	adenosine monophosphate		GXM	glucouroxylomannan
ANA	antinuclear antibody		HA	headache
AST	aspartate aminotransferase		HAV	hepatitis A virus
ATP	adenosine triphosphate		HBeAg	hepatitis B envelope antigen
BEA	bile esculin agar		HBsAG	hepatitis B surface antigen
BID	twice daily		HCV	hepatitis C virus
BP	blood pressure		Hct	hematocrit
BUN	blood urea nitrogen		HE	human granulocytic ehrlichiosis
BV	bacterial vaginosis		HIV	human immunodeficiency virus
C	Celsius		HLA	human leukocyte antigen haplotype
CAMP	cyclic adenosine monophoshate		HME	human monocytic ehrlichiosis
CDC	Centers for Disease Control		HR	heart rate
CGD	chronic granulomatous disease		HRCT	high-resolution CT scan
CIE	counter immune electrophoresis		HSV	herpes simplex virus
cm	centimeter		ICU	intensive care unit
CMV	cytomegalovirus		IgA	immunoglobulin A
CNS	central nervous system		IgE	immunoglobulin E
CSF	cerebrospinal fluid		IgG	immunoglobulin G
CT scan	computerized axial tomography scan		IgM	immunoglobulin M
CXR	chest roentgenogram		IL-6	interleukin-6
D	day		IL-8	interleukin-8
DFA	direct fluorescent antibody		IM	intramuscular
DIC	disseminated intravascular coagulation		IPV	inactive polio virus vaccine
DNA	deoxyribonucleic acid		IV	intravenously
DPT	diphtheria, pertussis, tetanus		IVDU	intravenous drug use
EBV	Epstein-Barr virus		IVIg	intravenous immunoglobulin
EF	edema factor		kg	kilogram
ELISA	enzyme-linked immunosorbent assay		KOH	potassium hydroxide
ER	emergency room		lbs	pounds

LDH	lactate dehydrogenase		PRN	as needed
LF	lethal factor		PYR	pyrrolidonyl-beta-naphthylamide
LFTs	liver function tests		q12h	every 12 hours
LGV	lymphogranuloma venereum		qD	once daily
LCR	ligase chain reaction		QID	four times daily
LP	lumbar puncture		RA	room air
LPS	lipopolysaccharide		RBC	red blood cells
MCV	mean corpuscular volume		RF	rheumatoid factor
MHA-TP	microhemagglutination assay for *Treponema pallidum*		RNA	ribonucleic acid
MHC	major histocompatability		RPR	rapid plasmin reagin
mg	milligram		RR	respiratory rate
MIC	minimum inhibitory concentration		RSV	respiratory syncytial virus
MRI	magnetic resonance imaging		STD	sexually transmitted disease
MRSA	methicillin-resistant *Staphylococcus aureus*		STI	sexually transmitted infection
NaCl	sodium chloride		T	temperature
NAD	nicotinamide adenine dinucleotide		TB	tuberculosis
NEJM	*New England Journal of Medicine*		TCR	T-cell receptor
NK	natural killer		Td	tetanus toxoid
O_2 sat	peripheral oxygen saturation		TID	three times daily
OPV	oral polio virus vaccine		TIG	tetanus immune globulin
PA	protective antigen		TMP-SMZ	trimethoprim-sulfamethoxazole
PCO_2	partial pressure of carbon dioxide		TNF-α	tumor necrosis factor-alpha
PCP	*Pneumocystis carinii* pneumonia		TPN	total parenteral nutrition
PcP	*Pneumocystis jiroveci* pneumonia		UA	urinalysis
PCR	polymerase chain reaction		URI	upper respiratory tract infection
PE	physical exam		UTI	urinary tract infection
PID	pelvic inflammatory disease		VRE	vancomycin-resistant enterococcus
po	by mouth		VZV	varicella-zoster virus
PO_2	partial pressure of oxygen		WBC	white blood cells
PPD	purified protein derivative		WM	white male
PPNG	penicillinase-producing *N. gonorrhoeae*		yo	year old

Normal Ranges of Laboratory Values

BLOOD, PLASMA, SERUM

Alanine aminotransferase (ALT, GPT at 30 C)	8–20 U/L
Amylase, serum	25–125 U/L
Aspartate aminotransferase (AST, GOT at 30 C)	8–20 U/L
Bilirubin, serum (adult) Total // Direct	0.1–1.0 mg/dL // 0.0–0.3 mg/dL
Calcium, serum (Ca^{2+})	8.4–10.2 mg/dL
Cholesterol, serum	Rec: < 200 mg/dL
Cortisol, serum	0800 h: 5–23 μg/dL // 1600 h: 3–15 μg/dL
	2000 h: ≤ 50% of 0800 h
Creatine kinase, serum	Male: 25–90 U/L
	Female: 10–70 U/L
Creatinine, serum	0.6–1.2 mg/dL
Electrolytes, serum	
Sodium (Na^+)	136–145 mEq/L
Chloride (Cl^-)	95–105 mEq/L
Potassium (K^+)	3.5–5.0 mEq/L
Bicarbonate (HCO_3^-)	22–28 mEq/L
Magnesium (Mg^{2+})	1.5–2.0 mEq/L
Ferritin, serum	Male: 15–200 ng/mL
	Female: 12–150 ng/mL
Follicle-stimulating hormone, serum/plasma	Male: 4–25 mIU/mL
	Female: premenopause 4–30 mIU/mL
	midcycle peak 10–90 mIU/mL
	postmenopause 40–250 mIU/mL
Gases, arterial blood (room air)	
pH	7.35–7.45
P_{CO_2}	33–45 mm Hg
P_{O_2}	75–105 mm Hg
Glucose, serum	Fasting: 70–110 mg/dL
	2-h postprandial: < 120 mg/dL
Growth hormone—arginine stimulation	Fasting: < 5 ng/mL
	provocative stimuli: > 7 ng/mL
Iron	50–70 μg/dL
Lactate dehydrogenase, serum	45–90 U/L
Luteinizing hormone, serum/plasma	Male: 6–23 mIU/mL
	Female: follicular phase 5–30 mIU/mL
	midcycle 75–150 mIU/mL
	postmenopause 30–200 mIU/mL
Osmolality, serum	275–295 mOsmol/kg
Parathyroid hormone, serum, N-terminal	230–630 pg/mL
Phosphate (alkaline), serum (p-NPP at 30 C)	20–70 U/L
Phosphorus (inorganic), serum	3.0–4.5 mg/dL
Prolactin, serum (hPRL)	< 20 ng/mL
Proteins, serum	
Total (recumbent)	6.0–7.8 g/dL
Albumin	3.5–5.5 g/dL
Globulin	2.3–3.5 g/dL
Thyroid-stimulating hormone, serum or plasma	0.5–5.0 μU/mL
Thyroidal iodine (^{123}I) uptake	8–30% of administered dose/24 h
Thyroxine (T_4), serum	5–12 μg/dL
Transferrin	221–300 μg/dL
Triglycerides, serum	35–160 mg/dL
Triiodothyronine (T_3), serum (RIA)	115–190 ng/dL
Triiodothyronine (T_3), resin uptake	25–35%
Urea nitrogen, serum (BUN)	7–18 mg/dL
Uric acid, serum	3.0–8.2 mg/dL

CEREBROSPINAL FLUID

Cell count	0–5 cells/mm^3
Chloride	118–132 mEq/L
Gamma globulin	3–12% total proteins
Glucose	40–70 mg/dL
Pressure	70–180 mm H$_2$O
Proteins, total	$<$ 40 mg/dL

HEMATOLOGIC

Bleeding time (template)	2–7 minutes
Erythrocyte count	Male: 4.3–5.9 million/mm^3
	Female: 3.5–5.5 million/mm^3
Erythrocyte sedimentation rate (Westergren)	Male: 0–15 mm/h
	Female: 0–20 mm/h
Hematocrit	Male: 41–53%
	Female: 36–46%
Hemoglobin A$_{1C}$	$\leq$ 6%
Hemoglobin, blood	Male: 13.5–17.5 g/dL
	Female: 12.0–16.0 g/dL
Leukocyte count and differential	
Leukocyte count	4500–11,000/mm^3
Segmented neutrophils	54–62%
Bands	3–5%
Eosinophils	1–3%
Basophils	0–0.75%
Lymphocytes	25–33%
Monocytes	3–7%
Mean corpuscular hemoglobin	25.4–34.6 pg/cell
Mean corpuscular hemoglobin concentration	31–36% Hb/cell
Mean corpuscular volume	80–100 μm^3
Partial thromboplastin time (activated)	25–40 seconds
Platelet count	150,000–400,000/mm^3
Prothrombin time	11–15 seconds
Reticulocyte count	0.5–1.5% of red cells
Thrombin time	$<$ 2 seconds deviation from control
Volume	
Plasma	Male: 25–43 mL/kg
	Female: 28–45 mL/kg
Red cell	Male: 20–36 mL/kg
	Female: 19–31 mL/kg

SWEAT

Chloride	0–35 mmol/L

URINE

Calcium	100–300 mg/24 h
Chloride	Varies with intake
Creatine clearance	Male: 97–137 mL/min
	Female: 88–128 mL/min
Osmolality	50–1400 mOsmol/kg
Oxalate	8–40 μg/mL
Potassium	Varies with diet
Proteins, total	$<$ 150 mg/24 h
Sodium	Varies with diet
Uric acid	Varies with diet

Microbiology

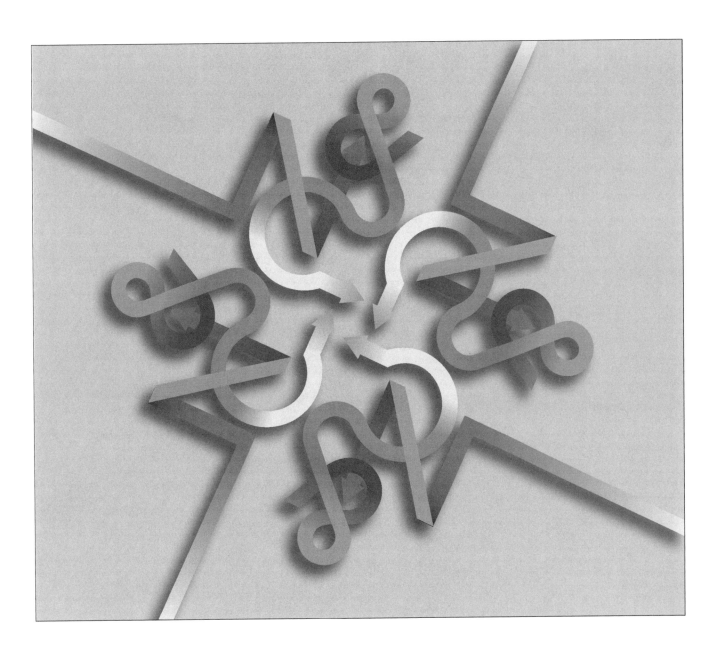

HPI: SA is a 70-year-old man who presents to the office with right knee swelling and pain. SA complains of increasing pain and swelling in his right knee after accidentally falling 1 week ago. He also reports 3 days of fevers and chills, along with fatigue and generalized weakness. SA denies any cough, shortness of breath, nausea, vomiting, chest pain, bowel or urinary symptoms, rash, or other joint problems.

PMH: SA has taken carbidopa-levodopa (Sinemet) for Parkinson's disease since 1992, lisinopril for hypertension, and glipizide for type II diabetes mellitus. No allergies to medications. Does not smoke; lives with wife.

PE: Temperature (T) 38.5°C, blood pressure (BP) 104/58, heart rate (HR) 75, respiratory rate (RR) 18, and oxygen saturation (SaO_2) on room air 96%.

SA was somnolent, but arousable. Neurologic exam notable for marked tremor in hands and rigidity of his extremities with passive movement. Heart exam revealed no murmurs and lungs were clear. His right knee had a 1-cm healing laceration on the surface with noticeable swelling, warmth, and tenderness to palpation. Range of motion of SA's knee was limited secondary to pain and swelling. No rashes on skin examination.

Labs: White blood cell count (WBC) 18.1 with 90% neutrophils. Glucose 278. Aspiration of knee fluid showed 290,000 WBC with 96% neutrophils, 450,000 red blood cell count (RBC), and a Gram stain with 4+ WBC, 2+ gram-positive cocci in clusters. Blood and knee fluid cultures grew out gram-positive cocci in clusters on the day following admission. Chest X-ray was clear.

Thought Questions

- How is *Staphylococcus* distinguished from the *Streptococcus* species?

- How are the different staphylococcal species distinguished?

- What are the key virulence factors of *Staphylococcus aureus?*

- What are the key clinical syndromes of the different staphylococci?

- What are treatment options for the staphylococci?

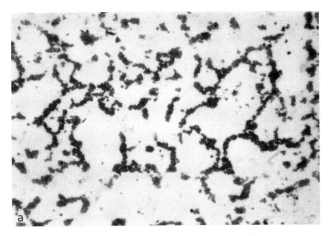

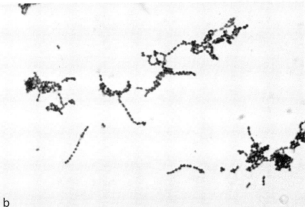

Basic Science Review and Discussion

Staphylococcus* versus *Streptococcus There are two main distinguishing features between the two groups of gram-positive cocci:

- **The staphylococcal organisms are catalase positive, whereas the streptococcal bacteria are catalase negative.** The catalase enzyme helps bacteria convert hydrogen peroxide (H_2O_2) into oxygen and water. The catalase test involves adding H_2O_2 to a culture sample; if the bacteria in question produce catalase, they will cause conversion of the H_2O_2 to oxygen gas and bubbles will form.

- Staphylococcal species are usually found in **grape-like clusters,** whereas the streptococci tend to form **pairs and chains** (see Figure 1-1).

Figure 1-1 Panel (a) shows the clustered gram-positive cocci typical of *Staphylococcus;* panel (b) shows the gram-positive cocci in pairs and chains typical of streptococcal species. (Image in public domain on Centers for Disease Control Public Health Image Library.)

Staphylococcal species The staphylococcal organisms of clinical interest include **S. aureus, S. epidermidis, S. saprophyticus,** and **S. lugdunensis.** S. aureus is distinguished from the other staphylococcal organisms mainly by its ability to produce **coagulase,** an enzyme that converts fibrinogen to fibrin in citrated plasma; **S. aureus is referred to as coagulase positive.** The other staphylococcal organisms usually do not produce this coagulase enzyme and are termed coagulase negative. The two main coagulase-negative staphylococcal species are distinguished by susceptibility to the antibiotic **novobiocin:** S. epidermidis is novobiocin susceptible and S. saprophyticus is novobiocin resistant. See Figure 1-2.

Staphylococcus aureus **S. aureus** has some of the following distinguishing features:

- Forms a **golden yellow colony** on agar
- Ferments **mannitol**
- Causes complete hemolysis (**β-hemolysis**) on blood agar
- Contains an **IgG-binding protein called protein A** in the cell wall
- Produces a **clumping factor** (different from coagulase) that binds fibrinogen

Microbiology labs either use the coagulase test (slide or tube) or watch for agglutination of latex beads coated with IgG, fibrinogen, and capsule-specific antibodies to distinguish S. aureus from the other staphylococcal species.

The clinical syndromes of S. aureus are multifarious and include **skin infections, abscesses, endocarditis, septic arthritis, osteomyelitis, sepsis, meningitis, pneumonia, food poisoning, and toxic shock syndrome.** S. aureus forms part of the normal flora in humans and is usually found in **nasal passages and on the skin.** Skin infections include impetigo, furuncles, carbuncles, cellulitis, paronychia, surgical wound infections, blepharitis, and breast mastitis. Endocarditis from S. aureus can occur on normal or prosthetic heart valves and can be quite destructive; **right-sided S. aureus endocarditis** (tricuspid or aortic valve involvement) is seen in intravenous drug users. Septic arthritis or osteomyelitis can occur from hematogenous spread or secondary to local trauma, as in the case of our patient. S. aureus pneumonia

is seen in postoperative patients or following viral respiratory infections, especially influenza. Staphylococcal abscesses can be seen in any organ, and often follow bacteremia. The syndromes of **food poisoning, toxic shock syndrome, and scaled skin syndromes are all "nonsuppurative" infections in that they are toxin mediated instead of a direct effect of bacterial replication.**

Virulence factors of *S. aureus* include

- **Enterotoxins** (six types, A-F), which cause the vomiting and watery diarrhea that characterize the food poisoning syndrome of *S. aureus.* The enterotoxin is preformed in foods and has a short incubation period (1–8 hr).
- **Toxic shock syndrome toxin** (TSST), which causes toxic shock, seen in individuals with wound infections or (in the past) menstruating women using tampons. TSST is indistinguishable from enterotoxin F and causes the release of large amounts of IL-1, IL-2, and TNF-α. Toxic shock syndrome is characterized by fever, hypotension, a desquamating rash, and multiorgan failure.
- **Exfoliatin,** which causes scaled skin syndrome, where the superficial layers of the epidermis are sloughed off.
- **Invasins** that promote bacterial spread through tissues (leukocidin, hyaluronidase, and fibrinolysin).
- **Surface factors** that inhibit phagocytic engulfment (capsule and protein A).

Coagulase-negative staphylococci Multiple coagulase-negative staphylococcal species exist in nature. The main species that are pathogenic in humans are *S. epidermidis, S. saprophyticus,* and *S. lugdunensis. S. schliferi,* and *S. haemolyticus* can also rarely cause disease in humans.

S. epidermidis is part of the normal flora on the skin and mucous membranes and forms a **glycocalyx** ("slime") layer that coats foreign surfaces. Hence, S. epidermidis is a frequent cause of **endocarditis on prosthetic heart valves** and of foreign body infections, including intravenous catheter and prosthetic implant infections. S. epidermidis can cause peritonitis in patients with renal failure undergoing peritoneal dialysis through an in-dwelling peritoneal catheter.

S. saprophyticus causes **urinary tract infections,** mainly in young sexually active women and elderly men. It is distinguished from the other coagulase-negative staphylococcal species by its resistance to novobiocin.

S. lugdunensis is increasingly reported as a cause of **infective endocarditis** (IE). S. lugdunensis causes a more virulent form of IE than the other coagulase-negative staphylococci, with high morbidity rates despite its in vitro susceptibility to penicillins and multiple other antibiotics. S. lugdunensis is frequently misidentified as *S. aureus,* as the former is also yellow pigmented, causes β-hemolysis on blood agar, and agglutinates with protein

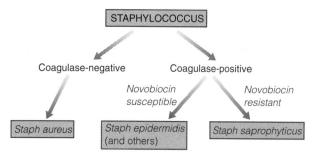

Figure 1-2 Classification scheme of *Staphylococci.*

A and the clumping factor. The two organisms are distinguished by the coagulase test. Of note, *S. lugdunensis* may be weakly coagulase positive on a slide test because it has a clumping factor that binds fibrinogen, but the organism will be clearly coagulase negative on the tube test.

Treatment　Ninety percent of *S. aureus* strains are **resistant to penicillin G** because of production of plasmid-derived β-**lactamases**. Such organisms can be treated with β-lactamase-resistant penicillins, such as nafcillin, dicloxacillin, or oxacillin, cephalosporins, or vancomycin. Adding a β-lactamase inhibitor (such as clavulanic acid) to a β-lactamase-sensitive penicillin (such as amoxicillin) will also treat β-lactamase-producing staphylococci. Some staphylococcal species are "**methicillin resistant**" (e.g., "nafcillin resistant") secondary to alteration in penicillin-binding proteins; such species are treated with **vancomycin or linezolid**. *S. epidermidis* infections are often highly antibiotic resistant and most likely will require vancomycin. *S. saprophyticus* urinary tract infections can be treated with trimethoprim-sulfamethoxazole (TMP-SMZ) or a quinolone.

Case Conclusion　SA's knee aspirate and blood cultures grew out methicillin-susceptible *S. aureus*. He was treated with appropriate antibiotics (nafcillin and then cefazolin) for a total of 4 weeks with clearance of his joint infection and bacteremia. A transesophageal echocardiogram showed no signs of infective endocarditis.

Thumbnail: *Staphylococcus aureus*

Organism	*S. aureus*
Type of organism	Gram-positive cocci in clusters; coagulase-positive
Diseases caused	Skin infections, abscesses, endocarditis, septic arthritis, osteomyelitis, sepsis, meningitis, pneumonia, food poisoning, and toxic shock syndrome
Epidemiology	Normal flora found mainly in nasal passages and on skin; right-sided endocarditis found mostly in intravenous drug users; compromised immune systems favor infection
Diagnosis	Culture of appropriate specimen
Treatment	Nafcillin, cephalosporins, amoxicillin-clavulanate for methicillin-susceptible species; vancomycin for methicillin-resistant species

Key Points

▶ Staphylococcal species are distinguished from streptococcal organisms by the presence of catalase and the formation of clusters instead of pairs and chains

▶ *S. aureus* is the only coagulase-producing staphylococcal species and is generally more virulent than the others, with multiple suppurative and toxin-mediated presentations

▶ The two main coagulase-negative staphylococcal species that cause human disease are *S. epidermidis* (foreign body infections) and *S. saprophyticus* (UTIs in sexually active women and elderly men)

▶ Methicillin-resistant *S. epidermidis* species are common, and methicillin-resistant *S. aureus* (MRSA) species are on the rise

Questions

1. Which of the listed antibiotics is the drug of choice for methicillin-sensitive staphylococci?
   - **A.** Vancomycin
   - **B.** Cefazolin
   - **C.** Linezolid
   - **D.** Ampicillin
   - **E.** Penicillin

2. What is the general carriage rate of methicillin-resistant *S. aureus* in the general population?
   - **A.** 1%
   - **B.** 10%
   - **C.** 25%
   - **D.** 80%
   - **E.** 100%

3. Which of the following is not a risk factor for the development of methicillin-resistant *S. aureus*?
   - **A.** Injection drug use
   - **B.** Dermatologic conditions
   - **C.** Frequent use of antibiotics
   - **D.** Diabetes mellitus
   - **E.** Nasal herpes

4. What is the rate of methicillin resistance in *S. epidermidis*?
   - **A.** 1%
   - **B.** 10%
   - **C.** 25%
   - **D.** 80%
   - **E.** 100%

> **HPI:** SP is a 21-year-old woman who presents with a 3-day history of a painful sore throat. She has pain with swallowing and even with talking. She also has felt feverish for the past 2 days and somewhat listless. She does not have a cough, runny nose, or shortness of breath. She just started a new job as a nanny and notes that the 18-month-old baby has been fussy, feverish, and not eating well.
> PMH: Had eczema as a child. Takes no medications and has no drug allergies. Not sexually active.
>
> **PE:** T 38.4°C HR 88 BP 100/70 RR 12
> On oropharyngeal examination, her posterior pharynx is erythematous, swollen, and coated with a whitish exudate. Bilateral tonsils are also edematous, red, and covered with a similar exudate. The lymph nodes in her neck are swollen and tender just beneath the angles of the mandible. Lung exam is clear.
>
> **Labs:** WBC 10.0 with 80% neutrophils. Throat culture pending.

Thought Questions

■ What are the leading organisms that cause acute pharyngitis?

■ How would you distinguish between the major bacterial etiologies in the lab?

■ What are some of the virulence factors of the relevant bacteria?

■ What are some long-term complications of these infections?

■ What are the best options for treating these organisms?

Basic Science Review and Discussion

Pharyngitis   Acute pharyngitis is an inflammatory disease of the pharynx and infectious causes include a multitude of viruses and bacteria. The most important viral etiology is **rhinovirus,** which is the most common agent of the common cold. The pharyngitis of a viral upper respiratory infection is often accompanied by a runny nose (called **coryza**), sneezing, and itchy eyes. Other viral etiologies of pharyngitis associated with the common cold are **coronavirus, parainfluenza virus, and adenovirus. Herpes simplex virus (HSV)** can cause pharyngitis, often with distinct vesicular ulcerations on the posterior pharynx. **Coxsackie virus** can cause herpangina, characterized by fever, sore throat, and tender vesicles in the oropharynx, as well as "hand, foot, and mouth disease," manifesting as a vesicular rash on the hands and feet and mouth ulcerations. **Epstein-Barr virus and cytomegalovirus** can lead to pharyngitis in the setting of the infectious mononucleosis syndrome, and the "flu" syndrome of influenza virus can include an inflamed pharynx. Finally, **primary human immunodeficiency (HIV)** infection can manifest with a host of nonspecific symptoms, including fever, rash, lymphadenopathy, pharyngitis, fatigue, myalgias/arthralgias, nausea, vomiting, diarrhea, night sweats, and oral and genital ulcers.

Bacterial causes   Bacterial etiologies of pharyngitis may include mixed anaerobic infections (called **Vincent's angina**). Sexually transmitted etiologies of pharyngitis include **Neisseria gonorrhoeae** and **Chlamydia trachomatis,** usually in the setting of orogenital contact. **Mycoplasma pneumoniae** and **Chlamydia pneumoniae** both cause atypical pneumonia syndromes, which can include a pharyngitis component. **Corynebacterium diphtheriae** was a frequent cause of bacterial pharyngitis prior to mass immunization of the populations of most industrialized nations with diphtheria toxoid. **The hallmark of diphtheria pharyngitis is a thick grayish exudate called a pseudomembrane.** Finally, *Arcanobacterium haemolyticum* (formerly called *Corynebacterium haemolyticum*) has been increasingly recognized as an agent of pharyngitis in young people, **almost always accompanied by a scarlatiniform rash.**

The most important bacterial etiology of acute pharyngitis, however, is the **group A β-hemolytic streptococcus, called** *Streptococcus pyogenes.* Strains of other serogroups of β-hemolytic streptococcus, especially **group C and group G,** are increasingly implicated in bacterial pharyngitis as well.

Streptococci   The **streptococci** species have been classified since 1919 into three different groups based on their hemolytic patterns on blood agar (see Figure 2-1). **α-hemolytic streptococci** create a greenish zone around their colonies on blood agar secondary to incomplete lysis of the red blood cells in the agar. **β-Hemolytic streptococci** form a clear zone around their colonies representing complete lysis of the red blood cells. γ-**Hemolytic** streptococci are generally nonhemolytic or variably hemolytic. A general classification scheme for the α-, β-, and γ-hemolytic streptococci is given in the following diagram, along with the appropriate laboratory tests to distinguish each organism

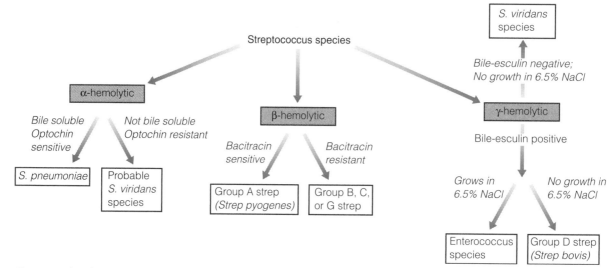

Figure 2-1 Classification scheme of *Streptococcus* species.

from one another within a hemolytic class. Of note, optochin and bacitracin are antibiotics to which different streptococcal species have varying susceptibility patterns, and a bile esculin-positive species hydrolyzes the esculin in bile esculin agar (BEA), resulting in a characteristic black discoloration.

The grouping of the **β-hemolytic streptococci** is based on antigenic differences in the **C carbohydrate** (located in the cell wall) from **Lancefield's** 1933 classification scheme; the distinct Lancefield groups A through U of the β-hemolytic streptococci are distinguished in the clinical laboratory by precipitin tests with specific antisera or by immunofluorescence. Additional methods of distinguishing the β-hemolytic streptococci include the diagnostic biochemical/antibiotic susceptibility tests in the chart above. For instance, group A streptococcus (*S. pyogenes*) is distinguished from the other β-hemolytic streptococcus by its susceptibility to **bacitracin.** The species name for group B streptococcus is **S. agalactiae,** which can colonize the female genital tract and cause neonatal meningitis and sepsis. **Group C streptococcus** species cause some of the same syndromes as group A streptococcus (e.g., pharyngitis and skin infections) and include *S. dysgalactiae* (rare in humans), *S. equisimilis* (most common group C streptococcus species in humans), and *S. zooepidemicus* (causes epidemic infections in domestic animals).

S. pyogenes   **Group A streptococcus (*S. pyogenes*)** is the most common bacterial cause of **pharyngitis,** and can resolve spontaneously or extend to otitis, sinusitis, mastoiditis, and meningitis if untreated. *S. pyogenes* can also produce **skin infections,** such as cellulitis, impetigo, erysipelas, necrotizing fasciitis, scarlet fever, or lymphangitis. The **M-protein** protrudes from the outer surface of the cell in *S. pyogenes* and is the most important **virulence factor** of group A streptococci; the factor impedes phagocytosis by host macrophages and polymorphonuclear leukocytes, and strains that do not express this protein are avirulent. Group A streptococci elaborate a number of extracellular products important in the pathogenesis of the organism. For instance, **erythrogenic toxin** causes the rash of **scarlet fever** and can lead to a toxic shock-like syndrome. Streptolysin O (oxygen-labile) and streptolysin S (oxygen-stable) are hemolysins that contribute to β-hemolysis when group A strains are grown on blood agar plates; antibody to the streptolysin O (called **ASO**) develops soon after group A infections, and its titer is important in the diagnosis of nonsuppurative complications (see below). Hyaluronidase degrades hyaluronic acid, which is the ground substance of subcutaneous tissue, facilitating spread of *S. pyogenes* in skin infections. **Streptokinase** activates plasminogen to form plasmin, dissolving the fibrin structure of clots.

Nonsuppurative disorders can follow acute infections with the group A streptococcus, and are usually caused by an immunologic response to streptococcal M-proteins that cross-react with human antigens. Nonsuppurative diseases include **poststreptococcal glomerulonephritis (PSGN)** and **acute rheumatic fever;** the group A strains that cause pharyngitis are more typically associated with rheumatic fever and the strains that cause scarlet fever are more likely to give PSGN. Most cases of PSGN resolve completely, but **rheumatic fever can lead to permanent aortic or mitral valve defects.** If streptococcal infections are treated within 8 days after onset, the complication of rheumatic fever is usually prevented, making early diagnosis and treatment of streptococcal pharyngitis important. **ASO titers and the anti-hyaluronidase Ab titers are usually elevated in the presence of poststreptococcal nonsuppurative complications** and aid in diagnosis.

Diagnosis and Treatment Diagnosis of group A pharyngitis is usually made by **throat culture,** and there has never been a reported case of penicillin-resistant *S. pyogenes.* Hence, **penicillin is the drug of choice** in the treatment of streptococcal infections, given its safety, narrow spectrum, low cost, and efficacy in the prevention of acute rheumatic fever. Penicillin can either be administered as a single dose of **benzathine penicillin G intramuscularly** (1.2 million units IM given once) or as a 10-day course of **oral penicillin** (penicillin V 500 mg PO two to three times a day for 10 days). **Amoxicillin is usually easier to administer in children** for group A streptococcus, as its liquid formulation tastes better than the oral suspension of penicillin. Other antibiotics (such as second- or third-generation cephalosporins) may be administered in short courses with equal efficacy. **Erythromycin is the drug of choice in penicillin-allergic patients.**

Case Conclusion SP's throat culture was positive for β-hemolytic streptococcus that was bacitracin susceptible. She was given a 10-day course of oral penicillin, with resolution of her symptoms within 2 days of starting antibiotics. The baby under her care was also positive for group A streptococcal pharyngitis and received a 10-day course of oral amoxicillin.

Thumbnail: Streptococcal Pharyngitis

Organism	*S. pyogenes* (group A streptococcus)
Type of organism	Gram-positive cocci in pairs and chains; catalase negative; β-hemolytic; bacitracin-susceptible
Diseases caused	Pharyngitis, skin infections (including scarlet fever), nonsuppurative complications (poststreptococcal glomerulonephritis and rheumatic fever)
Epidemiology	Most common cause of bacterial pharyngitis; disease primarily occurs among children ages 5 to 15; spread by direct person-to-person contact, usually through saliva or nasal secretions
Diagnosis	Throat culture
Treatment	Intramuscular benzathine penicillin or 10-day course of oral penicillin or amoxicillin; erythromycin for penicillin-allergic patients; can use azithromycin, cefuroxime, cefixime, and cefpodoxine for 5-day courses

---

Key Points

▶ Group A streptococcus is the most frequent etiology of acute bacterial pharyngitis

▶ Group A streptococcus is a β-hemolytic streptococcus and can usually be distinguished from the other β-hemolytics by its bacitracin susceptibility or by precipitation with specific antisera (against its "Lancefield antigen")

▶ Group A streptococcal infections can lead to nonsuppurative complications following acute *S. pyogenes* infection, including poststreptococcal glomerulonephritis and rheumatic fever

▶ The treatment of choice for *S. pyogenes* is penicillin

Questions

1. Which of the following substances contribute to the complete lysis of red blood cells on blood agar plates by the β-hemolytic streptococcus?

   A. Streptokinase

   B. M-protein

   C. Erythrogenic toxin

   D. Streptolysin O

   E. Hyaluronidase

2. Which of the following features do not help distinguish group A streptococcus from other streptococcal species?

   A. Bacitracin susceptibility

   B. Most likely infection to trigger immunologic disorders, such as rheumatic fever and acute glomerulonephritis

   C. Catalase negativity

   D. M-protein is a virulence factor

   E. Species name of *S. pyogenes*

HPI: SV is a 48-year-old man with a history of mitral valve regurgitation who presents to your office with a 10-day history of fatigue, fever, and generalized malaise. He also notes some reddish lesions on his palms, which he has never noticed before. He denies any cough, but has mild new shortness of breath with exertion and with lying down flat at night in bed. SV is generally in good health except for a root canal approximately 3 weeks previously.
PMH: History of mitral valve regurgitation thought secondary to rheumatic fever as a child

PE: T 38.6°C HR 115 BP 110/78 RR 12
Heart examination is notable for a loud systolic murmur best heard at the left sternal border with radiation over to the left axilla. Lungs are clear and abdominal examination is normal. Skin examination is significant for several scattered reddish lesions over his palms and soles that are not painful when palpated.

Labs: WBC 14.8 with 86% neutrophils; blood cultures grew out gram-positive cocci in chains that are α-hemolytic on blood agar.

Thought Questions

- Which species of gram-positive cocci are α-hemolytic?

- What syndromes does *Streptococcus pneumoniae* cause?

- What are the treatment options for *S. pneumoniae*?

- How are the *Streptococcus viridans* species classified?

- How is *S. viridans* endocarditis treated?

Basic Science Review and Discussion

α-Hemolytic Streptococci   The classification of streptococcal species has been reviewed elsewhere in this text (see Case 2: *S. pyogenes*) and the **α-hemolytic streptococci** flowchart (Figure 3-1) is replicated here. α-hemolytic streptococci create a greenish zone around their colonies on blood agar secondary to incomplete lysis of the red blood cells in the agar. The two main species of α-hemolytic streptococci are **S. pneumoniae** and the **S. viridans** group.

Streptococcus pneumoniae
Properties   Gram-positive **lancet-shaped cocci** arranged in pairs or short chains. As indicated above, *S. pneumoniae* is lysed by bile and growth is inhibited by optochin. Pneumococci possess a prominent polysaccharide capsule and over 80 antigenically distinct types of pneumococci exist.

Transmission and epidemiology   There is no animal reservoir for the pneumococcus. Immunocompromised patients, HIV-infected patients, and alcoholics are predisposed to disseminated pneumococcal illness. Splenectomized patients lack the ability to develop specific antibody to opsonize the organism's polysaccharide capsule and these patients are susceptible to overwhelming pneumococcal sepsis.

Clinical   *S. pneumoniae* causes a variety of clinical syndromes, including pneumonia (usually lobar), bacteremia, meningitis, otitis media, sinusitis, and bronchitis. Immunocompromised patients are more prone to the overwhelming pneumococcal sepsis syndrome.

Diagnosis   Typical pneumococcal species (lancet-shaped gram-positive cocci in pairs and short chains) should be seen on Gram stains of sputum, cerebrospinal fluid (CSF), or blood. Culture can confirm the diagnosis. See Figure 3-2.

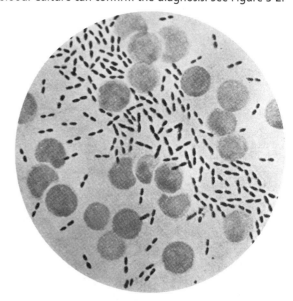

Figure 3-2 Gram stain showing lancet-shaped diplococci typical of *S. pneumoniae*. (Image in public domain on Centers for Disease Control Public Health Image Library.)

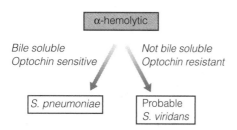

Figure 3-1 Classification of α-hemolytic streptococci.

Table 3-1 MIC ranges of penicillin susceptibility in the pneumococcus and prevalence in a city hospital

MIC to penicillin	Level of resistance	Rate at SFGH
< 0.1 μg/mL	Penicillin susceptible	84.5%
0.1 μg/mL to 1 μg/mL	Intermediate resistance	11.6%
≥2 μg/mL	Highly resistant	3.9%

Modified from Winston LG, Perlman JL, Rose DA, Gerberding JL. Penicillin-nonsusceptible *Streptococcus pneumoniae* at San Francisco General Hospital [SFGH]. Clin Infect Dis 1999;29:580–585.

Treatment Although penicillin was formerly the drug of choice for the pneumococcus, there is emerging **penicillin resistance** within this species. The minimal inhibitory concentration (MIC) is a measure of antibiotic sensitivity and is defined as the lowest concentration of drug that inhibits the growth of the organism. A pneumococcal species is considered highly penicillin susceptible if the MIC to penicillin is less than 0.1 μg/mL. Intermediate resistance of a pneumococcal strain to penicillin is defined as having an MIC of between 0.1 and 1 μg/mL. A strain is highly resistant to penicillin if the MIC is greater than or equal to 2 μg/mL. The rate of intermediate- and high-level penicillin resistance varies by institution, with cumulative rates of up to 20% to 30% in some parts of the U.S.

Table 3-1 summarizes the MIC cut-offs for determination of penicillin resistance in the pneumococcus. The rates of penicillin resistance given in the table are rates reported from a major public institution in San Francisco in 1999.

Penicillin-resistant strains of the pneumococcus tend to also have high rates of resistance to other antibiotics. Ceftriaxone can be used for strains of pneumococcus with intermediate resistance to penicillin for most infections, but vancomycin is usually required for high-level resistance to penicillin, especially in the setting of meningitis.

Classification of *S. viridans* Species Viridans streptococci are part of the normal flora of the upper respiratory tract, oral cavity, gastrointestinal tract, and female genital tract. These organisms are generally of low virulence, but the most common syndrome of *S. viridans* is **infective endocarditis** or **subacute bacterial endocarditis** in patients with underlying valvular heart disease. Subacute bacterial endocarditis often follows a history of dental work, as the latter causes transient viridans streptococcal bacteremia that may seed abnormal valvular tissue. Viridans streptococci have rarely also been associated with meningitis, pneumonia, and abscess formation. Organisms in the *S. milleri* group have a proclivity for forming localized purulent collections.

The classification of viridans streptococci species has undergone multiple revisions, given that the viridans group is composed of a number of disparate α-hemolytic and sometimes nonhemolytic species of streptococcal organisms. The current *S. viridans* taxonomy is shown in the following table (see Table 3-2).

Treatment Most viridans streptococci are **highly penicillin susceptible** with an MIC to penicillin of less than 0.1 μg/mL. Some species of streptococci are nutritionally variant, defined by their requirement for pyridoxal or thiol group supplementation for growth. These streptococcal species are less susceptible to penicillin than other species of streptococcus, with MICs ranging from 0.2 to 1 μg/mL. Although these nutritionally variant streptococci were formerly classified under the viridans streptococci group of organisms, they have recently been reclassified into their own genus called **Abiotrophia** (main species are *Abiotrophia adjacens* and *A. defectiva*).

The treatment for *S. viridans* endocarditis is as follows:

For penicillin-susceptible streptococcal species (MIC < 0.1 mg/mL):

> Penicillin, 12–18 million units intravenously (IV) total per day for 4 weeks

Table 3-2 Names of strepviridans species (current taxonomy)

Current taxonomic name	
S. mitis	
S. oralis	
S. sanguis	
S. gordonii	
S. crista	
S. salivarius	
S. mutans group[1]	
S. intermedius	
S. constellatus	*S. intermedius* group
S. anginosus	
S. vestibularis	
S. parasanguis	

[1]*S. mutans* group strongly associated with dental caries.

or penicillin plus gentamicin, 1 mg/kg IV every 8 hours for 2 weeks

or ceftriaxone, 2 g IV every day for 4 weeks

or vancomycin, 30 mg/kg IV total per day for 4 weeks (in penicillin-allergic patients)

For penicillin intermediate resistance streptococcal species (e.g., *Abiotrophia* species; MIC > 0.1 and ≤ 1 μg/mL):

Penicillin, 18 million units intravenously (IV) total per day plus gentamicin for 4 weeks

or vancomycin, IV for 4 weeks

Case Conclusion SV's blood cultures were confirmed as positive for viridans streptococci (*S. salivarius* species) and his cardiac echocardiogram showed a vegetation on the mitral valve. He was given the diagnosis of *S. viridans*-infective endocarditis. As the MIC of the *S. viridans* species to penicillin was less than 0.1 μg/mL, SV was treated with penicillin and gentamicin for a 2-week course, with complete resolution.

Thumbnail: Subacute Bacterial Endocarditis

Organism	Species of viridans streptococci group
Type of organism	Catalase-negative gram-positive cocci in pairs and chains
Diseases caused	Infective endocarditis on heart valves with underlying defects; rarely, pneumonia, meningitis, and abscess
Epidemiology	Part of normal flora in oral cavity, gastrointestinal tract, respiratory tract, and female genital tract; pathogens are of low virulence and usually require damaged heart valve prior to causing endocarditis
Diagnosis	Gram stain to look for gram-positive cocci in pairs and chains; α-hemolytic; insoluble in bile and resistant to optochin
Treatment	Penicillin

Key Points

▶ α-hemolytic streptococci include S. *pneumoniae* and species in the viridans streptococci group

▶ *S. pneumoniae* species are developing increasing penicillin resistance

▶ Viridans streptococci species cause infective endocarditis on structurally damaged valves

▶ Viridans streptococci are highly penicillin susceptible; nutritionally variant streptococci (*Abiotrophia* genus) often have intermediate resistance to penicillin

---

Questions

1. Nutritionally variant streptococci will grow under the following conditions:
   A. On sheep blood agar
   B. Around a *Staphylococcus aureus* streak on a blood agar plate
   C. In tryptic soy broth
   D. Around a *Streptococcus pneumoniae* streak on a blood agar plate
   E. On a charcoal yeast extract agar plate

2. The erythematous painless lesions on SV's palms in the setting of infective endocarditis are called
   A. Osler's nodes
   B. Roth's spots
   C. Splinter hemorrhages
   D. Janeway lesions
   E. Palpable purpura

HPI: A 63-year-old male is admitted to the hospital overnight for pacemaker placement. He is discharged the following day with no problems. At his follow-up appointment a week later, he complains of pain at the pacemaker insertion site.

PE: T 38.4°C BP 116/76 HR 80 paced RR 18
The pacemaker pocket is warm, erythematous, and tender. There is a 2/6 systolic murmur on the cardiac exam.

Labs: Labs and blood cultures are drawn in the office. WBC 12.2 with a left shift. He is admitted to the hospital and put on vancomycin and gentamicin. The following day, his blood cultures grow gram-positive cocci in chains.

Thought Questions

- What laboratory tests help distinguish *Enterococcus* from related species?

- What are the mechanisms of drug resistance in *Enterococcus*?

- What parameters for the use of antibiotics can reduce the incidence of vancomycin-resistant enterococci (VRE)?

Basic Science Review and Discussion

Originally classified in the 1930s as group D streptococci, enterococci possess a group D-specific cell wall carbohydrate (glycerol teichoic acid linked to the cytoplasmic membrane). In 1984, hybridization studies showed a more distant relationship to streptococci, and enterococci were officially given their own genus. **Enterococci are facultatively anaerobic, nonmotile, gram-positive, spherical bacteria, which grow in pairs or short chains.** Enterococci are catalase negative and have complex nutritional requirements. **They are able to grow in high concentrations of salt** (termed **halotolerant) and bile acids,** both adaptive to their ecological niche in the intestinal environment.

In the laboratory, colonies of *Enterococcus* are white in color and are typically nonhemolytic, but may be α- or β-hemolytic. They can be distinguished from other species of streptococci by their growth on **bile esculin agar (BEA)** slants with blackening of the medium due to hydrolysis of esculin; production of acid from several sugars, including glucose, maltose, and lactose; growth in **SF broth** (*Streptococcus faecalis* broth) with production of acid; resistance to **optochin** (differentiates from *S. pneumoniae*); and hydrolysis of **pyrrolidonyl-β-naphthylamide** (PYR; differentiates from *S. pneumoniae*). See Figure 2-1 (Case 2) for a general classification of streptococcal species.

Although not considered to be highly virulent, the **intrinsic resistance and ability to develop resistance** to several types of broad-spectrum anti-infectives allow the enterococci to cause superinfections in patients already receiving antimicrobial therapy. Infections containing enterococcal species are often **polymicrobial** and may contain anaerobes, such as *Bacteroides* species.

Currently, enterococcal infections account for 12% of all nosocomial infections, second only to *Escherichia coli* infections. Enterococcus can cause complicated abdominal infections, skin and skin structure infections, urinary tract infections, infections of the bloodstream, and subacute bacterial endocarditis. **Risk factors for enterococcal infections include urinary or intravascular catheterization, long-term hospitalization, and use of broad-spectrum antibiotics.**

There are two species of enterococci that cause the majority of human infections: *E. faecalis* (which accounts for 80% of enterococcal infections) and *E. faecium* (which accounts for 10% of enterococcal infections). Clinical isolates of *E. faecium* are becoming increasingly common, which is a particular concern due to its high resistance to antibiotics, especially in nosocomial settings (e.g., intensive care units). In a study conducted between 1995 and 1997, data were collected from over 15,000 *Enterococcus* isolates. Of those, less than 2% of *E. faecalis* were found to be resistant to ampicillin and vancomycin, whereas 83% of the *E. faecium* isolates were resistant to ampicillin and 52% were resistant to vancomycin.

Vancomycin-resistant enterococci (VRE) emerged first in Europe in 1988 and became one of the most important nosocomial pathogens of the 1990s. Broad-range multidrug antibiotic resistance is **mediated by R plasmids** that are promiscuously spread between bacteria—both within species and across species.

There are five described **phenotypes of vancomycin resistance.** VanA and VanB are the most common phenotypes associated with clinical isolates of *E. faecium*. VanC is the intrinsic phenotype of *E. gallinarum* and *E. casseliflavus/E. flavescens.* Less common are the acquired VanD and VanE phenotypes. **The mechanism of resistance is alteration of the terminal dipeptide of the precursors of the peptidoglycan cell wall from D-ala-D-ala to D-ala-D-lactate (in VanA, VanB, and VanD) or to D-ala-D-serine (in VanB and VanE).** With the incorporation of these new dipeptides, the binding affinity of vancomycin is greatly reduced.

E. faecium is the most frequently isolated species of VRE in hospitals and typically produces high vancomycin MICs

(>128 μg/mL). These isolates typically contain *vanA* genes. A *vanB*-containing isolate typically produces lower level resistance to vancomycin (MICs 16–64 μg/mL).

Newer agents, such as quinupristin-dalfopristin and linezolid, have been developed with activity against VRE.

Enterococci are also **intrinsically resistant to aminoglycosides,** but the addition of a β-lactam antibiotic (e.g., ampicillin) allows entry of the aminoglycoside into the bacterial cell, producing a synergistic combination that results in cell death. Enterococci that are highly resistant to aminoglycosides pose an important clinical problem, as these organisms are resistant to synergistic killing by β-lactam/aminoglycoside combinations. The resistance is due to the production of plasmid-mediated aminoglycoside-modifying enzymes.

Case Conclusion   Our patient's pacemaker is removed, and the wires are culture positive for *Enterococcus.* His blood cultures from admission are speciated as *E. faecalis,* with an MIC to ampicillin of 64 μg/mL and to vancomycin of 4 μg/mL. A transthoracic echocardiogram demonstrates a small vegetation on his mitral valve. After his pacemaker is removed, he is treated for 6 weeks with vancomycin and gentamicin for endocarditis and a new pacemaker is placed without complication.

Thumbnail: *Enterococcus*

Organisms	*Enterococcus faecalis, Enterococcus faecium*
Type of organism	Gram-positive cocci in chains; group D streptococci
Diseases caused	Urinary and biliary tract infections, septicemia, endocarditis, wound infection, intra-abdominal abscesses complicating diverticulitis or appendicitis
Epidemiology	Normal flora of the gastrointestinal tract
Diagnosis	Isolation of organism from sterile site; distinguished from other streptococci in the laboratory by ability to grow in 6.5% NaCl and ability to hydrolyze bile esculin
Treatment	β-lactam (e.g., ampicillin) plus aminoglycoside (e.g., gentamicin), vancomycin, quinupristin-dalfopristin, linezolid

Key Points

▸ Enterococci have high levels of resistance to salt and bile acids, making them particularly well suited to their environment in the human gastrointestinal and biliary tracts

▸ Increasing rates of vancomycin resistance are common in hospital settings, and treatment is difficult

Questions

1. According to the CDC guidelines for the appropriate use of vancomycin, which of the following cases would be considered appropriate use?
   A. Primary treatment of antibiotic-associated colitis
   B. Continued use in a patient with methicillin-sensitive *S. epidermidis*
   C. Once a week treatment in a hemodialysis patient with a streptococcal infection
   D. Methicillin-sensitive *S. aureus* endocarditis in a patient with a history of anaphylaxis to penicillin
   E. Attempt to eradicate MRSA colonization in a patient on chronic hemodialysis

2. The *Enterococcus* phenotype that expresses high-level vancomycin resistance is:
   A. VanA
   B. VanB
   C. VanC
   D. VanD
   E. VanE

HPI: NA is a 65-year-old woman who presents to your clinic with a 2-week complaint of cough and shortness of breath. The cough is described as occasionally productive of greenish sputum, although it is mostly dry. NA also complains of low-grade fevers, worse at night, accompanied by night sweats. Her recent history is significant for a diagnosis of temporal arteritis—a medium and large vessel vasculitic syndrome that can lead to blindness—5 weeks ago, for which she has been treated with corticosteroids. She denies any abdominal pain, nausea, vomiting, diarrhea, constipation, or urinary symptoms.

PMH: Temporal arteritis diagnosed 5 weeks ago as above; NA also has a history of adult-onset diabetes mellitus and hypertension. Medications include prednisone at a dose of 40 mg orally per day currently, two antihypertensive medications, and an oral hypoglycemic medication. NA has no known drug allergies and does not smoke.

PE: T 38.3°C BP 150/95 HR 90 RR 18 SaO$_2$ on room air 92%
NA is generally a chronically ill-appearing woman who looks older than her stated age. The main findings on her physical examination are crackles in the right upper lobe with egophany changes in that area. Moderate soft tissue swelling is noted over her right scapular area. No rashes. Heart, lung, and neurologic examination are all normal.
WBC 8.5 with a normal differential; chest roentgenogram shows a large, cavitating nodule in the right upper lobe with surrounding pneumonitis; Gram stain of the sputum sample shows branching, slender, gram-positive rods.

Thought Questions

- What is a classification scheme for the gram-positive rods?

- Which gram-positive rods are filamentous and how are they distinguished?

- What are the clinical syndromes caused by the filamentous gram-positive rods?

- How should these infections be treated?

Basic Science Review and Discussion

Classification of Gram-Positive Rods The diagram (Figure 5-1) shows a classification scheme for gram-positive rods.

Filamentous gram-positive rods The filamentous gram-positive rods are in the **Nocardia** and **Actinomyces** genera.

Nocardia *Nocardia* is a genus of **aerobic** actinomycetes and its main species include *N. asteroides, N. brasiliensis, N. farcinica, N. otitidiscaviarum,* and *N. transvalensis.*

Properties *Nocardia* species are filamentous, branching, beaded, gram-positive rods. These organisms also stain weakly positive with a modified **acid-fast** bacteria (AFB) stain, which is a distinguishing characteristic of *Nocardia* from *Actinomyces* species.

Transmission and epidemiology *Nocardia* species are ubiquitous **environmental** saprophytes, living in soil, organic matter, and water. Human infection usually arises from direct inoculation of the skin or soft tissues or by inhalation of the organism.

Clinical *Nocardia* infections tend to occur in immunocompromised hosts (e.g., patients on steroids, organ transplant recipients, or patients with advanced HIV infection). The three main clinical syndromes of *Nocardia* infection are

1) **Skin/soft tissue infections and mycetoma:** *N. asteroides* tends to cause self-limited skin infections; *N. brasiliensis* is the most common cause of progressive cutaneous and lymphocutaneous (*sporotrichoid*) disease.

   Mycetoma (**madura foot**) is a local, chronic, slowly progressive, often painless destructive infection that begins in the subcutaneous tissue and spreads to contiguous structures. Causative organisms from plant debris or soil are inoculated into the subcutaneous tissue by minor trauma. A defining characteristic of mycetoma is the presence of tiny grains seen in the drainage from **sinus tracts** (representing clumps of organisms). Mycetoma can be caused by two groups of organisms: (1) **actinomycetoma** is caused by filamentous, aerobic branching bacteria (such as *Nocardia brasiliensis, Nocardia asteroides, Streptomyces somaliensis, Actinomadura madurae,* and *Actinomadura pelletierii*); (2) **eumycetoma** is caused by soil fungi (such as *Pseudoallescheria boydii, Madurella mycetomatis, Madurella grisea, Fusarium, Acremonium,* and *Corynespora*).

2) **Respiratory infections:** Pulmonary disease is the prominent clinical finding of nocardiosis, with more than 90% of such cases caused by *N. asteroides.* Pulmonary nocardiosis has manifold manifestations, including suppurative pneumonia, lung abscess, and **cavitary disease** with contiguous extension to surrounding areas, causing

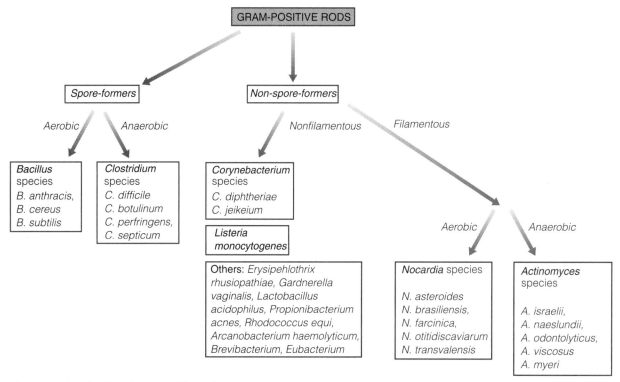

Figure 5-1 Classification of gram-positive rods.

pleural effusion, empyema, and overlying soft tissue swelling.

3) **Neurologic infections:** central nervous system (CNS) manifestations of nocardiosis often accompany respiratory disease, and include distinct granulomas or abscesses in the brain. Neurologic manifestations can progress very slowly and result in a chronic, debilitating neurologic syndrome. Diagnosis of nocardial infection in the brain lesion is usually made by biopsy or aspiration.

Diagnosis Nocardia can be isolated from respiratory secretions, skin biopsies, or brain lesion aspirations. Direct smears should show gram-positive, beaded, branching filaments that are usually acid fast.

Treatment The mainstay of treatment for nocardial infections is **sulfonamides. Trimethoprim-sulfamethoxazole (TMP-SMZ)** is the formulation most often used for these agents, although sulfadiazine and sulfisoxazole demonstrate equal efficacy in the treatment of nocardiosis. Alternative agents in the face of sulfa allergies include amikacin, imipenem, and minocycline.

Actinomyces Actinomycosis is an indolent infection caused by the following **anaerobic** or microaerophilic bacterial species: *Actinomyces israelii, Actinomyces naeslundii, Actinomyces odontolyticus, Actinomyces viscosus,* and *Actinomyces myeri.*

Properties When *Actinomyces* organisms invade tissue, they form tiny but visible grains called **"sulfur granules"** because of their yellow color. Classic features of actinomycosis infections include extension to contiguous structures by crossing anatomic boundaries with the formation of fistulae and sinus tracts.

Transmission and epidemiology *Actinomyces* species are part of the **endogenous human flora** that normally colonize the mouth, colon, and vagina. The peak incidence of actinomycosis is reported to be in the mid-decade with a male-to-female predominance, thought to be secondary to poorer oral hygiene in this age group. No person-to-person transmission has been documented and immunocompromise is not a precondition for actinomycosis infections.

Clinical The major clinical syndromes of *Actinomyces* include the following:

1) **Orocervicofacial disease:** soft tissue swelling, abscesses, or mass lesions in the head and neck area, especially the **angle of the jaw,** are the most common manifestations of actinomycosis. Chronic, recurring abscesses and spread to adjacent structures are common. Extension of orofacial actinomycosis can lead to brain abscesses.

2) **Thoracic involvement:** indolent infection usually involving a combination of the pulmonary parenchyma and

pleural space, with spontaneous drainage of an empyema through the chest wall serving as a diagnostic clue.

3) **Abdominal and pelvic disease:** actinomycosis in these regions most often manifests as an abscess or hard mass lesion with fistula and sinus tract formation to contiguous structures and through the overlying skin.

4) **Musculoskeletal disease:** actinomycotic infection of the bone is usually a result of adjacent soft tissue infection and can involve prosthetic joints.

Diagnosis As *Actinomyces* infections are exquisitely sensitive to antibiotics, aspiration of the involved tissue for Gram stain and culture should be performed prior to the administration of antibiotics. Branching, gram-positive, filamentous rods should be cultured out under anaerobic conditions. A diagnostic clue to actinomycosis is the presence of visible sulfur granules in the pus or tissue from a biopsy.

Treatment **Penicillin** is the mainstay of treatment. Use tetracycline or erythromycin for penicillin-allergic patients.

Case Conclusion Modified acid-fast staining and culture of the organism from NA's sputum confirmed *Nocardia asteroides* and she was treated with an 8-week long course of TMP-SMZ with complete resolution. Her steroid therapy was also tapered off.

Thumbnail: Pulmonary Nocardiosis

Organism	*Nocardia asteroides*
Type of organism	Branching, beaded, filamentous gram-positive rod that is acid-fast positive
Diseases caused	Skin and soft tissue infections, including mycetoma, respiratory infections such as cavitary nodules, and brain abscesses
Epidemiology	Respiratory, neurologic, and disseminated infections usually occur in immunocompromised hosts; actinomycetoma occurs from inoculation of *Nocardia* (usually *N. brasiliensis*) from soil into skin of foot through minor trauma
Diagnosis	Gram stain to look for typical morphology and modified acid-fast stain; culture
Treatment	Sulfonamides (usually TMP-SMZ)

Key Points

▶ Gram-positive rods can be divided initially into spore-forming rods and non-spore-forming rods, with the latter being divided into filamentous and nonfilamentous rods

▶ The filamentous gram-positive rods include *Nocardia* species (aerobic; soil organisms) and *Actinomyces* species (anaerobic; endogenous flora)

▶ The main clinical findings of nocardiosis are skin and soft tissue infections, including mycetoma, and respiratory and neurologic infections in immunocompromised hosts

▶ The treatment of choice for nocardial infections is sulfonamides

---

Questions

1. The most common site of *Actinomyces* abscesses is the
   A. Brain
   B. Perimandibular region
   C. Tongue
   D. Maxillary sinus
   E. Pleural cavity

2. *Listeria* is a common etiology of meningitis in
   A. Neonates
   B. Adults
   C. Patients with complement deficiencies
   D. Patients after a neurosurgical procedure
   E. Splenectomized patients

HPI: BA is a 54-year-old male presenting with a 2-day history of shortness of breath and fever. He was in his usual state of good health until 6 days ago when he started experiencing fatigue, mild fever, a nonproductive cough, and some frontal chest pain with deep breathing or coughing. He now complains of worsening shortness of breath and high fevers, with a severe headache. He has mild abdominal pain, but no nausea or vomiting. He denies any diarrhea or pain with urination.

PMH: Hypertension, well controlled on medication. Has no allergies to medications. Lives with his wife and teenage son. BA works in a postal office in Washington, DC.

PE: T 38.9°C HR 109 BP 98/45 RR 20
The patient is clearly short of breath during examination and is unable to complete full sentences without panting. His lung sounds are significant for decreased breath sounds in the left base. He is somnolent, although the rest of his neurologic examination is nonfocal. There are no rashes on skin exam.

Labs: WBC 16.8 with 85% neutrophils. Liver function tests and chemistry panel within normal limits. Chest X-ray shows a widened mediastinum without any pulmonary infiltrates and a left-side pleural effusion.

The health department is notified.

Thought Questions

- What is the infection that you are most worried about in this patient?

- What is the microbiology of this organism?

- What are the risk factors for acquiring this infection?

- What are the typical clinical manifestations of this infection?

- What are some treatment options for this infection?

Basic Science Review and Discussion

The most likely organism causing BA's illness is **Bacillus anthracis,** given the constellation of symptoms, the risk factor of being a postal worker in the era of recent **bioterrorist events** in the U.S., and the typical chest X-ray finding of a **widened mediastinum.**

Microbiology *B. anthracis* is **a gram-positive, spore-forming, aerobic rod** that can afflict many species. The organism can usually be identified in the clinical laboratory by the **presence of a capsule, lack of motility, catalase positivity, lack of hemolysis, and penicillin sensitivity,** although **penicillin-resistant "designer strains"** of *B. anthracis* have been developed for purposes of bioterrorism. The gram stain reveals **large, gram-positive rods** in chains, sometimes described as **"boxcar-like"** (see Figure 6-1). The *B. anthracis* spores are usually not visualized in smears of exudates.

The key virulence factors of *B. anthracis* are **protective antigen (PA), edema factor (EF), and lethal factor (LF).** The PA toxin binds to the edema and lethal factors extracellularly, and the complex is then transported into the cytoplasm of eukaryotic cells. EF generates cyclic adenosine monophosphate (cAMP) within the eukaryotic cell and inhibits neutrophil phagocytosis via ATP depletion, in a process similar to the toxin of *Bordetella pertussis.* LF is sufficient to kill laboratory animals and is thought to be the mediator of anthrax mortality in infected humans. Although the exact mechanism of lethality is unclear, in vitro LF is known to induce the death of macrophages via activation of cytokines, such as interleukin-1 (IL-1) and tumor necrosis factor (TNF), and oxygen radicals. Antibodies to IL-1 and TNF are protective against the lethal challenge of LF in mice, as is pre-exposure depletion of macrophages.

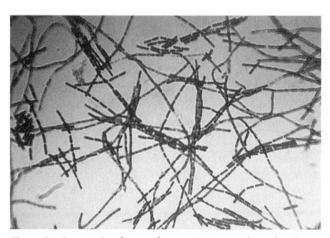

Figure 6-1 Gram stain of smear from cutaneous anthrax showing large "boxcar-like" gram-positive rods. (Image in public domain on Centers for Disease Control Public Health Image Library.)

Epidemiology   **B. anthracis is the agent of anthrax, a** largely zoonotic gastrointestinal illness in herbivores (goats, sheep, and cattle) following ingestion of spores in the soil. Prior to the wide implementation of animal vaccination in 1957, anthrax was the scourge of the livestock industry. **Human cases of anthrax were traditionally linked to exposure to animals,** either in the setting of agriculture, abattoir work, or other industrial settings involving animal products such as hide, wool, or hair, or laboratories. **Humans are infected from direct skin contact, inhalation, or ingestion of the B. anthracis spores,** leading to the clinical manifestations of **cutaneous anthrax, inhalational anthrax, and gastrointestinal anthrax,** respectively. Since vaccination for *B. anthracis* in animals has become routine, naturally occurring cases of anthrax in humans have decreased dramatically. **Outbreaks of anthrax have become rare in the industrialized world,** but still occur in resource-poor settings in Africa and Asia. **Human-to-human transmission has not been documented.**

Given the airborne nature of the spores, *B. anthracis* can be harvested as an **agent of bioterrorism,** and **22 cases of confirmed or suspected anthrax (with five deaths) occurred in the U.S. in the fall of 2001.** These anthrax cases were linked to exposure to *B. anthracis* spores in letters sent from Trenton, New Jersey, **through the U.S. mail.** As the last natural case of inhalation anthrax in the U.S. occurred in 1978, any single case of anthrax in the industrialized world is suspicious for bioterrorist activity and should be investigated accordingly.

Clinical manifestations   **Cutaneous anthrax** is the most common form of natural disease (>90% of cases) and has a 15% to 20% mortality if left untreated, and a 1% mortality if treated. The incubation period for this disease is 1 to 12 days. The cutaneous form of this infection begins as a papule, and then progresses through a vesicular stage to a **depressed black necrotic eschar** (Figure 6-2). **Edema is a**

prominent feature of this condition and regional lymphadenopathy is often observed.

Inhalational anthrax (also called Woolsorter's disease) occurs in 5% of natural cases and is the most important infection from a bioterrorist point of view given its high mortality rate. Left untreated, **the mortality of inhalational anthrax is approximately 85% to 95%;** the mortality of treated inhalational anthrax is around 60%. High-level spore exposure is required (4000–80,000 spores) for infection and the incubation period is between 2 and 43 days. The spores are inhaled, ingested by pulmonary macrophages, and transported to hilar and mediastinal nodes where the spores germinate and produce toxin. The edematous necrotic mediastinal nodes lead to a **hemorrhagic mediastinitis and an enlarged mediastinum on chest roentgenogram** (Figure 6-3). **Pleural effusion** can also accompany the enlarged mediastinum, but parenchymal abnormalities are unusual. The bacilli can rapidly disseminate, with ensuing bacteremia and death. **Anthrax meningitis** can accompany any case of disseminated anthrax; it was the discovery of a boxcar-shaped, grampositive rod in the CSF that led to the diagnosis of anthrax in the index case of the bioterrorist events in 2001. *B. anthracis* meningitis is characterized by subarachnoid hemorrhage and marked leptomeningeal edema.

Gastrointestinal anthrax occurs in 5% of natural cases, although it has not been reported in the U.S. This condition

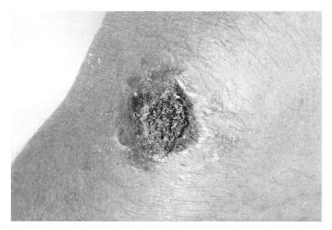

Figure 6-2 Black necrotic eschar of cutaneous anthrax. (Image in public domain on Centers for Disease Control Public Health Image Library.)

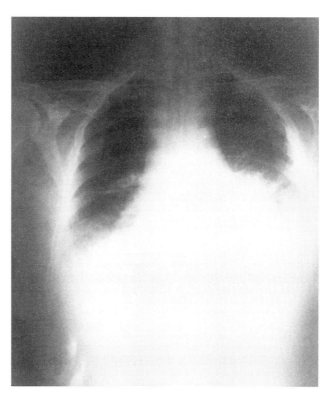

Figure 6-3 Chest X-ray of pulmonary anthrax showing widened mediastinum. (Image in public domain on Centers for Disease Control Public Health Image Library.)

occurs 2 to 5 days after the consumption of meat contaminated with *B. anthracis* spores. Spore germination and toxin production can occur anywhere in the gastrointestinal (GI) tract, including the throat. The **pharyngeal presentation** of this disease entails ulcerative lesions in the oropharynx and neck swelling. The **GI presentation** of anthrax includes the symptoms of diarrhea, hematemesis, hematochezia, melena, ascites, and severe abdominal pain. A gastrointestinal site of entry is associated with rapid bacillary dissemination and a mortality rate of 25% to 60%.

Diagnosis and Treatment   The diagnosis of *B. anthracis* is usually made on a smear of a cutaneous lesion or blood cultures. Standard blood cultures in the presence of disseminated disease should be positive in 6 to 24 hours for *B. anthracis*'s characteristic gram-positive rods. **Colonies on solid media produce long chains of square-ended bacteria, giving an appearance of swirling hairs (called "medusa head" colonies).** Microbiologic identification can be confirmed by specific polymerase chain reaction (PCR) primers.

Bacillus anthracis displays a natural antimicrobial resistance to third-generation cephalosporins, trimethoprim, and sulfa-based regimens. **Although natural species of *B. anthracis* are susceptible to penicillin, human-made resistance to penicillins has been reported.** *B. anthracis* is susceptible to fluoroquinolones, tetracyclines, chloramphenicol, clindamycin, rifampin, and vancomycin. **In the bioterrorist or military setting, ciprofloxacin is the first-choice regimen, and doxycycline is the second-choice regimen for anthrax.** Additional antimicrobials may be added according to the severity of illness in the patient. The addition of rifampin may reduce the mortality rate of inhaled disease and treatment is most effective if initiated prior to the disseminated phase of the disease. **Postexposure *B. anthracis* vaccination in conjunction with antibiotic prophylaxis** affords the best protection against the development of disease, although vaccine supplies are currently limited. **Postexposure antibiotics should be continued for 60 days given the long incubation period of inhalational anthrax.**

Case Conclusion   BA was admitted to the hospital and started immediately on ciprofloxacin 400 mg IV every 12 hr and rifampin 300 mg PO twice a day. Within 12 hours of admission, he entered a state of hemodynamic shock, requiring endotracheal intubation and the use of vasopressor agents. Despite efforts at resuscitation, BA expired. The health department initiated an immediate shutdown and investigation of the postal office where BA was formerly employed.

Thumbnail: Anthrax

Organism	*Bacillus anthracis*
Type of organism	Gram-positive rod in chains ("boxcar-like"); aerobic, spore-forming, nonhemolytic, catalase-positive, nonmotile
Diseases caused	Cutaneous anthrax, inhalational anthrax, gastrointestinal anthrax, disseminated anthrax, anthrax meningitis
Epidemiology	Natural form of disease acquired by contact with animals or animal products; anthrax can also result from dissemination and aerosolization of *B. anthracis* spores with bioterrorist intent; no human-to-human transmission
Diagnosis	Smear of lesion, blood or CSF culture ("medusa head" colonies), PCR confirmation
Treatment	Penicillin if sensitive; ciprofloxacin or doxycycline in a bioterrorist or military setting; postexposure vaccination and prophylaxis with 60 days of appropriate antibiotics

Key Points

- *Bacillus anthracis* is a large, gram-positive rod that forms spores under aerobic conditions
- Natural infection is linked to exposure to animals or animal products, but the airborne nature of the spores makes this agent subject to dissemination by bioterrorists
- *B. anthracis* is susceptible to penicillin in nature, but human-made resistance has been documented, so ciprofloxacin or doxycycline should be the antibiotics of choice in the military or bioterrorist setting
- Postexposure vaccination and antimicrobial prophylaxis for 60 days should follow a possible exposure

Questions

1. Which of the following agents should be considered for additional antimicrobial therapy with ciprofloxacin in the setting of bioterrorist-related inhalational anthrax?
   A. Ceftazidime
   B. Aztreonam
   C. Vancomycin
   D. Ceftriaxone
   E. Trimethoprim-sulfamethoxazole

2. Antimicrobial prophylaxis following a significant exposure to anthrax spores should be continued for how long?
   A. 2 days
   B. 12 days
   C. 45 days
   D. 60 days
   E. 100 days

HPI: A 60-year-old woman is brought into the emergency room by her husband complaining of muscle spasms and difficulty swallowing. The symptoms began yesterday when she noticed a tight feeling in her jaw (trismus) and difficulty swallowing solid food (dysphagia). Over the next 24 hours, she has developed stiffness and pain in her neck, back, and shoulders, and has noticed painful muscle spasms in her back and neck. She has felt sweaty, but has not taken her temperature. On further questioning, she recalls cutting her right hand on a sharp wire fence while gardening in her back yard 1 week earlier.

PMH: She has hypertension, well controlled with atenolol 25 mg once daily, and has been taking hormone replacement therapy with estrogen since a hysterectomy 6 years earlier for benign uterine fibroids.

PE: T 38.2°C BP 108/60 HR 46 RR 20
She is clammy and has a pronounced grimace. Her cardiac exam is tachycardic but regular, with no murmurs. Lungs are clear. Abdomen is firm but nontender. She has generalized increased muscle tone in her face, back, abdomen, neck, shoulders, and proximal lower extremities. Her deep tendon reflexes are increased, but the remainder of the neurologic exam, including mentation, is normal. She has no rashes, but there is a 2-cm cut on the palm of her right hand with no erythema.

Labs: WBC 13.6, normal differential. All other labs are within normal limits.

Thought Questions

- What is the organism that causes lockjaw?

- How does it cause disease?

- What complications from the disease is this patient at risk for?

- What treatment(s) is of most benefit in this case?

- How might this disease have been prevented?

Basic Science Review and Discussion

Tetanus Tetanus, or lockjaw, is caused by a neurotoxin produced by *Clostridium tetani,* an **anaerobic, spore-forming gram-positive rod.** Because of the asymmetric terminal spore, the organism resembles a **drumstick** on Gram stain (see Figure 7-1). Spores are very hearty, may survive in the environment for years, and are resistant to many disinfectants and heating.

The toxin, **tetanospasmin,** is produced only by vegetative cells. When released, it binds to peripheral α-motor neurons, where it is internalized and travels in a retrograde fashion up the axon to the nerve cell body in the brain stem and spinal cord. The toxin then migrates across the synapse to block the release of the inhibitory neurotransmitters glycine and gamma aminobutyric acid (GABA) from the presynaptic terminal. This loss of inhibition leads to increased firing of the motor neurons with resultant muscle spasm. It may also affect preganglionic sympathetic neurons in the lateral gray matter of the spinal cord to produce sympathetic hyperactivity. The toxin is very potent, and a lethal dose for humans is about 150 nanograms.

Symptoms of tetanus usually begin about 1 week after an injury, which inoculates the wound with *Clostridium* spores. The wound may be fairly minor, and patients do not always seek medical attention for the initial injury. The spores germinate best under anaerobic conditions with low oxidation-reduction potential such as in devitalized tissue or in the presence of foreign bodies. As the vegetative cells elaborate toxin, the patient first notices **trismus,** or increased tone of the masseter muscles of the jaw. Soon after, **dysphagia** may

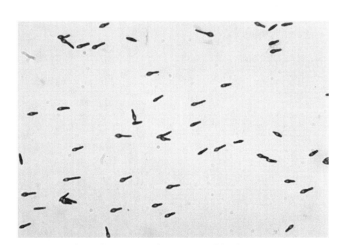

Figure 7-1 *Clostridium tetani.* (Image in public domain on Centers for Disease Control Public Health Image Library, phil.cdc.gov, courtesy of Dr. George Lombard.)

occur, along with increased tone and spasm of other muscle groups—particularly the neck, back (where spasm may lead to an arched back called **opisthotonos**), and proximal limb muscles. Distal limb muscles are usually spared. Spasm of facial muscles produces a characteristic grimace (**risus sardonicus**). Autonomic instability may result in profuse sweating, fever, or labile hemodynamic vital signs.

Complications such as bone fractures or muscle rupture may occur with forceful muscle paroxysms, and rhabdomyolysis may occur with prolonged spasm. Ventilation may be threatened during periods of generalized spasm, and apnea or laryngospasm may necessitate intubation. Ileus resulting from intestinal muscle paralysis may make parenteral nutrition imperative. The autonomic instability associated with tetanus may result in periods of bradycardia and hypotension, but these are usually easily reversed with physical stimulation.

The diagnosis of tetanus is initially made on the basis of clinical findings. *C. tetani* may be cultured out of an infected wound (only in 30% of cases), but it may also be cultured out of wounds of patients without clinical tetanus. The major diagnostic procedure is inoculation and **demonstration of toxin production in mice.** Electromyograms show continuous discharge of motor neurons with shortening of the silent interval that normally follows an action potential.

Treatment of tetanus depends on supportive care, cessation of ongoing toxin production, neutralizing circulating toxin, and preventing muscle spasm until patient recovery. Recovery is usually complete but may take several months. During acute tetanus, cardiopulmonary monitoring is imperative and intubation may be necessary for airway protection. Wounds should be debrided and cultured. Antibiotic therapy is of questionable benefit, but often penicillin is administered at 10–12 million units daily. Clindamycin, metronidazole, and macrolide antibiotics are acceptable alternatives in penicillin-allergic patients.

Tetanus immune globulin (TIG) should be administered immediately at a dose of 3000–6000 units IM in divided doses. Because of its long half-life, a single dose of TIG is all that is required. TIG acts to neutralize unbound toxin.

Minimizing external stimuli reduces the frequency and intensity of muscle contraction. Benzodiazepines such as diazepam, lorazepam, and midazolam, which are GABA agonists, may be used to control muscle spasms. Dantrolene, baclofen, barbiturates, and chlorpromazine may also be used for this purpose. In severe cases, neuromuscular blockade with vecuronium or a similar agent may be necessary.

As adjunctive therapy, patients with tetanus should begin active immunization with **tetanus toxoid (Td)** because the small amount of toxin that produces disease is insufficient to induce immunity. All unimmunized adults, as well as those with active disease, should receive a primary series of three doses of vaccine (given combined with diphtheria toxoid adsorbed as Td in persons age 7 or greater), given at 0, 2, and 8 months. A booster is required every 10 years to maintain immunity.

Prevention of active disease may be accomplished with passive immunization with TIG and/or active immunization with Td. Tetanus immunizations are begun in infancy as a series of DPT shots (diphtheria, pertussis, and tetanus). Boosters are given to teenagers and older adults as Td shots (adult tetanus and diphtheria) or singly as just tetanus shots.

Proper management of those individuals at risk for tetanus with a possible wound exposure can successfully preclude clinical tetanus. For clean wounds, Td is given if (1) history of tetanus immunization is unknown; (2) fewer than three doses of Td have been given in the past; or (3) the last dose of Td was given more than 10 years ago. The recommendations for unclean wounds are identical, except that a dose of Td is given if the last dose of tetanus toxoid was given more than 5 years ago. TIG is not given for clean wounds, but is given for all other wounds if the vaccination history indicates unknown or incomplete immunization. The dose of TIG used is 250 units IM. TIG and Td should be given in separate locations using separate syringes to avoid inactivation of the toxoid by the immune globulin.

Generalized tetanus carries a 25% to 50% mortality without supportive care and appropriate therapy.

Case Conclusion   This woman was treated for tetanus with Td, 3000 units IM in divided doses, as well as penicillin 12 million units a day for 10 days. She also immediately began tetanus vaccination with the first of three doses of Td. She was admitted to the ICU for observation but did not require intubation. Her muscle spasms were treated with diazepam and baclofen with good response. After 10 days, she was transferred to a skilled nursing facility for rehabilitation, and she had complete recovery by 4 months.

Thumbnail: Tetanus

Organism	*Clostridium tetani*
Type of organism	Anaerobic, spore-forming, motile, gram-positive rod
Disease caused	Tetanus (lockjaw)
Epidemiology	Sporadic cases worldwide among unimmunized or partially immunized persons after exposure to organism or spores in contaminated wound
Diagnosis	Clinical; inoculation with demonstration of toxin production in mice; may culture organism from infected wounds
Treatment	Tetanus immune globulin (TIG); tetanus toxoid (Td); supportive care; antibiotics are of possible but unproven benefit

Key Points

▶ Tetanus only occurs in unimmunized or partially immunized persons

▶ Tetanus may be prevented by proper administration of TIG and/or Td at the time of injury

▶ The important points of treating acute tetanus are preventing further toxin production (wound debridement and antibiotics), supportive care (monitoring, nutrition, and intubation as needed), and preventing complications (antispasmodics)

Questions

1. A 45-year-old man comes to the ER after being cut by an old saw blade on a construction site where he works. He does not remember when his last tetanus shot was. Which of the following are appropriate to administer to him on this visit:

   A. Tetanus and diphtheria toxoids adsorbed (Td) only
   B. Tetanus immune globulin (TIG) only
   C. Both Td and TIG
   D. Oral penicillin only
   E. No treatment is necessary

2. Which of the following is true of *Clostridium tetani,* the causative organism of tetanus?

   A. It is a gram-negative rod
   B. It forms spores that are heat resistant
   C. It is an obligate intracellular organism
   D. It is best cultured on Thayer-Martin agar
   E. It grows best at 42°C

3. Which of the following organisms does *not* produce a toxin as a mechanism of its pathogenesis?

   A. *Vibrio cholerae*
   B. *Clostridium tetani*
   C. *Clostridium botulinum*
   D. *Plasmodium falciparum*
   E. *Escherichia coli* O157:H7

HPI: A 64-year-old farmer is brought to the ER by his wife who returned home earlier today after visiting relatives in another state to find her husband mildly dysarthric. She was concerned that he had suffered a stroke. The patient notes slight dizziness and blurred vision. He has a history of hypertension, well controlled on an ACE inhibitor. Because of a history of diet-controlled type II diabetes, he had been eating home-canned vegetables and free-range chicken from their farm during his wife's 3 day absence.

PE: T 36.8°C BP 158/90 HR 88 RR 12
He is alert and oriented, but somewhat anxious. Oral mucus membranes are dry and no gag reflex is present. There is mild ptosis and pupillary reflexes are sluggish. There is a right third cranial nerve palsy. The remainder of the exam is normal.

Labs: Routine labs are completely within normal limits and an emergent brain MRI shows no abnormality.

Thought Questions

■ What is the major determinant of pathogenesis of this organism?

■ What characteristics of the organism are associated with the epidemiology of the disease?

■ How does the organism produce disease?

Basic Science Review and Discussion

Botulism Botulism is a paralytic disease caused by the **neurotoxin** of *Clostridium botulinum,* an **anaerobic, spore-forming, gram-positive rod.** The spores are the most resistant of any anaerobe, surviving several hours at 100°C, 10 minutes at 120°C, freezing to −190°C, and irradiation.

The clinical effects of botulism are attributable to the toxin of *C. botulinum,* which is one of the most potent toxins known. There are eight distinct toxin types, each of which may cause disease in animals; humans are susceptible to types A, B, E, and F. **The toxins act by blocking the release of acetylcholine in peripheral nerve terminals.**

There are four categories of human disease that relate to the mode of acquisition of the organism and/or toxin:

1) **Food-borne botulism** results from ingestion of pre-formed toxin in foodstuffs contaminated with the organism. Depending on the size of the inoculum, clinical disease may be mild (needing no treatment) to severe (resulting in death within 24 hours). Incubation period usually ranges from 18 to 36 hours. It is associated primarily with home-canned vegetables and fruit.

2) **Wound botulism** occurs when *C. botulinum* spores in contaminated wounds germinate and produce toxin. Incubation period is longer (up to 15 days), as the organism must germinate before toxin is produced. Cases are typically associated with traumatic wounds contaminated with soil, and outbreaks have been associated with skin popping of black tar heroin among drug abusers. The wounds often appear clinically unremarkable.

3) **Infant botulism,** the most common form of botulism, occurs when *C. botulism* spores are ingested by the infant, leading to an overgrowth of toxin-producing *C. botulinum* in the microbiologically immature gastrointestinal tract. In infants, the disease may present as simple failure to thrive or as rapidly progressive paralysis with respiratory failure. Some experts implicate it as a cause of sudden infant death syndrome.

4) **Adult infant botulism** (also called adult enteric infectious botulism) is etiologically analogous to infant botulism and occurs when toxin is produced in the intestine of colonized individuals.

Finally, some cases of clinical botulism are without identifiable cause.

Clinical botulism in adults presents similarly regardless of etiology. It is characteristically a **symmetric descending paralysis** beginning with **cranial nerve involvement.** Initial symptoms include diplopia, dysarthria, or dysphagia. The symptoms progress to involve other cranial nerves and subsequently muscles of the head, neck, arms, and trunk. Respiratory muscle paralysis may ensue. Mental status is typically unaffected. In progressive disease, paralytic ileus, constipation, and urinary retention may occur.

Clinical botulism may be confused with other causes of paralysis, including myasthenia gravis (which may be distinguished by electromyography), Guillain-Barré syndrome (which presents with *ascending* paralysis), and the Miller-Fisher variant of Guillain-Barré (which is a descending paralysis and, thus, particularly difficult to distinguish).

The demonstration of toxin in serum by a **bioassay in mice** is definitive and is performed at specialized laboratories under the direction of public health authorities. Toxin may also be demonstrated in stool and contaminated food. Isolation of the organism in a wound or stool leads to presumptive diagnosis.

Treatment for botulism must begin prior to definitive diagnosis, as immediate administration of **trivalent**

equine antitoxin may be life saving. Supportive care is also of critical importance, including mechanical ventilation in the case of respiratory failure. Antibiotics are of no proven value, but the organism is susceptible to penicillin, which is often given to eradicate contaminated wounds of *C. botulinum*.

Case Conclusion   The patient's symptoms progress during his stay in the ER to include dysphagia and bilateral arm weakness. He vomits once. A presumptive diagnosis of botulism is made and the state health department is called. Two vials of polyvalent antitoxin is administered after a skin test for hypersensitivity to horse serum is negative. He is monitored in the ICU as weakness progresses over the next 2 days. As hypercarbia develops, he is intubated on day 3. After a prolonged ICU course and several months of rehabilitation, he recovers completely. Several days into his ICU course, specimens sent to the state lab from the ER demonstrate the presence of botulism toxin type B.

Thumbnail: *Clostridium botulinum*

Organism	*Clostridium botulinum*
Type of organism	Anaerobic, spore-forming, gram-positive rod
Disease caused	Botulism
Epidemiology	Four types: (1) food-borne botulism; (2) infant botulism; (3) wound botulism; (4) adult infant botulism; primarily in northern hemisphere; often occurs in outbreaks with consumers of home-canned food or users of contaminated drugs (black tar heroin)
Diagnosis	Bioassay of serum for toxin; cultures of wounds, stool, or food for *C. botulinum*; electromyography can differentiate botulism from myasthenia gravis
Treatment	Antitoxin; supportive care, including mechanical ventilation when necessary; antibiotics are of unproven value

Key Points

▶ Botulism must be considered in any afebrile patient with symmetric descending paralysis, and treatment must be initiated immediately

▶ Botulinum toxin is a very potent neurotoxin that blocks acetylcholine release from presynap-

tic nerve terminals in the peripheral nervous system

▶ Respiratory muscle paralysis is a common complication of botulism, requiring mechanical ventilation

Questions

1. Which of the following is true of botulinum toxin?
   A. It is an endotoxin
   B. It acts on the postsynaptic membrane of peripheral nerves to block acetylcholine receptors
   C. It is a neurotoxin, which primarily affects the central nervous system
   D. It is a relatively weak neurotoxin
   E. It is used therapeutically to treat conditions unrelated to botulism

2. Which of the following public health measures is helpful in preventing infant botulism?
   A. Do not feed honey to infants less than 12 months of age
   B. Administration of prophylactic penicillin to siblings of an index case
   C. Respiratory precautions for the index case
   D. Vaccination with attenuated toxin at 6 and 12 months of age
   E. Breast-feeding

HPI: A 49-year-old man recently fell while hiking. He scraped his leg and was unable to clean the wound properly at the time. Several days later, he developed a low-grade fever, and erythema and swelling around the wound. He was diagnosed with cellulitis, and as he is allergic to penicillin, he was prescribed a 10-day course of clindamycin. His cellulitis promptly resolved, but he returns to his primary care doctor 1 week later with low-grade fever, abdominal pain, and nonbloody diarrhea. He denies any recent travel or suspicious meals. No one else at home has diarrhea.

PE: T 38.0°C BP 130/70 HR 85 RR 12
The patient appears well. There is no rash. Mucous membranes are moist. Heart and lung exam are normal. Abdominal exam shows diffuse mild tenderness, but no peritoneal signs. There are no masses or hepatosplenomegaly. Rectal exam shows trace guaiac-positive brown stool. The patient's cellulitis has completely resolved, with no erythema, exudate, or edema.

Labs: WBC 12, normal differential. Hematocrit is 47. Platelets are 350.
Stool cultures show no pathogens. A test for *C. difficile* toxin in the stool is positive.

Thought Questions

■ What bacteria can cause infectious diarrhea?

■ What predisposed this patient to get *C. difficile* colitis?

■ Why should this patient not receive antimotility agents to relieve his symptoms?

Basic Science Review and Discussion

Clostridium species are anaerobic, spore-forming gram-positive rods that can be found in soil, and in certain cases, as intestinal colonizers. They can cause a wide variety of **toxin-mediated illnesses**, including gas gangrene (*C. perfringens*), tetanus (*C. tetani*), botulism (*C. botulinum*), food poisoning (*C. perfringens*), and pseudomembranous colitis (*C. difficile*).

Antibiotic use is frequently associated with diarrhea, because of alterations in the bowel flora. Most of these cases will resolve once the antibiotics are withdrawn, but about 10% to 30% of antibiotic-associated diarrhea is due to *C. difficile* colitis, one of the serious **complications of antibiotic use.** (Other complications of antibiotic use include allergic reactions, renal or hepatic toxicity, systemic fungal infections, and creation of antibiotic-resistant pathogens.) For an expanded discussion of bacterial causes of infectious diarrhea, see Case 11.

Pseudomembranous colitis is caused by overgrowth of *C. difficile* after antibiotics have disrupted the normal ecology of the gut. Even a single dose of virtually any antibiotic can lead to *C. difficile,* although clindamycin and the third-generation cephalosporins are the classic offenders. Once the gut ecology has been altered, *C. difficile* colonization occurs through fecal-oral transmission of the organism. Toxogenic strains of *C. difficile* elaborate two toxins, A and B, which inactivate Rho small GTP signaling proteins and lead to intestinal epithelial cell death. The symptoms of *C. difficile* colitis are fever, abdominal pain, and diarrhea. On endoscopic exam, the colon mucosa is covered with a yellow coating, known as a **pseudomembrane.** If untreated, *C. difficile* colitis can lead to **toxic megacolon,** which can be life threatening if bowel necrosis or perforation occur. To avoid precipitating toxic megacolon, antimotility agents are relatively contraindicated.

C. difficile is rarely diagnosed via endoscopy. More commonly, stool is sent for an assay that detects *C. difficile* toxin either through a cytotoxicity assay or with an enzyme-linked immunosorbent assay (ELISA). Culture for *C. difficile* is more sensitive, but many strains of *C. difficile* do not produce toxins and are subsequently not virulent, so the test is less specific.

To underscore that *C. difficile* colitis is due to ecological disruption in the colon, the infection can actually be treated by enemas containing stool from a healthy person. A more palatable and commonly used treatment consists of a course of antibiotics that kill *C. difficile* in the intestinal lumen. **Oral metronidazole** is the treatment of choice. Oral vancomycin will also work, but it is expensive and runs the risk of selecting for vancomycin-resistant enterococci in the patient's gut. If the patient is unable to take oral medication, IV metronidazole can be secreted into the gut, and has some efficacy. Oral supplements of *Lactobacillus* or *Saccharomyces* have been used to try to restore ecological order in the gut, but these treatments remain unproven. If at all possible, the broad-spectrum antibiotics that precipitated the *C. difficile* infection should be withdrawn.

> **Case Conclusion** The patient is treated with a 10-day course of metronidazole and his diarrhea resolves.

Thumbnail: Clostridial Infections

Organism	*Clostridium difficile*	*Clostridium perfringens*	*Clostridium tetani*	*Clostridium botulinum*
Type of organism	Anaerobic, spore-forming, motile, gram-positive rod	Anaerobic, spore-forming, nonmotile, gram-positive rod	Anaerobic, spore-forming, motile, gram-positive rod	Anaerobic, spore-forming, gram-positive rod
Disease caused	Pseudomembranous colitis	Gas gangrene (also can cause enterotoxin-mediated food poisoning)	Tetanus (lockjaw)	Botulism
Epidemiology	Illness follows antibacterial antibiotic treatment	Organism is ubiquitous in soil and common in stool; infection usually follows traumatic injury	Sporadic cases worldwide among unimmunized or partially immunized persons after exposure to organism or spores in contaminated wound	Infection via contaminated food (particularly infants fed honey), or via wounds
Diagnosis	Stool assay for *C. difficile* toxin; pseudomembranes visualized on endoscopy	Clinical diagnosis; presence of gas or creptitus in wounds; gram-positive rods on gram stain of exudate	Clinical; may culture organism from wound	Clinical; may culture organism or detect toxin from samples of serum, stool, or implicated food or wound
Treatment	PO metronidazole; PO vancomycin; IV metronidazole	Emergent surgical debridement; penicillin; hyperbaric oxygen	Penicillin; tetanus immune globulin (TIG); tetanus toxoid (Td); supportive care	Antitoxin immune globulin; penicillin; wound debridement

Key Points

▶ *C. difficile* colitis is a potentially lethal complication of antibiotic use

▶ The treatment of choice is oral metronidazole; oral vancomycin or IV metronidazole are alternatives

Questions

1. Which antibiotic is least likely to cause *C. difficile* colitis?
- **A.** Clindamycin
- **B.** Ceftriaxone
- **C.** Metronidazole
- **D.** Cefoxitin
- **E.** Cefotaxime

2. What is the life-threatening complication of *C. difficile* infection?
- **A.** Gas gangrene
- **B.** Toxic megacolon
- **C.** Sepsis
- **D.** Pneumonia
- **E.** Appendicitis

HPI: NM is a 19-year-old female college student who presents to the emergency department with a 1-day history of high fever, headache, stiff neck, rash, and fatigue. She was observed to have a characteristic rash upon presentation to the ER and was quickly moved to an isolation room. Blood cultures were drawn, NM was started on antibiotics, and a lumbar puncture to obtain CSF was performed.

PMH: NM has no significant past medical history and takes no medications. She has no allergies. She is not sexually active and lives in the sophomore dormitory at her college with two roommates.

HPI: T 39.5°C HR 135 BP 85/58 RR 20
NM is acutely ill in appearance. Notable physical findings include photophobia, stiff neck, and a diffuse rash composed of multiple large purpura and petechiae, which looked like she was bleeding underneath her skin.

Labs: WBC 24.0 with 95% neutrophils.

Thought Questions

- What is the most likely diagnosis in this patient?
- Why was she moved into an isolation room?
- What are some risk factors for this condition?
- Should her roommates be contacted?
- What is the treatment for this condition?

Basic Science Review and Discussion

The most likely diagnosis in this patient is meningococcemia with *Neisseria meningitidis* meningitis.

Characteristics *Neisseria meningitidis* is a **gram-negative coccus** with a prominent polysaccharide capsule and at least 13 different serologic types. The most important serologic groups of *N. meningitidis* (based on their capsular polysaccharides) are the A, B, C, Y, and W-135 groups. The **endotoxin** in the cell wall of the gram-negative *N. meningitidis* is a **lipopolysaccharide** similar to that found in gram-negative rods, with a corresponding ability to cause a **sepsis-like syndrome.** Both *N. meningitidis* and *Neisseria gonorrhoeae* species require culture on heated sheep blood agar (called "**chocolate agar**"), and they are both **oxidase positive.**

Transmission and Epidemiology *N. meningitidis* organisms are transmitted from person to person by **airborne respiratory droplets,** after which time they can temporarily colonize the **nasopharynx** in the exposed individual (although carriers are usually asymptomatic). The organism then enters the bloodstream from the nasopharynx and is disseminated either widely or just to the meninges. Approximately **5% of the population are chronic carriers** of *N. meningitidis* and serve as a source of infection to others.

Epidemics of meningococcal disease still occur around the world, especially in **sub-Saharan Africa.** Infection in the U.S. is associated with individuals living in close contact, such as among **military recruits and college students living in dormitories.** The spleen is important for opsonization of the polysaccharide-enclosed organism as an initial defense mechanism. Hence, **splenectomized patients** have an increased susceptibility to *N. meningitidis* infection. Individuals with complement deficiencies, particularly in the **late-acting complement components (C5–C9),** also have an increased incidence of severe meningococcal disease.

Clinical The two most important clinical manifestations of *N. meningitidis* infection are **meningitis and meningococcemia.** *N. meningitidis* and *S. pneumoniae* are the most common etiologies of bacterial meningitis in adults. *N. meningitidis* causes the typical symptoms of a bacterial meningitis, including fever, headache, stiff neck, photophobia, and **polymorphonuclear pleocytosis** in the CSF. Meningitis can occur alone or with the syndrome of meningococcemia.

Meningococcemia can be quite severe in its presentation, including high fever, shock-like symptoms, **wide-spread purpura and petechiae, disseminated intravascular coagulation** (DIC), and **adrenal insufficiency** caused by hemorrhagic necrosis of the adrenal glands **(Waterhouse-Friderichsen syndrome)** usually in the setting of DIC and septic emboli. The massive DIC and septic emboli can lead to the worse case scenario of digit and extremity gangrene (Figure 10-1). Meningococcemia can occur either alone or with the syndrome of meningitis. *N. meningitidis* bacteremia without the syndrome of sepsis can also occur and is usually manifested by a low-grade fever and an upper respiratory illness. The serum level of bacteremia is low in this condition (e.g., 22–325 organisms/mL of blood in one small series in children).

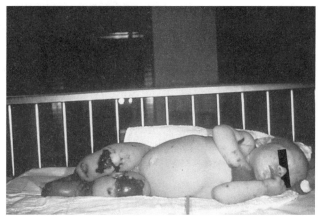

Figure 10-1 Four-month-old infant with petechiae and gangrene of lower extremities of meningococcemia. (Image in public domain on Centers for Disease Control Public Health Image Library, phil.cdc.gov.)

Therapy **Penicillin or ampicillin** were the former mainstays of treatment for *N. meningitidis,* but there has been increasing **penicillin resistance** with the meningococcus, mainly secondary to the alteration of penicillin-binding proteins or high-level β-lactamase production. Hence, **high-dose ceftriaxone** is the initial therapy of choice for serious meningococcal infections until the susceptibility of the organism to penicillin can be determined.

Chemoprophylaxis for close contacts of the index patient is indicated to eliminate the nasal carriage of the *N. meningitidis* organism and prevent further infection and transmission. Individuals qualifying for chemoprophylaxis include household and close contacts, fellow children and adults in a day care facility, individuals in a closed population such as a boarding school, dormitory, or military unit, and only hospital personnel who had close contact with the patient's respiratory secretions (e.g., respiratory technologist or physician who intubated the patient). In addition, the index patient will require chemoprophylaxis before he or she leaves the hospital to clear the nasal carriage of *N. meningitidis* if solely treated with penicillin (or chloramphenicol, which is mainly used in nonindustrialized settings), which does not reliably eliminate nasal carriage. Adequate chemoprophylaxis regimens include **rifampin** 600 mg twice a day for 3 days, a single 500 mg dose of **ciprofloxacin,** or 250 mg of **intramuscular ceftriaxone** administered once.

The **meningococcal vaccine** contains the capsular polysaccharides of **groups A, C, Y, and W-135 strains, but not group B,** which is a major cause of disease, but poorly immunogenic. Groups qualifying for the vaccine are military personnel, individuals with travel to endemic regions, splenectomized patients, and individuals with C5–9 or properidin deficiency. College freshmen are often offered the vaccination upon entry to college depending on the institution.

Case Conclusion NA quickly entered a full septic shock syndrome and was intubated and continued on high-dose ceftriaxone. She died 18 hours after admission despite vigorous attempts to reverse the syndrome of septic shock. All close contacts and fellow dormitory dwellers underwent chemoprophylaxis with single doses of ciprofloxacin administered within several days of NA's presentation.

Thumbnail: Meningococcemia

Organism	*Neisseria meningitidis*
Type of organism	Gram-negative cocci, oxidase-positive
Diseases caused	Meningitis; meningococcemia with sepsis-like syndrome, widespread purpura and petechiae, DIC, adrenal insufficiency; bacteremia without sepsis
Epidemiology	Common cause of meningitis in adults; can occur in epidemic form, especially in sub-Saharan Africa; outbreaks in military recruits and college students in dormitories; splenectomy and late complement deficiencies are risk factors
Diagnosis	Blood and CSF culture; gram-negative cocci, oxidase-positive, only grows on chocolate agar; capsular polysaccharide (five important serotypes)
Treatment	High-dose ceftriaxone until susceptibilities available (then high-dose penicillin if susceptible)

Key Points

▶ *N. meningitidis* causes meningitis and meningococcemia, often accompanied by septic shock with widespread purpura and petechiae

▶ Risk factors for *N. meningitidis* infection include close, crowded conditions, splenectomy, and late complement and properdin deficiencies

▶ Increasing rate of penicillin resistance in the meningococcus, necessitating initial treatment with ceftriaxone

▶ Chemoprophylaxis indicated for close contacts of the index patient to eliminate nasal carriage of *N. meningitidis* and further transmission and infection. Meningococcal vaccination is indicated for patients with the risk factors listed above

Questions

1. Which of the following side effects occurs commonly with the administration of rifampin for *N. meningitidis* chemoprophylaxis?

   A. Liver failure
   B. Renal failure
   C. Orange discoloration of secretions
   D. Anemia
   E. Leukopenia

2. Which of the following organisms is also a gram-negative coccus?

   A. *Pseudomonas aeruginosa*
   B. *Listeria monocytogenes*
   C. *Streptococcus pneumoniae*
   D. *Chlamydia trachomatis*
   E. *Moraxella catarrhalis*

HPI: SS is a 34-year-old woman normally in good health who presents to your office with a 3-day history of diarrhea. She first started having small amounts of brown, watery stools 3 days ago, and noted blood and mucus in her stool over the past 2 days. SS also reports 2 days of fever and severe abdominal cramping, which is often relieved by defecation. She does not have any cough, shortness of breath, nausea, vomiting, pain with urination, or rash. She has been trying to keep fluids down, but has not eaten much over the past 3 days. One of her children had a 2- to 3-day history of watery diarrhea last week without accompanying blood in the stool or fever.

PMH: Had appendectomy at age 14; SS does not take any regular medications and has no drug allergies. Married with two children (ages 4 and 6).

PE: T 38.6°C HR 116 BP 98/68 RR 12

SS's abdomen is diffusely tender to palpation and no masses are appreciated. Bowel sounds are present. Rectal examination significant for brownish-green stool with streaks of blood and mucus. No rashes. Lung and heart exam within normal limits.

Labs: WBC 13.5 with 90% neutrophils; all other lab tests within normal limits.

Thought Questions

- How would you distinguish between an upper gastrointestinal (GI) syndrome and a lower gastrointestinal syndrome?

- What are the types of organisms that cause either upper or lower gastrointestinal syndromes?

- What are the bacterial etiologies of diarrhea?

- Which of these bacterial organisms tend to cause bloody diarrhea?

Basic Science Review and Discussion

The major clinical manifestations of **upper gastrointestinal infections (gastroenteritis)** are usually nausea, vomiting, and watery diarrhea. A number of pathogens and pre-formed toxins can lead to such syndromes. The most common viral pathogens that cause upper GI infections are Norwalk virus, calcivirus, astrovirus, and rotavirus; **Norwalk virus** infection is characterized mainly by nausea and vomiting and **rotavirus** is the most common cause of pediatric diarrhea worldwide.

The **toxin-mediated** upper GI infections are usually caused by enterotoxin-producing strains of *S. aureus, Bacillus cereus,* or *Clostridium perfringens.* The mean time to illness from ingestion of preformed *S. aureus* toxin is 2 to 7 hours and the staphylococcal food poisoning syndrome is characterized mainly by vomiting with occasional mild diarrhea. *B. cereus* strains can produce two different toxins: a heat-stable toxin that can result in diarrhea after 2 to 7 hours, and a heat-labile toxin that can result in disease manifestations 8 to 14 hours after ingestion. The classic food

associated with *B. cereus* poisoning is reheated fried rice. Finally, the enterotoxin of *C. perfringens* is heat labile and usually results in clinical manifestations 8 to 14 hours after food consumption. The syndrome of enterotoxigenic *C. perfringens* is usually dominated by mild to moderate diarrhea with abdominal cramping; vomiting is less common with *B. cereus* and *C. perfringens* infections.

Lower gastrointestinal syndromes (enterocolitis) are manifested mainly by the symptom of diarrhea, and the responsible pathogens can be bacterial, viral, or parasitic. The most common viral agent of diarrhea in immunocompetent children is **rotavirus,** although this infection is rarely seen in adults. Rotavirus infections are major causes of dehydration and mortality in children in the developing world. **Adenoviruses** are increasingly recognized as agents of pediatric diarrhea as well, especially in industrialized regions.

In terms of **protozoal** causes of diarrhea, *Cryptosporidium* has been associated with water-borne outbreaks of diarrhea in both immunocompetent and immunocompromised hosts. *Cyclospora* is increasingly reported in food-borne diarrhea outbreaks, especially associated with imported berries. *Giardia lamblia* infection can manifest as both an acute and chronic syndrome: acute giardiasis presents with loose foul-smelling stools accompanied by flatulence, abdominal cramping, bloating, nausea, anorexia, and malaise. Chronic giardiasis can present just with malaise and diffuse epigastric abdominal discomfort without diarrhea. *Entamoeba histolytica* infection usually presents as **dysentery** (bloody diarrhea mixed with mucus) accompanied by lower abdominal cramping, tenesmus, fever, and flatulence. The differential for acute diarrhea in the immunocompromised host broadens to include a host of other viral and parasitic pathogens.

In terms of **bacterial** etiologies of diarrhea, the most common agents are enteric gram-negative rods. These syndromes are typically divided into **invasive** infections and **noninvasive** infections, with the former more likely to cause bloody diarrhea. Noninvasive enteric bacterial infections are typically caused by enterotoxigenic *E. coli* (ETEC), enteropathogenic *E. coli* (EPEC), and enteroaggregative *E. coli* (EAggEC) strains, all acquired from ingestion of contaminated water or food. Other bacterial etiologies of noninvasive enterocolitis include *Vibrio cholerae* (cholera), *Clostridium difficile* toxin (antibiotic-associated diarrhea that can also lead to an invasive syndrome), *Salmonella enteritidis* (a fast-growing organism with a fairly short time period of 14 to 21 hours from ingestion to symptoms), and *Vibrio parahaemolyticus* (usually acquired from ingestion of contaminated undercooked or raw seafood). The cholera toxin is an enterotoxin that is found in many other bacterial species that cause watery diarrhea, either alone or in combination with mucosal invasion. This enterotoxin ribosylates GTP-binding protein and causes a sustained increase in adenylate cyclase activity and intracellular accumulation of cyclic AMP, triggering a molecular cascade that ultimately manifests in the symptom of diarrhea.

Table 11-1 presents some of the distinguishing characteristics of bacterial organisms in the U.S. that can lead to mucosal invasion and dysentery.

Table 11-1 Bacterial organisms

Organism	Source of infection	Pathogenesis	Syndrome	Comments
Shigella dysenteriae, S. flexneri, S. boydii (mostly in travelers); *Shigella sonnei* (most common in U.S.— more mild disease)	Transmitted by the "4-F"s: food, finger, feces, and flies	Organism invades mucosa of distal ileum and colon; also has a cholera toxin-like enterotoxin	Fever, crampy abdominal pain, diarrhea—watery at first, but then with blood and mucus	Low infectious dose (ingestion of as few as 100 organisms causes disease)
Salmonella typhi, Salmonella para-typhi A, B, and C; *Salmonella choleraseuis*	Ingestion of fecally contaminated food or water	Enterocolitis characterized by invasion of small and large intestinal tissue	Variety of syndromes: typhoid fever has few GI symptoms, with constipation predominating; enterocolitis causes abdominal pain and diarrhea, with or without blood (mostly *S. typhimurium*)	Infectious dose is 10^4 to 10^5 organisms
Campylobacter jejuni	Contaminated water and raw food (especially poultry); domestic animals (cattle, chickens, and dogs) serve as a source of human transmission	Organism often invades intestinal mucosa, but also has cholera toxin-like enterotoxin	Enterocolitis begins as a watery, foul-smelling diarrhea followed by bloody stools, severe abdominal pain, and fever	*C. jejuni* GI infection is associated with Guillain-Barré syndrome; organism is a comma- or S-shaped gram-negative rod
Enteroinvasive *E. coli* (EIEC)	Ingestion of contaminated food and water	Plasmid-mediated invasion of epithelial cells	Fever, cramping, watery diarrhea as initial syndrome, followed by scant bloody stools	Common in travelers returning from Europe and Latin America
Enterohemorrhagic *E. coli* (EHEC), including the O157:H7 serotype	Ingestion of contaminated food (e.g., undercooked hamburger) and water	Verotoxin (called this because it's toxic to Vero [monkey] cells in culture), which blocks protein synthesis	Diarrhea is bloody, but often without leukocytes; fever is uncommon; severe cases can lead to hemolytic-uremic syndrome, hallmarked by microangiopathic hemolytic anemia, thrombocytopenia, and acute renal failure	Antibiotic treatment of children with *E. coli* O157: H7 infection seems to increase the risk of the hemolytic-uremic syndrome[1]

[1]Wong CS, Jelacic S, Habeeb RL, et al. The risk of the hemolytic-uremic syndrome after antibiotic treatment of *Escherichia coli* O157:H7 infections. N Engl J Med 2000;342:1930–1936.

Case Conclusion Stool culture from SS revealed *Shigella sonnei,* a non-lactose-fermenting gram-negative rod. She was treated with fluids and given a 5-day course of ciprofloxacin for treatment. Her child's diarrhea had resolved completely, so he was not given any treatment. SS's diarrhea, fever, and abdominal pain resolved 2 days after starting the antibiotics.

Thumbnail: Bloody Diarrhea

Organism	*Shigella (S. dysenteriae, S. flexneri, S. boydii, S. sonnei)*
Type of organism	Non-lactose-fermenting gram-negative rods
Diseases caused	All cause an acute lower gastrointestinal syndrome after an incubation period of 1 to 4 days; symptoms begin with abdominal cramps followed initially by watery diarrhea and then diarrhea mixed with blood and mucus; fever is common
Epidemiology	*S. dysenteriae, S. boydii,* and *S. flexneri* are usually only seen in recently returned travelers from abroad; *S. sonnei,* which causes a more mild disease than the others, is isolated from approximately 75% of all individuals with shigellosis in the U.S.; *Shigella* has a very low infectious dose, with only about 100 organisms required to produce illness in 25% of exposed patients
Diagnosis	Stool culture
Treatment	The main treatment for shigellosis is fluid and electrolyte replacement; antibiotics are not needed in mild cases, but may reduce the duration of symptoms in more severe cases; ciprofloxacin is now the drug of choice given increasing TMP-SMZ resistance in the organism; antiperistaltic agents may prolong the excretion of the organism and prolong the symptoms of fever and diarrhea

Key Points

▶ Upper gastrointestinal syndromes are accompanied by nausea, vomiting with or without watery diarrhea, and are usually caused by viral infections or bacteria-derived enterotoxins such as *S. aureus* toxin, *B. cereus* toxin, and *C. perfringens* toxin

▶ Lower GI syndromes can be caused by adenoviral or rotaviral infections, intestinal protozoa, or bacteria; latter infections can be either noninvasive or invasive, leading to bloody diarrhea in the latter

▶ Main bacterial etiologies of bloody diarrhea in the U.S. include *Shigella, Salmonella, Campylobacter,* enteroinvasive *E. coli* (EIEC), and enterohemorrhagic *E. coli* (EHEC)

▶ *Shigella* species are non-lactose-fermenting gram-negative rods that cause dysentery with a very low infectious dose of 100 organisms; accompanying symptoms include fever and abdominal cramping

Questions

1. Which of the following pathogens are associated with watery diarrhea after an incubation period of 8 to 14 hours?
   A. Rotavirus and Norwalk virus
   B. *Shigella* and *Salmonella*
   C. EIEC and EHEC
   D. *S. aureus* and *Bacillus cereus*
   E. *Bacillus cereus* and *Clostridium perfringens*

2. If SS's stool culture showed comma- or S-shaped gram-negative rods, which of the listed agents is the most likely etiology of her diarrhea?
   A. *Giardia lamblia*
   B. *Salmonella typhi*
   C. *Bacillus cereus*
   D. *Campylobacter jejuni*
   E. *Shigella dysenteriae*

HPI: PA is an 18-year-old female with cystic fibrosis who presents to the emergency department with 2 days of worsening shortness of breath and cough. Her cough is productive of greenish sputum and she also complains of a low-grade fever. PA denies any abdominal pain, nausea, or vomiting. She has chronic diarrhea controlled by pancreatic enzymes, which has not changed in any way. PA is usually admitted to the hospital two or three times a year for pneumonia and worsening pulmonary function in the setting of her chronic lung disease.

PMH: As above, PA has cystic fibrosis with a history of multiple pneumonias and hospital admissions. Chronic medications include pancrease enzymes and various bronchodilators. No allergies to medications.

PE: T 38.4°C HR 118 BP 95/60 RR 20 SaO$_2$ on room air 89%
PA is generally thin and chronically ill in appearance. Her lung exam is significant for diffuse crackles and wheezing throughout both lung fields.

Labs: WBC 11.5 with 80% neutrophils. Sputum shows slender gram-negative rods on Gram stain and the chest x-ray shows patchy pneumonia in both lower lobes on top of PA's chronic lung disease.

Thought Questions

- What is the most likely etiology of PA's pneumonia?
- What are the characteristics of this organism?
- What kind of infections does this organism cause?
- How would you diagnose this infection?
- How would you treat this infection?

Basic Science Review and Discussion

The most likely etiology of PA's pneumonia is a *Pseudomonas* species given the fact that cystic fibrosis patients are susceptible to pseudomonal infections and given the characteristic Gram stain.

Characteristics *Pseudomonas* species are **aerobic** gram-negative rods that do not ferment glucose for energy. These organisms are called **nonfermenters** as compared to the *Enterobacteriaceae,* which ferment glucose for energy. *Pseudomonas* species derive their energy by oxidation of sugars rather than fermentation, so they are **oxidase positive.** *Pseudomonas aeruginosa* is one of the major species in the *Pseudomonas* genus and derives its name from the production of various pigments, including **pyoverdin,** a yellow-green pigment, and **pyocyanin,** a blue or green pigment. *P. aeruginosa* is motile, nutritionally versatile, and can grow at a variety of temperatures (optimally at 37°C, but can also grow at 42°C).

Transmission and Epidemiology *P. aeruginosa* is found in soil, water, plants, and animals, and can be found in various **water supplies,** including disinfectants, in the hospital setting. Given its minimal nutritional requirements,

P. aeruginosa can exist in a number of different environmental settings and is a major etiology of nosocomial infections. *P. aeruginosa* can also compose part of the normal microbial flora of humans, with rates of colonization enhanced in hospitalized patients.

Although *P. aeruginosa* is ubiquitous in the environment, pseudomonal infections are mainly **opportunistic and affect compromised hosts.** For instance, **patients with extensive burns** have impaired skin host defense mechanisms, predisposing them to *P. aeruginosa* invasion. **Cystic fibrosis patients** or other patients with chronic lung disease have impaired respiratory clearance mechanisms, predisposing them to *P. aeruginosa* colonization and subsequent disease.

Clinical Syndromes *P. aeruginosa* can cause a variety of clinical syndromes, including:

1) **Respiratory infections:** *P. aeruginosa* pneumonia occurs almost exclusively in patients with compromised lung function or systemic immunocompromise. Exposure to the hospital environment, especially in ICUs, **endotracheal intubation, and prior use of antibiotics** increases the likelihood of *P. aeruginosa* pneumonia. Other risk factors for this condition include cystic fibrosis, chronic bronchiectasis or other chronic lung diseases, **neutropenia,** administration of cancer chemotherapy, and **AIDS.** Cystic fibrosis patients tend to develop lower respiratory tract infections with **mucoid strains** of *P. aeruginosa.*

2) **Urinary tract infections:** *P. aeruginosa* infections of the urinary tract are often nosocomial, iatrogenic, and related to prolonged **urinary tract catheterization.** *Pseudomonas* urinary tract infections (UTIs) occur frequently in chronic care facilities and frequently plague spinal cord injury victims. *P. aeruginosa* UTIs are often

recurrent and clearance may require removal of urinary tract catheters.

3) **Skin and soft tissue infections:** *Pseudomonas* bacteremia can produce distinctive skin lesions called **ecthyma gangrenosum,** which involve local hemorrhage, necrosis, surrounding erythema, and vascular invasion by the *Pseudomonas* bacteria. Bacteremia can also be associated with subcutaneous nodules, deep abscesses, cellulitis, bullae, necrotizing fasciitis, and vesicular or pustular lesions. Primary *P. aeruginosa* skin and soft tissue infections can be also be localized or diffuse, and predisposing factors include burns, trauma, decubitus ulcers, dermatitis, and **frequent swimming or exposure to water.**

4) **Ear infections:** *P. aeruginosa* is the predominant bacterial pathogen of **external auditory canal otitis** and is usually associated with injury, meatal maceration, inflammation,

chronic humid conditions in the ear, and swimming (**"swimmer's ear"**). This infection is manifested by an itchy or painful ear with discharge and edema and is treated with **topical application of antibiotic-** and steroid-containing otic solutions. **"Malignant" external otitis** is defined by locally invasive *P. aeruginosa* infections of the external auditory canal, with destruction of underlying soft tissues. This condition occurs mainly in **elderly diabetic patients** and requires **systemic therapy.**

5) **Other:** other *P. aeruginosa*-associated conditions include endocarditis, meningitis, brain abscess, eye infections, **bone and joint infections,** and **necrotizing enterocolitis,** especially in young infants and **neutropenic cancer patients.**

Diagnosis   Diagnosis of *P. aeruginosa* infections is made by Gram stain and culture. *P. aeruginosa* grows as **non-lactose-fermenting, oxidase-positive colonies,** and these gram-negative rods have a **typical slender morphology** (Figure 12-1).

Treatment   *P. aeruginosa* is resistant to a number of antibiotics. The four classes of antibiotics that are most commonly used against *Pseudomonas* species are listed below (Table 12-1).

Serious infections often require combination therapy among these classes of antibiotics.

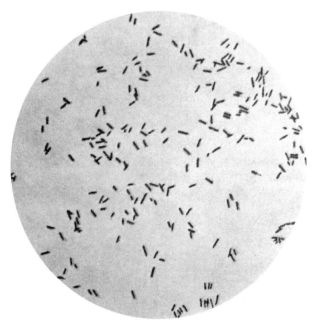

Figure 12-1 Slender gram-negative rods typical of *Pseudomonas aeruginosa.* (Image in public domain on Centers for Disease Control Public Health Image Library, phil.cdc.gov.)

Table 12-1 Antibiotic classes effective for *Pseudomonas*

Drug class	Examples
1. Aminoglycosides	Gentamicin, tobramycin
2. Fluoroquinolones	Ciprofloxacin
3. Antipseudomonal penicillins	Ticarcillin, piperacillin,
4. Third- and fourth-generation cephalosporins	Ceftazidime and cefepime, respectively
Other active agents include	
5. Aztreonam (monobactam)	
6. Imipenem-cilastatin	

Case Conclusion   Culture of PA's sputum grew out a mucoid strain of *P. aeruginosa.* She was treated with a combination of piperacillin and tobramycin in-house and discharged on a course of oral ciprofloxacin with gradual improvement.

Thumbnail: *P. aeruginosa* Pneumonia

Organism	*Pseudomonas aeruginosa*
Type of organism	Oxidase-positive, aerobic, gram-negative rod
Diseases caused	Respiratory tract infections, especially in patients with cystic fibrosis and chronic lung disease, urinary tract infections, external otitis and malignant external otitis, bacteremia, ecthyma gangrenosum, skin and soft tissue infections, bone and joint infections, eye infections, and necrotizing enterocolitis in young infants and neutropenic patients
Epidemiology	*P. aeruginosa* mainly causes disease in hosts with impaired immune function, impaired respiratory tracts, and impaired skin defenses; major cause of nosocomial infections; found ubiquitously in soil and water, including water supplies in hospital environment
Diagnosis	Oxidase-positive, non-lactose-fermenting, slender, gram-negative rod seen on Gram stain of affected tissue
Treatment	Fluoroquinolones; aminoglycosides; antipseudomonal penicillins; third- and fourth-generation cephalosporins, and imipenem; serious infections may require combination therapy with an aminoglycoside and an appropriate β-lactam antibiotic

Key Points

▸ *Pseudomonas aeruginosa* is an oxidase-positive, aerobic, non-lactose-fermenting gram-negative rod with minimal nutritional requirements and the ability to live in hospital water supplies

▸ Major cause of infection in nosocomial settings and in compromised hosts

▸ Major clinical syndromes are respiratory, skin and soft tissue, UTIs, bone and joint infections, and eye and ear infections

▸ Resistant to multiple antibiotics, and mainstays of treatment are fluoroquinolones, aminoglycosides, antipseudomonal penicillins, and third- and fourth-generation cephalosporins

Questions

1. Which of the following combinations would be most appropriate for a serious *P. aeruginosa* pneumonia with bacteremia in a bone marrow transplant recipient?

   A. Penicillin and gentamicin
   B. Cefepime and tobramycin
   C. Cefepime and piperacillin
   D. Ciprofloxacin and cefuroxime
   E. Imipenem and ticarcillin

2. Which of the following is a risk factor for *P. aeruginosa*-associated necrotizing enterocolitis?

   A. Use of prior antibiotics
   B. Mesenteric ischemia
   C. Neutropenia
   D. Ulcerative colitis
   E. Pseudomembranous colitis

HPI: A previously healthy 5-year-old boy is brought to the ER by his mother because of fever, sore throat, hoarseness, and difficulty swallowing for 1 day.

PE: T 38.6°C BP 110/78 HR 118 RR 22
The patient is very anxious, sitting on the side of the bed and leaning forward. He is drooling. His voice is weak and hoarse. Stridor is present.

Thought Questions

- What is the most common cause of this disease?

- By what mechanism(s) does this organism become resistant to antibiotics, and how does this resistance affect treatment?

- What factors account for the epidemiology of this organism?

Basic Science Review and Discussion

Haemophilus influenzae (*H. flu*) is a **gram-negative pleomorphic short rod or coccobacillus.** Both encapsulated and unencapsulated strains exist, although invasive disease is most often caused by **encapsulated** strains.

All species of *Haemophilus* require either one or both of the growth factors designated **V-factor (nicotinamide adenine dinucleotide [NAD])** and **X-factor (hemin).** These factors may be added to media to differentiate *Haemophilus* species. *H. flu* requires both V- and X-factor, as do *H. aegyptius* and *H. haemolyticus*. Other species, such as *H. aphrophilus* and *H. ducreyi* require only the X-factor. Still other species require only the V-factor—these are all designated by the prefix "*para-*," such as *H. parainfluenzae, H. parahaemolyticus, H. paraphrophilus,* and *H. paraphrophohaemolyticus*.

Staphylococcus aureus produces V-factor, allowing satellite colonies of *H. flu* to grow around *S. aureus* colonies on routine blood agar (which contains X-factor). This property is useful for identifying *H. flu* in routine respiratory specimens plated onto blood agar.

There are six **capsular serotypes** of *H. flu* (a–f), with **H. influenza serotype b (Hib)** being the most commonly isolated in human disease.

H. flu is part of the **normal flora of the upper respiratory tract** in humans. No nonhuman reservoirs have been identified. *H. flu* passes between cells of the respiratory epithelium to invade and cause disease. The **capsule** acts as an important virulence factor, protecting the organism from the complement system and phagocytosis. *H. flu* has a potent lipopolysaccharide **endotoxin** that acts to cause CSF inflammation and many of the signs associated with sepsis. *H. flu* also produces human

IgA proteases, which cleave IgA (the antibody most commonly found at mucosal surfaces, the entry point of *H. flu*) and help the organism evade the immune system.

Clinically, *H. flu* causes a range of diseases including **upper and lower respiratory tract infections** (otitis media, sinusitis, tracheobronchitis, and pneumonia). *H. flu* is the major cause of acute **epiglottitis**. It is also the most common cause of **meningitis** among children from 3 months to 3 years old. Children of this age are particularly vulnerable to *H. flu* infections due to their relative state of humoral immunodeficiency: maternal antibodies protect the infant early in life, but fade by 2 to 3 months, and a mature humoral response is not fully developed until after a few years of life. Other infections caused by *H. flu* include pyarthrosis, cellulitis, pericarditis, endocarditis, osteomyelitis, empyema, cholecystitis, obstetric infections, and UTIs.

Diagnosis is typically made by growth of the organism on **chocolate agar** (which contains both V- and X-factor). Blood cultures are often positive in invasive disease such as meningitis and epiglottitis. **Gram stain** of specimens from sterile sites, such as CSF, may allow for presumptive diagnosis. **Antigenic detection** methods such as counter immune electrophoresis (CIE), latex particle agglutination, and ELISA provide rapid presumptive diagnosis as well.

Antibiotic treatment of *H. flu* infections varies by site and likelihood of resistance. Ampicillin or amoxicillin may be used for less serious infections such as otitis or sinusitis, where resistance is not suspected. Overall, about 20% of strains of *H. flu* isolated in the U.S. are now resistant to ampicillin. The most common mechanism of resistance is production of a **β-lactamase,** although some resistant strains have modified penicillin-binding proteins or outer membrane proteins. Cases of ampicillin resistance may be treated with addition of β-lactamase inhibitors (e.g., ampicillin/sulbactam or amoxicillin/clavulanate), TMP-SMZ, quinolones (although quinolone resistance is emerging), or chloramphenicol. Third-generation cephalosporins such as ceftriaxone and cefotaxime have good CSF penetration and are commonly used in *H. flu* meningitis therapy.

With prompt care, most *H. flu* infections can be successfully treated. In the case of meningitis, long-term neurologic sequelae, including hearing loss and developmental delay, are common. The medical management of suspected epiglottitis must include immediate airway assessment—any delay in securing an airway may mean the difference between life and death. Diagnostic tests such as lateral X-rays of the neck, CT scans, or direct laryngoscopy should be delayed until airway is secured.

With the widespread use of the new conjugate **Hib vaccine,** the incidence of invasive *H. flu* disease in the U.S. has declined dramatically. In regions of the world where the vaccine is not used, Hib infections still account for significant morbidity and mortality, particularly among children.

Case Conclusion The boy was taken to X-ray for soft tissue films of his neck. While still in the X-ray suite, his stridor acutely worsened, making him unable to maintain an adequate airway. A code was called. Attempts at oral intubation failed due to extreme laryngeal edema, and an emergency tracheostomy was performed. Once his airway was secured, he stabilized and was transferred to the ICU where he was started on ampicillin/sulbactam. The lateral neck X-rays taken just before he coded showed an enlarged epiglottis (the classic "**thumb sign**" of acute epiglottitis). Subsequently, blood cultures were positive for *H. influenzae,* serotype b. After several days on the ventilator and antibiotics, he was able to be extubated and completed his course of antibiotics without complication. The patient completely recovered.

Thumbnail: *Haemophilus influenzae*

Organism	**Haemophilus influenzae**
Type of organism	Pleomorphic gram-negative coccobacillus
Diseases caused	Meningitis, otitis media, epiglottitis, sinusitis, tracheobronchitis, pneumonia, cellulitis, or bacteremia
Epidemiology	Commonly part of normal respiratory flora; most common cause of meningitis in children aged 3 months to 3 years; Hib vaccine has dramatically reduced the incidence of disease
Diagnosis	Culture of infected site (CSF, blood, joint fluid, respiratory secretions, ear fluid, etc.); typical appearance on Gram stain in proper clinical setting should lead to presumptive diagnosis; direct antigen detection in body fluids
Treatment	Antibiotic resistance increasing; ampicillin or amoxicillin; in cases of β-lactamase-mediated resistance, a β-lactamase inhibitor may be added; other options include TMP-SMZ, quinolones, and chloramphenicol; use third-generation cephalosporins in cases of meningitis

Key Points

▶ *H. influenzae* requires both V-factor and X-factor for growth in the laboratory

▶ β-lactamase-mediated resistance is increasing and may affect choice of therapy

▶ Improper diagnosis and management of serious *H. influenzae* infections, such as meningitis and epiglottitis, may result in serious long-term sequelae or death

Questions

1. Blood cultures from a patient with suspected endocarditis turn positive on day 6 of incubation in the microbiology lab. Gram stain shows short, gram-negative rods. The organism grows well on chocolate agar in 10% CO_2. It is demonstrated to require V-factor, but not X-factor for growth. What is the organism?
   A. *Streptococcus sanguis*
   B. *Haemophilus influenzae*
   C. *Haemophilus parainfluenzae*
   D. *Haemophilus aphrophilus*
   E. *Pseudomonas aeruginosa*

2. Which of the following statements about the pathogenesis of *Haemophilus influenzae,* serotype b (Hib) is correct?
   A. Transplacental transfer of antibody protects infants from Hib disease in the first 3 months of life
   B. Most Hib is acquired from contact with mammalian reservoirs other than humans
   C. Immunity to Hib infection is primarily determined by strong cellular immune responses elicited by vaccination
   D. The most common portal of entry is the gastrointestinal tract
   E. Hib relies on capsular antigens for transport across cellular membranes of epithelial cells for invasion

HPI: While working as a Peace Corps volunteer in Zimbabwe, you see a 31-year-old man who presents to your clinic with a painful penile lesion, which has been present for 5 days. He admits to sex with a commercial sex worker 2 weeks ago.

PE: Afebrile. Single 1- by 2-cm indurated, sharply defined ulcer with undermined edges is present on the distal shaft of his penis. The base of the ulcer is yellow and friable and bleeds easily. It is moderately painful. There are 2-cm lymph nodes in the right inguinal region that are boggy and tender. One of the lymph nodes has ulcerated through the skin. There is no urethral discharge.

Thought Questions

- What is the differential diagnosis of genital ulcers?
- What is the best treatment for this disease?

Basic Science Review and Discussion

The differential diagnosis of **genital ulcer disease** should always include consideration of **syphilis** and **herpes simplex virus (HSV)**. The chancre of primary syphilis, caused by *Treponema pallidum,* is usually painless and indurated. Lymph nodes, if enlarged, are nonsuppurative. The incubation period after exposure is 9 to 90 days. In contrast, the ulcers of HSV are usually multiple, may be preceded by vesicles, and are usually exquisitely tender. The incubation period for HSV is 3 to 5 days.

Other infectious diseases in the differential diagnosis of genital ulcer disease are chancroid, granuloma inguinale, and lymphogranuloma venereum (LGV). The painful ulcers of chancroid may be indurated and are often associated with **suppurative unilateral inguinal lymphadenopthy.** Granuloma inguinale, or Donovanosis, is caused by infection with *Calymmatobacterium granulomatis,* which produces painless, beefy-red ulcers. LGV is caused by *Chlamydia trachomatis* serovars L1, L2, and L3. The ulcers of LGV are painless and heal rapidly and are characteristically found in association with prominent, suppurative lymphadenopathy.

In the U.S., syphilis and herpes are the common etiologies of genital vicer disease. LGV and Donovanosis are more prevalent in developing countries. Chancroid is endemic in developing countries with a tropical climate and occurs sporadically in the U.S.

This patient has chancroid, caused by *Haemophilus ducreyi.* This organism is difficult to grow in culture. When seen on Gram stain, it appears as a **gram-negative bacillus in chains,** a typical "**railroad cars**" appearance. (See Figure 14-1.)

H. ducreyi invades via a break in the surface epithelium. After an incubation period of 4 to 7 days, a small painless papule surrounded by an erythematous halo develops over an area of indurated skin. It ruptures in 2 to 4 days, leaving a sharply defined ulcer with a yellow, friable base that bleeds easily. Painful unilateral inguinal lymphadenopathy develops in over half of patients. The lymph nodes may form buboes, suppurate, and rupture, leaving inguinal ulcers. In women, the most common site for the primary ulcer is at the entrance to the vagina, as well as the fourchette, labia, vestibule, and clitoris.

First line of treatment for chancroid is erythromycin 500 mg PO four times a day for 7 days. Other regimens include azithromycin 1 g PO once, ceftriaxone 250 mg IM once,

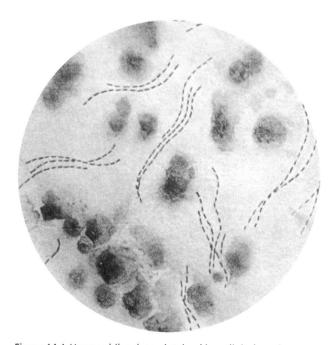

Figure 14-1 *Haemophilus ducreyi* stained in a clinical specimen. (Image in public domain on Centers for Disease Control Public Health Image Library, phil.cdc.gov.)

ciprofloxacin 500 mg PO twice a day for 3 days, or TMP-SMZ (Septra) DS 1 tablet PO twice a day for 5 days. Testing for other sexually transmitted diseases (STDs) should be part of the evaluation, as multiple infections may be transmitted at once. Chancroid has been implicated as a **cofactor for HIV transmission** in Africa.

Case Conclusion   This patient was treated for chancroid with erythromycin. His ulcer responded well to treatment and resolved. He also tested positive for HIV.

Thumbnail: Chancroid

Organism	*Haemophilus ducreyi*
Type of organism	Gram-negative bacillus in chains
Disease caused	Chancroid
Epidemiology	More common in less developed, tropical countries but may occur anywhere
Diagnosis	Mostly clinical; Gram stain is insensitive and nonspecific; culture requires special media and is insensitive
Treatment	Erythromycin 500 mg four times a day for 7 days; azithromycin 1 g PO once; ceftriaxone 250 mg IM once; ciprofloxacin 500 mg twice a day for 3 days

Key Points

▶ Chancroid usually presents as a painful ulcer with unilateral, possibly suppurative, tender inguinal lymphadenopathy

▶ When treating one STD, testing for all other STDs (including HIV) should be considered

Questions

1. A 23-year-old commercial sex worker in Nairobi, Kenya, presents with a painful ulcer on her outer labia with painful, swollen inguinal lymph nodes on the right side. Testing for HIV antibodies is negative. Serology for *Chlamydia* is negative. Repeated rapid plasma reagin test (RPR) is negative. Viral and bacterial culture of the ulcer is negative. What is the most likely diagnosis?
   A. Primary syphilis
   B. Secondary syphilis
   C. Lymphogranuloma venereum
   D. Donovanosis
   E. Chancroid

2. Of the following, the best treatment for chancroid is:
   A. Penicillin
   B. Erythromycin
   C. Acyclovir
   D. Atovaquone
   E. No antibiotic treatment is necessary

HPI: An 86-year-old woman is brought in to the emergency room by her family because of sudden onset of confusion. She has no past medical history, other than hypertension, and had been living independently before admission. Review of systems is positive for fevers, nausea and vomiting, back pain, dysuria, and urinary frequency and urgency. There are no focal neurologic symptoms and she has no history of syncope or seizure.

PE: T 38.0°C BP 120/70 HR 105 RR 18
An elderly woman, toxic appearing, oriented to her name only. While the doctor is examining her, she has an episode of violent shaking chills. The patient's mucous membranes are dry; the oropharynx has no exudate. The neck is supple without lymphadenopathy. Lungs are clear. Heart exam has a 1/6 systolic ejection murmur and an S4. Abdominal exam shows mild diffuse tenderness, but no masses or hepatosplenomegaly. There are no peritoneal signs. Back exam shows no spinous tenderness, but exquisite tenderness at the left costovertebral angle. Extremities have no edema. There is no rash. A neurological exam is nonfocal.
A head CT, done in the ER, is negative for acute bleed or stroke.

Labs: White count is 18, with 90% neutrophils, and bands present. Hematocrit is 38. Platelets are 190. A chemistry panel shows a sodium of 148, blood urea nitrogen of 32, and creatinine of 0.9. A urine dipstick shows pH 8.0, specific gravity 1.028, no glucose, 1+ ketones, 4+ nitrates, and 4+ leukocyte esterase. The microscopic urinalysis shows no epithelial cells, 0–2 red blood cells, and 50–100 white blood cells per high-power field, as well as many bacteria. The bacteria are gram-negative rods on Gram stain. After two blood cultures and a urine culture are sent, the patient is started on ciprofloxacin.

Thought Questions

- Which aspects of the urinalysis indicate infection?

- Which laboratory tests indicate dehydration?

- How can lower UTIs and pyelonephritis be distinguished?

- What routes can bacteria take to infect a kidney?

- Which is most likely in this case?

- Which bacteria are most likely to cause UTIs?

Basic Science Review and Discussion

Epidemiology Urinary tract infections (UTIs) can be divided into lower **(cystitis)** and upper **(pyelonephritis).** Most cases of pyelonephritis are caused by ascension of bacteria from the bladder to the kidney via the ureter. Less commonly, bacteremia can lead to hematogenous seeding of the kidney. The distinction between lower and upper UTIs can be a difficult one to make, but it is important because pyelonephritis is a life-threatening infection that requires more reliable antibiotic regimens given for longer durations. Lower UTIs manifest with **dysuria,** urinary **frequency,** and urinary **urgency.** Any symptoms such as high fever, rigors, hypotension, nausea or vomiting, mental status changes, and costovertebral angle tenderness suggest pyelonephritis. Women are more prone to UTIs than men because their urethras are shorter and it is easier for bacteria to reach the bladder. Men with UTIs, or any patient with repeated episodes of pyelonephritis, need evaluation for possible anatomic abnormalities allowing bacteria to spread to normally sterile areas of the body.

Species involved The organisms that cause UTIs tend to come from gut flora. Gram-negative rods that may cause community-acquired urinary tract infection include *Escherichia coli (E. coli), Proteus, Morganella,* and *Providencia,* all members of the family Enterobacteriaceae. Gram-positive cocci, such as *Staphylococcus saprophyticus* and enterococcal species, are other common causes of these infections. Because *E. coli* is the most common cause of UTIs, antibiotic coverage is tailored to the antibiotic resistance profile of community isolates of this organism. If rates of resistance to sulfa drugs are low, then TMP-SMZ is an excellent empiric choice for lower UTIs. If sulfa resistance rates are high, then fluoro-quinolones, nitrofurantoin, or cephalexin may be preferred. (Although cephalexin is most often used for its gram-positive coverage, it does cover many community isolates of *Proteus mirabilis, E. coli,* and *Klebsiella.)*

After *E. coli, Proteus* species are the second most common cause of community UTIs. *Proteus* is notable for its ability to split urea in the urine, leading to an alkaline urine pH. This can predispose patients to the development of **struvite** kidney stones, which in turn can lead to a vicious cycle of repeat infections. *Proteus* is also a highly motile organism, and it will quickly spread over the entire surface of a culture plate. *Morganella morganii* and *Providencia* are gram-negative rods closely related to *Proteus,* but often with a greater degree of antibiotic resistance.

Other gram-negative rods common in nosocomial UTIs include *Pseudomonas, Klebsiella, Citrobacter, Serratia,* and *Enterobacter.* Many of these organisms have considerable resistance to β-lactams and cephalosporins. Because of resistance problems, and because patients with nosocomial infections are frequently quite ill, broad empiric coverage is often given for infections with these organisms until sensitivities are determined.

Diagnosis Urinalysis (UA) is a common initial diagnostic test for UTIs. Table 15-1 lists some of the characteristics present in UAs in the presence of a UTI.

Urine cultures are usually plated on two selective media. One, such as **CNA** (colistin nalidixic acid), is selective for

gram-positive cocci. The other, such as **MacConkey** agar, is selective for gram-negative rods. MacConkey also distinguishes between lactose fermenters, such as the *Enterobacteriaciae,* which are purple, and lactose nonfermenters, such as *Pseudomonas,* which are pale pink. Once the bacteria have grown on the plate, the number of colonies per mL of urine is calculated. Counts as low as 10^2/mL of a single species are probably significant in a symptomatic patient, but for practical reasons, laboratories usually use higher counts, such as 10^5/mL, as a test for significance. The bacteria, if present in significant amounts, can be further speciated using combinations of biochemical tests (either done by hand with multiple tubes or a test strip, or in an automated machine).

Table 15-1 Understanding the urinalysis in urinary tract infections

Measurement	Comes from	Interpretation in this case
pH	Can reflect the patient's acid-base metabolism; in the present case, the urine is alkaline due to splitting of urea in the urine by *Proteus*	More evidence of *Proteus* infection
Specific gravity	Degree of urine concentration	The patient is dehydrated due to vomiting
Glucose	Glucose in urine comes from high blood glucose levels	If present, would suggest diabetes, which can predispose to UTIs
Ketones	Ketones in urine come from ketones in blood	Suggests the patient is in a fasting state due to vomiting
Nitrates	Made by bacterial metabolism	Evidence of bacteria in the urine, consistent with UTI
Leukocyte esterase	Made by white blood cells	Evidence of a host response to infection, consistent with UTI
Bacteria	May be due to bacteria in the urine when it was collected, or may be a contaminant since collection	Evidence of UTI; more than 10^5 colonies/mL on culture is usually significant
Epithelial cells	Skin of genitalia during collection	Their presence would raise suspicion of an improperly collected sample contaminated by skin flora
White cells	Host response to infection	Confirms the dipstick result of a positive leukocyte esterase; More than five per high power field are probably significant
Red cells	Extravasation into the urinary tract at any level from kidney to bladder to urethra	Their presence may be due to infection, but could also indicate kidney stones, trauma, or tumor

Case Conclusion After a dose of ciprofloxacin, the patient has a dramatic overnight improvement in her mental status; her fever, nausea, and vomiting resolve. The urine culture grows out greater than 10^5 colonies/mL of *Proteus mirabilis.* Two of two blood cultures grow *Proteus mirabilis* as well. The culture plates have the classic appearance of *Proteus:* because of swarming motility, bacteria have moved away from individual colonies and have covered the entire surface of the normally shiny agar with a thin coating of bacteria. The patient is discharged from the hospital 2 days later, to finish a 2-week course of ciprofloxacin.

Thumbnail: UTIs

Type of organism	Aerobic, gram-negative rod organism: *Proteus mirabilis*
Diseases caused	UTIs; abdominal infections
Epidemiology	Normal bowel flora, which may cause infection if normal gastrointestinal barriers are breached, or if transmitted to the genitourinary tract
Diagnosis	Culture
Treatment	Fluoroquinolones; cephalexin, nitrofurantoin, or TMP-SMZ for outpatient treatment of lower UTIs

Key Points

▶ Community-acquired UTIs are usually due to organisms from the gut flora; empiric antibiotic coverage should be tailored to *E. coli* resistance patterns in the community

▶ The presence of high fever, rigors, nausea, and vomiting, or costovertebral angle tenderness are all concerning for pyelonephritis, rather than simple cystitis

Questions

1. A urine Gram stain in a patient with a UTI shows thick gram-negative rods. Which is the most likely organism?
   A. *Staphylococcus aureus*
   B. *Staphylococcus saprophyticus*
   C. *Corynebacteria*
   D. *Escherichia coli*
   E. *Enterococcus faecalis*

2. Which of the following symptoms and signs is most commonly seen in uncomplicated cystitis?
   A. Rigors
   B. Dysuria
   C. Costovertebral angle tenderness
   D. Vomiting
   E. Gross hematuria

3. Which antibiotic is a reasonable choice for a healthy young woman diagnosed with an uncomplicated lower urinary tract infection?
   A. Imipenem
   B. Azithromycin
   C. Nitrofurantoin
   D. Trovafloxacin
   E. Metronidazole

HPI: A 23-year-old man is a Peace Corps volunteer in Ecuador. Yesterday he suddenly developed voluminous diarrhea; he has already had over 20 watery stools. There is no blood or pus in the stools. He feels profoundly fatigued. He has no fever. Upon further questioning, he admits that after the first few months in Ecuador, he has become less careful about his food and water: recent meals have included raw shellfish and fruit drinks with ice cubes. He denies any recent antibiotic use that could predispose him to *C. difficile* colitis.

PE: T 37.9°C BP 100/50 HR 110 RR 24
Vital signs are repeated with the patient standing, and blood pressure falls to 85/40 with an increased heart rate of 135. He appears uncomfortable and weak and apologizes as he rushes out of the room to use the toilet. Skin is clammy with poor turgor. Mucous membranes are dry. His heart is tachycardic but regular, with no murmurs. Lungs are clear, but he is breathing rapidly. Abdomen has mild diffuse tenderness with increased bowel sounds. He is still alert and oriented, and a neurologic exam is nonfocal.

Labs: White blood count of 15, with a normal differential. Electrolytes show a sodium of 128, potassium of 3.0, chloride of 93, bicarbonate of 10, BUN of 30, and creatinine of 0.8.
A stool sample has the appearance of "rice water" due to flecks of mucus and epithelial cells in the otherwise watery stool.

Thought Questions

■ What is the difference in pathogenesis between watery and bloody diarrhea?

■ Which infectious agents cause diarrhea?

■ Why did this patient not receive antibiotics?

■ How can people stand to eat raw shellfish?

Basic Science Review and Discussion

Cholera is spread through contaminated water and food. *Vibrio cholerae* is a motile, gram-negative rod with one polar flagellum. The organism is ingested and then colonizes the small intestine. It is noninvasive and causes disease by producing an **exotoxin**. Producing cholera toxin confers a selective advantage to the organism, because the diarrhea it causes helps the organism spread to new hosts. The cholera toxin causes **ADP-ribosylation of the Gs subunit** of the G protein of intestinal cells. This prevents the G protein from being turned off, and results in excess production of cAMP. (Pertussis toxin also results in excess production of cAMP, but acts by binding and inactivating the Gi subunit instead.) Table 16-1 gives examples of other toxin-mediated diarrheal illnesses. Figure 16-1 schematicizes the mechanism of action of the cholera and pertussis toxins.

The cholera toxin results in excess secretion of calcium ions into the intestinal lumen. Water, sodium, potassium, and bicarbonate all follow due to concentration and electrical gradients. This causes watery diarrhea classically described as **"rice-water stools."** Because the organism is not invasive, and the toxin does not kill the intestinal cells, the diarrhea usually does not contain blood or pus. The diarrhea causes hypovolemia, hyponatremia, hypokalemia, and metabolic acidosis. Untreated cholera can be rapidly fatal, due to profound **dehydration** and electrolyte abnormalities, which can cause shock, cardiac arrhythmias, or brain damage. Table 16-2 lists the differences between secretory diarrhea and invasive disease (i.e., dysentery).

Table 16-1 Examples of toxins causing diarrhea

Name	Biochemical mechanism	Clinical effect
Cholera toxin	Adenylation of Gs subunit, causing irreversible G protein activation and cAMP production	Watery diarrhea due to uncontrolled secretion by intestinal epithelial cell
E. coli heat-labile toxin	Adenylation of Gs subunit, causing irreversible G protein activation and cAMP production	Watery diarrhea due to uncontrolled secretion by intestinal epithelial cell.
E. coli heat-stable toxin	Activates guanylate cyclase	Watery diarrhea due to uncontrolled secretion by intestinal epithelial cell.
Shiga toxin (*Shigella* and *E. coli* O157:H7)	Blocks protein synthesis by cleaving 28S ribosomal RNA	Bloody diarrhea due to cell death
Aerolysin (*Aeromonas*)	Binds glycophorin and causes pore formation	Bloody diarrhea due to cell death
C. difficile toxins A and B	Binds Rho, a small G protein	Diarrhea and pseudomembrane formation in colon

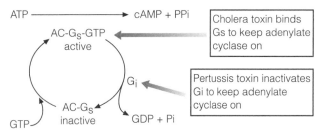

Figure 16-1 Adenylate cyclase activation by cholera and pertussis toxins.

There is partial host immunity to *Vibrio cholerae,* as children are more affected than adults by outbreaks in endemic areas. Immunity is likely due to secreted IgA antibodies in the gut mucosa. The cholera toxin itself is a poor antigen, so immunization with a toxoid (as is done for tetanus) is not effective. Efforts are still under way to develop a more efficacious vaccine.

Treatment   The cornerstone of cholera treatment is replacement of lost fluids and electrolytes (sodium, potassium, and chloride) with rehydration. Oral rehydration solution also contains sugar to help with absorption of the other components in the gut. **Oral rehydration therapy** is preferred over IV hydration in developing countries because oral solutions are much cheaper and do not require sterilization. Although some antibiotics, such as tetracyclines or quinolones, may modestly shorten the duration and severity of diarrhea, they are usually not prescribed for cholera. The most effective way of combating cholera is by improving sanitation standards and water quality.

Table 16-2 Diarrhea syndromes

	Secretory diarrhea	Dysentery
Syndrome	Watery stools	Stools with blood or pus; fever, abdominal pain, tenesmus
Anatomic location	Small intestine	Colon
Pathogenesis	Toxin causing increased secretion of electrolytes into gut lumen	Toxin causing damage to cells of intestinal epithelium, or direct invasion by microorganism
Examples	Enterotoxigenic *E. coli*, cholera	*E. coli* O157:H7, *Shigella*, *Campylobacter jejuni*, amebiasis

Case Conclusion   The patient is given intravenous hydration with 6 L of normal saline with added potassium. He is then given packets of a salt and sugar mix (e.g., oral rehydration therapy) to dissolve in water and drink to replete electrolytes lost in his diarrhea. Although timely rehydration produced a complete recovery in our patient, untreated cholera can cause up to 50% mortality by dehydration within hours to days. Afterward, he is reminded to be more careful about avoiding contaminated food and water with the rule: **"open it, boil it, cook it, peel it, or forget it."**

Thumbnail: Cholera

Organism	***Vibrio cholerae***
Type of organism	Gram-negative rod; facultative anaerobe; motile with single polar flagellum
Disease caused	Cholera
Epidemiology	Epidemic spread through contaminated water supply
Diagnosis	Clinical; may culture organism from stool
Treatment	Supportive rehydration—either intravenous or oral; antibiotics usually not necessary; immunization available but not recommended, as it protects less than 50% of travelers for 3 to 6 months

Key Points

▶ Cholera is the prototype for secretory diarrhea, caused by a toxin that constitutively activates G protein signaling in intestinal epithelial cells

▶ The disease kills because of dehydration

▶ The major intervention is supportive care with oral or IV rehydration

▶ The classic advice to prevent traveler's diarrhea is "open it, boil it, cook it, peel it, or forget it"

Questions

1. A 32-year-old man returns from a vacation to Central America with frequent bloody stools. Which organism is unlikely to cause this syndrome?
   A. *E. coli*
   B. *Shigella*
   C. *Salmonella*
   D. *Vibrio cholerae*
   E. *Vibrio parahaemolyticus*

2. The most useful of the following measures against cholera is:
   A. Vaccination before travel
   B. Avoiding soups made without bottled water when traveling
   C. Starting ciprofloxacin once cholera has been diagnosed
   D. Decontamination of the gut with oral neomycin
   E. Ingesting a mixture of water, salt, and sugar

HPI: A 45-year-old man presents to his primary care physician complaining of several weeks of sharp, burning epigastric pain, which occurs 2 hours after eating. The pain is relieved with antacids and is diminished immediately after eating. He has had two similar episodes of epigastric pain over the past 5 years, each lasting about 1 month and resolving without medical intervention. He sought attention for this episode because it has lasted longer than his previous ones. He has had no hematemesis, melena, weight loss, fevers, or chills. He drinks 2 to 3 beers only on weekends and smokes one pack of cigarettes per day.

PMH: Hypertension, well controlled with salt restriction and hydrochlorothiazide 50 mg once daily; hyperlipidemia, on simvastatin 20 mg once daily; diet-controlled type II diabetes mellitus.

PE: T 36.2°C BP 140/86 HR 86 RR 16
Abdominal exam demonstrates tenderness in the right upper quadrant and epigastrium. He has no rebound or guarding. No masses can be palpated. His stool is brown and tests positive for occult blood. He is not jaundiced. The remainder of the exam is normal.

Labs: Hemoglobin 13.6; hematocrit 40.2; MCV 88. AST, ALT, bilirubin, amylase, and lipase are all within the normal range for the laboratory.
Endoscopy demonstrates a normal esophagus and stomach, but shows a single 2-cm ulcer in the first portion of the duodenum.

Thought Questions

- Infection with what organism has been associated with duodenal ulcers?

- What tests are available to diagnose this infection? How do these tests work?

- What are the options for treatment of this infection?

- What are the indications for treatment?

Basic Science Review and Discussion

Infection with the **multiflagellated, curved, gram-negative rod** *Helicobacter pylori* has been found in **60% to 80% of patients with gastric ulcers and greater than 90% of those with duodenal ulcers.** The organism is best cultured on blood agar plates at 37°C in a microaerobic atmosphere with 5% to10% CO_2. *H. pylori* has large amounts of the enzyme **urease,** which hydrolyzes urea to ammonia and CO_2. This serves as the basis for the diagnostic urea breath test.

Most transmission of *H. pylori* occurs in children and young adults through oral and gastric secretions and by the fecal-oral route. Rates are increased in poor socioeconomic environments. Infections typically persist for decades if untreated, although most patients with colonization by *H. pylori* remain asymptomatic.

Patients with *H. pylori* infection are more likely to develop **acute and chronic gastritis, gastric ulcers, and duodenal ulcers.** Ulcers may be asymptomatic, but commonly produce epigastric pain, often localized to the right of midline. Complications of gastric or duodenal ulcers include bleeding, gastric outlet obstruction, perforation, and carcinoma.

There are many tools for the diagnosis of *H. pylori* infection related to duodenal ulcers. Noninvasive tests include the relatively inexpensive serology (sensitivity and specificity 85%–95%), a stool antigen test, and the urea breath test. To perform the **urease breath test,** the subject ingests a meal containing ^{13}C- or ^{14}C-urea. After 1 hour, a breath sample is analyzed for $^{13}CO_2$ or $^{14}CO_2$, the presence of which indicates activity of the urease enzyme and the presence of *H. pylori*. Because it relies on metabolically active organisms, the urease breath test is useful as a test of cure, unlike serology, which remains positive even after successful eradication of infection.

Invasive diagnosis of *H. pylori* infection at the time of endoscopy can be achieved by a rapid urease test, culture of the organism from tissue samples (the least sensitive of the diagnostic tools), demonstration of the organism on histologic examination of biopsy specimens (on Gram stain, Giemsa stain, or silver stain), or PCR.

Eradication of *H. pylori* from gastric and duodenal ulcers is associated with healing of the ulcers and a lower rate of ulcer recurrence than patients in whom the organism is not treated. Single-agent therapy for *H. pylori* is ineffective due to the emergence of resistance. Several regimens including **combinations of antibiotics, bismuth, and proton pump inhibitors** are effective. FDA-approved regimens are listed in the Thumbnail section.

Treatment is generally prescribed for 2 weeks. A test of eradication (usually the urease breath test) should be considered in those in whom symptoms persist. Resistance of *H. pylori* to most of these individual agents has been described.

H. pylori has also been demonstrated to be a risk factor for carcinoma of the distal (but not proximal) stomach. It has also been associated with **gastric non-Hodgkin's lymphoma** (gastric MALToma), where eradication of the organism is associated with tumor regression.

Because only a minority of persons with *H. pylori* infection develop symptoms or complications of the infection and because of problems with *H. pylori* treatment (resistance or medication side effects), not all cases of *H. pylori* infection should be treated. Definite indications for treatment are in cases of gastric non-Hodgkin's lymphoma and diagnosed peptic ulcer disease. Other cases in which eradication of *H. pylori* may be considered include those with a family history of gastric cancer, atrophic gastritis, gastric or intestinal metaplasia or dysplasia, and after resection of an early gastric carcinoma. Nonulcer dyspepsia is not an indication for antimicrobial therapy.

Case Conclusion   A diagnosis of *H. pylori* was made in this patient by demonstrating the organism on Giemsa stain of a biopsy specimen of the duodenal ulcer taken at the time of endoscopy. He was treated with 2 weeks of clarithromycin, metronidazole, and omeprazole with improvement of his symptoms. Urease breath test performed 6 weeks after completion of therapy was negative for active infection.

Thumbnail: Gastric and Duodenal Ulcer Disease

Organism	*Helicobacter pylori*
Type of organism	Gram-negative curved bacillus with multiple flagella
Diseases caused	Acute and chronic gastritis, gastric ulcers, duodenal ulcers; associated with carcinoma of the distal stomach and gastric non-Hodgkin's lymphoma
Epidemiology	Ubiquitous; infection occurs early in life and persists for decades if untreated; transmission is by oral and gastric secretions and the fecal-oral route; an estimated 60% of the world's population is infected
Diagnosis	Noninvasive: serology, stool antigen test, or urease breath test; invasive: tissue culture, histology (Gram stain, Giemsa stain, or silver stain), rapid urease test, or PCR
Treatment	Eradication rates up to 90% with multiple FDA-approved regimens given for 2 weeks, including: 1) tetracycline + metronidazole + bismuth subsalicylate + H$_2$ blocker 2) amoxicillin + clarithromycin + protease pump inhibitor (PPI) 3) metronidazole + clarithromycin + PPI 4) amoxicillin + metronidazole + PPI

Key Points

▶ Infection with *H. pylori* is very common; however, most individuals remain asymptomatic and should not be treated

▶ Indications for treatment of documented infection include peptic ulcer disease and gastric non-Hodgkin's lymphoma; consideration should be given to treatment of those with a family history of gastric cancer, successful resection of early gastric carcinoma, atrophic gastritis, or gastric or intestinal metaplasia/dysplasia; treatment of nonulcer dyspepsia should not include attempts at *H. pylori* eradication

▶ Multiple methods of diagnosis and multiple treatment regimens are available

▶ Test for cure after treatment is optional; can be determined using the urease breath test

▶ Serology, while useful in diagnosis, has no role in test of cure

Questions

1. A 48-year-old man is diagnosed with gastric non-Hodgkin's lymphoma. Treatment of which of the following microorganisms is most likely to result in tumor regression?

   A. *Treponema pallidum*
   B. *Giardia lamblia*
   C. Hepatitis B virus
   D. Epstein-Barr virus
   E. *Helicobacter pylori*

2. Which of the following is the best test of *H. pylori* eradication following treatment?

   A. Culture
   B. Urease breath test
   C. Serology
   D. Stool PCR
   E. CAMP test

3. A 40-year-old woman with complaints of epigastric pain and sour taste in her mouth has a positive serology for *H. pylori.* Endoscopy is normal. Which of the following is the best treatment?

   A. Ranitidine only
   B. Omeprazole + metronidazole + clarithromycin
   C. Bismuth + tetracycline + metronidazole
   D. Ciprofloxacin only
   E. Omeprazole + ciprofloxacin

HPI: FT is a 23-year-old male who presents to your office with a 1 week history of "feeling flu-like" with fever, fatigue, generalized malaise, mild myalgias, and arthalgias. FT also complains of swollen lymph nodes that are painful around his right elbow and armpit. He does not have any cough, shortness of breath, abdominal pain, diarrhea, constipation, problems with urination, or rash. FT is a construction worker by trade, but is an avid rabbit hunter and spent the last 10 days hunting in the woods surrounding his home. He shot and skinned several rabbits over this period, although he has not yet consumed the meat. When asked about tick exposure during the hunting expedition, he states "critters were all over the place in the woods and that includes my body." FT also states that his father accompanied him on all his hunting trips and has a similar illness. No one else in the house is sick.

PMH: FT has been generally healthy. He takes no medications and has a penicillin allergy manifested by rash. Lives with his parents and grandparents in a rural area of Missouri.

PE: T 38.0°C HR 96 BP 128/88 RR 12
Mildly ill-appearing young man in no respiratory distress. Main findings on exam are a 1 by 1 cm erythematous ulceration on his right palm with several swollen lymph nodes in the right epitrochlear region (just above the elbow and medial in location) and axillary region that are extremely painful to palpation. Heart, lung, and abdominal examination are all within normal limits.

Labs: WBC 13.0 with 88% neutrophils; all other laboratory tests within normal limits.

Thought Questions

- What is the most likely mode of transmission of FT's infectious illness?

- What are some of the bacterial infections associated with animal exposure in humans?

- What is the epidemiology of these infections?

- How would you distinguish some of these bacteria in the laboratory?

- Do any of these agents have a potential for bioterrorist exploitation?

Basic Science Review and Discussion

The most significant aspect of FT's history is the temporal relation of his syndrome to exposure to rabbit hides and the woods, as well as the development of a similar illness in his father who had the same exposures. Both aspects suggest a **zoonotic** transmission of the described illness. The paragraphs and summary table below describe some of the major zoonotic gram-negative rod bacterial infections in humans.

Francisella tularensis
Properties   *F. tularensis* is a small pleomorphic gram-negative rod.

Epidemiology   *F. tularensis* can occur in a wide variety of animals and is endemic in animals (enzootic) in every state, although most human cases of the disease are reported from rural areas in Arkansas and Missouri. Although the organism has been isolated from a number of different wild animals, the most important animals in terms of human transmission are **rabbits,** deer, and a variety of rodents. The bacteria are transmitted among these animals by various vectors, including **ticks,** especially the ***Dermacentor*** and ***Amblyomma*** ticks.

Transmission   Humans can acquire tularemia by having skin contact with the animal during removal of its hide or by being bitten by the transmitting vector (e.g., tick). Gastrointestinal tularemia can rarely occur from ingestion of contaminated meat and spontaneous tularemia pneumonia can occur from inhalation of the organism.

Clinical   Tularemia patients usually present with an acute influenza-like syndrome or a low-grade fever with adenopathy. The "**ulceroglandular type**" of tularemia results in ulceration at the site of organism entry into the skin accompanied by swollen and painful regional lymph nodes. Spontaneous acquisition of tularemia pneumonia is rare and presentation of this disease should trigger a suspicion of **bioterrorism.** A weapon using airborne tularemia would likely result in an outbreak of acute, undifferentiated febrile illness with pneumonia, pleuritis, and hilar lymphadenopathy.

Diagnosis   Given the risk to laboratory workers for inhalation of the organism, culture is rarely undertaken. Acute and convalescent serum samples for serology is the standard method of diagnosis.

Treatment   Standard treatment is intravenous streptomycin.

Yersinia pestis

Properties   *Y. pestis* is a small gram-negative rod with bipolar staining on Gram stain (resembles a **safety pin**). *Y. pestis* is one of the most virulent organisms in nature and exposure to only 1–10 organisms can cause disease.

Epidemiology   Most of the cases of plague occur in Southeast Asia because of endemicity in wild rodents throughout most of this region. However, the plague bacillus has also entered the wild rodent population in the U.S., especially in the western states, and is carried by prairie dogs.

Transmission   **Fleas** transmit infection from infected rodents to humans.

Clinical   *Y. pestis* organisms are inoculated to the human at the time of the flea bite and spread to regional lymph nodes, which become swollen and tender; these nodes are known as **buboes,** leading to the nickname of "**bubonic plague**" for the syndrome of *Y. pestis* infection. See Figure 18-1.

From the buboes, the organism can spread to the bloodstream and form abscesses in multiple organs, as well as cause the syndromes of DIC, sepsis, and cutaneous hemorrhages (leading to the nickname of "**black death**" for the plague). High fever, myalgias, and prostration are frequent accompanying symptoms. **Pneumonic plague** is caused by inhalation of the *Y. pestis* organisms and is hallmarked by fever, dyspnea, cough, purulent sputum, and hemoptysis in most cases. Clinical findings are those of a rapidly progressive bronchopneumonia and patients who do not receive specific therapy within 18 hours of the onset of respiratory symptoms are unlikely to survive. Given the high mortality

with this illness, aerosolized *Y. pestis* is also a listed agent of **bioterrorism.**

Diagnosis   Smear and culture of the blood or pus from the bubo is the best diagnostic procedure and should show a typical safety pin bipolar staining of the organism (best appreciated on Giemsa or Wayson stain). Given the highly infectious nature of the organism, a safer procedure for diagnosis is fluorescent antibody staining in tissues. See Figure 18-2.

Treatment   Streptomycin or gentamicin. Alternatives are ciprofloxacin or tetracycline.

Brucella species

Properties   Small gram-negative rods without a capsule. The three main human pathogens are *B. abortus* (cattle), *B. melitensis* (goats and sheep), and *B. suis* (pigs). (*B. canis* is a rare cause of human disease and is found in dogs.)

Epidemiology   Infections usually seen in abattoir workers, meat inspectors, animal handlers, veterinarians, and laboratory workers.

Transmission   *Brucella* organisms are commonly transmitted through skin abrasions when humans handle infected mammals or animal products. Infection can also occur through the ingestion of contaminated milk and dairy products. For instance, imported cheese made from **unpasteurized goat's milk** from either Mexico or the Mediterranean has been a source of *B. melitensis* infection in the U.S. Given the highly infectious nature of the organism, laboratory workers handling *Brucella* are also at risk for infection.

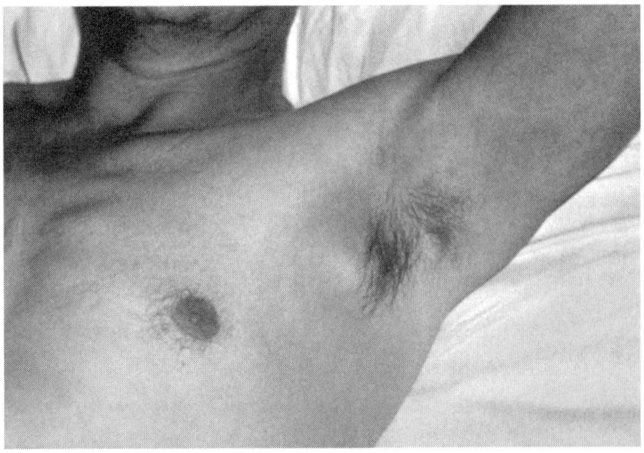

Figure 18-1 Bubo in axillary lymph node (regional adenopathy with edema). (Image in public domain on Centers for Disease Control Public Health Image Library, phil.cdc.gov.)

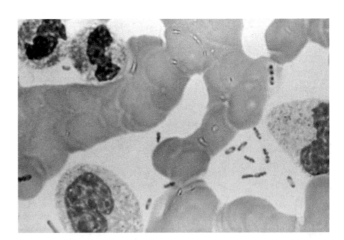

Figure 18-2 Stain of peripheral blood smear of a patient with septicemic plague demonstrating bipolar, safety pin staining of *Yersinia pestis*. (Image in public domain on Centers for Disease Control Public Health Image Library, phil.cdc.gov.)

Clinical Brucellosis has multiple clinical syndromes, including a nonspecific influenza-like syndrome in the acute setting with fevers, sweats, malaise, anorexia, headache, myalgias, and back pain. In the recurring form of the disease (called "**undulant fever**" and defined as occurring less than 1 year from illness onset), symptoms include cyclical fevers, **arthritis,** and orchiepididymitis (males). In the chronic form (more than 1 year after exposure), arthritis and a syndrome of chronic fatigue can occur. Other sequelae of *Brucella* infection include **endocarditis,** granulomatous hepatitis, spondylitis, uveitis, meningitis, and optic neuritis.

Diagnosis *Brucella* can be cultured on enriched media and incubation at 10% CO_2. However, the diagnosis of brucellosis is most often made serologically.

Treatment Doxycycline (or tetracycline) plus gentamicin.

Pasteurella multocida
Properties Gram-negative coccobacillus.

Epidemiology and transmission *P. multocida* inhabits the oral cavity and gastrointestinal tracts of many animals. Human infections are most commonly caused by bites from **cats or dogs.**

Clinical The most common clinical syndrome of *P. multocida* bites is a localized **cellulitis,** although complications can include bone and joint infections, bacteremia, sepsis, subcutaneous abscesses, pneumonia, meningitis, endocarditis, and intra-abdominal infections. Approximately 15% to 20% of dog bites and 50% of cat bite wounds will become infected with this organism without treatment.

Diagnosis Culture.

Treatment Penicillin was the former drug of choice for this infection. However, as plasmid-mediated β-lactamase production has been described in some *P. multocida* strains isolated from animals, amoxicillin-clavulanate is currently the drug of choice. Fluoroquinolones can be used in penicillin-allergic patients.

Capnocytophaga Species
Properties Thin, delicate, fusiform, gram-negative rods with tapered ends. Grow best in 5% to 10% CO_2 and are yellow pigmented.

Epidemiology and transmission *C. canimorsus* and *C. cynodegmi* are found in the oral cavity of dogs; *C. ochracea, C. sputigena,* and *C. gingivalis* are found in the oral cavity of humans. The canine species of *Capnocytophaga* cause infections after **dog bites** or scratches.

Clinical Although the main clinical syndrome of *Capnocytophaga* is a localized **cellulitis** at the site of the bite, severe disease can occur, particularly in **splenectomized** patients, alcoholics, patients with liver disease, and patients on steroids. This infection can lead to DIC, sepsis, meningitis, endocarditis, pneumonia, and septic arthritis.

Diagnosis Culture.

Treatment Penicillin or amoxicillin-clavulanate are the recommended agents for treating *Capnocytophaga.* The organism is also susceptible to clindamycin, macrolides, doxycycline, and fluoroquinolones.

Table 18-1 summarizes the main features of the zoonotic organisms described above.

Table 18-1 Summary of zoonotic gram-negative rods

Organism	Disease	Source of human infection	Mode of transmission from animal to human	Diagnosis
Francisella tularensis	Tularemia	Rabbits, deer, variety of rodents, ticks	Contact with infected animal's tissues; bites from ticks (especially *Dermacentor* ticks that feed on the blood of wild rabbits); consuming infected meat (rarely); inhaling organisms	Serology (can also culture in the lab, but high risk of infection to lab workers)
Yersinia pestis	Plague	Rodents	Bite from infected rat flea	Smear and culture of fluid or pus from the bubo (also dangerous for lab workers) or immunofluorescence
Brucella species (*B. abortus, B. melitensis, B. ovis, B. suis, B. canis*)	Brucellosis	Pigs, cattle, goats, sheep	Contact with animal tissues; ingestion of contaminated milk products	Serology
Pasteurella multocida	Cellulitis	Cats, dogs	Bite from cat or dog	Culture of wound
Capnocytophaga (*C. canimorsus* and *C. cynodegmi*)	Cellulitis	Dogs; *C. ochracea, C. sputigena,* and *C. gingivalis* are species found in the human mouth	Bite from dog (or human)	Culture of wound

Case Conclusion   *F. tularensis* was the suspected diagnosis for FT, and acute and convalescent serology confirmed this suspicion in both FT and his father. They were treated with streptomycin with complete resolution of symptoms.

Thumbnail: Tularemia

Organism	*Francisella tularensis*
Type of organism	Small, pleomorphic gram-negative rod
Diseases caused	Acute influenza-like syndrome or a low-grade fever with adenopathy; ulceroglandular tularemia: ulceration at the site of entry into the skin accompanied by swollen and painful regional lymph nodes; tularemia pneumonia is an acute pneumonia with pleuritis and hilar lymphadenopathy
Epidemiology	Exposure to rabbits, deer, or wild rodents; transmitted usually through skinning animals or from animal-associated ticks
Diagnosis	Serology
Treatment	Intravenous streptomycin or gentamicin

Key Points

▶ Zoonotic gram-negative rods are a rare cause of human infection in the U.S., but occur more commonly in nonindustrialized regions

▶ *Tularemia* pneumonia and pneumonic plague should raise a suspicion for bioterrorism

▶ *F. tularensis* can be found in a wide variety of animals in the U.S., although animal-to-human transmission is most often associated with rabbits, deer, and wild rodents

▶ The major clinical syndrome of tularemia is an ulcer at the site of organism entry with regional painful, swollen lymph nodes; tularemia can be treated with aminoglycosides

Questions

1. Which of the following zoonotic gram-negative rods can be commonly acquired by ingestion?
   A. *Brucella melitensis*
   B. *Pasteurella multocida*
   C. *Capnocytophaga canimorsus*
   D. *Yersinia pestis*
   E. *Francisella tularensis*

2. Which of the following conditions is a major risk factor for sepsis and death with exposure to *Capnocytophaga*?
   A. HIV
   B. Splenectomy
   C. Eczema
   D. Iron overload
   E. Complement deficiencies

HPI: A 27-year-old man returns from a 2-week trip to India with a fever and abdominal pain. He also complains of constipation. The patient had full immunizations, including typhoid and hepatitis A, before leaving on his trip. He took mefloquine for malaria prophylaxis during the trip, and used insect repellent. His friend did not become ill on the trip. He has no past medical history. He works as a prep cook in a salad bar restaurant.

PE: T 40.0°C BP 120/70 HR 85 RR 16
A toxic looking man in no acute distress. The skin of his trunk shows some faint salmon-colored macules. His oropharynx is benign. He has some mild cervical and axillary lymphadenopathy. Lungs are clear. Heart is regular in rhythm, but the relatively slow heart rate for his fever is noted. His belly is diffusely tender, but there are no peritoneal signs. There is mild hepatosplenomegaly but no masses. No peripheral edema; no embolic stigmata on the extremities.

Labs: His complete blood count shows a leukopenic white count of 2.1, anemia with a hematocrit of 38, and thrombocytopenia with platelets of 95.
Thick blood smears are negative for malaria.
Dengue serologies are negative. An HIV test is negative.
One of two blood cultures, a stool culture, and a skin biopsy of his rash grow out *Salmonella typhi.*

Thought Questions

- What are common causes of fever to consider in a returning traveler?

- What clinical syndromes can *Salmonella* cause?

- Why is the patient's occupation important in this case?

Basic Science Review and Discussion

See Table 45-1 (p. 130) for a differential of fever in a traveler. **Typhoid fever** is a febrile illness caused by *Salmonella typhi,* a gram-negative rod. It is spread through fecal-oral transmission. It should not be confused with unrelated but similarly named febrile illnesses collectively known as **typhus,** caused by rickettsial species: Murine typhus (*Rickettsia typhi*), scrub typhus (*Orientia tsutsugamushi*), and epidemic typhus (*Ricketsia prowazekii*) are all spread by arthropod vectors.

Salmonella strains can be distinguished on the basis of serological and biochemical tests. They can cause two clinical presentations. **Gastroenteritis** is caused by strains such as *S. enteritidis* and *S. typhimurium,* along with others collectively known as the nontyphoidal salmonellae. This self-limited illness is characterized by nausea, vomiting, non-bloody diarrhea, along with fevers and abdominal cramping. The other presentation, **typhoid fever,** is caused by *S. typhi* and *S. paratyphi.* Typhoid fever is more serious than *Salmonella* gastroenteritis; about 10% of untreated patients die. Patients commonly suffer high fevers and abdominal

pain. Although diarrhea can occur, constipation is actually more common. Patients often manifest **relative bradycardia**—their heart rate does not increase in proportion to their body temperature. One third of patients have **rose spots,** a faint salmon-pink maculopapular rash, usually over the trunk. Blood counts often show leukopenia, anemia, and thrombocytopenia. Typhoid fever causes swelling of gut-associated lymphoid tissue, which can result in intestinal perforation or necrosis.

Typhoid fever is diagnosed by culture of *Salmonella* from blood, stool, urine, or skin biopsy of a rose spot. Bone marrow and duodenal cultures are more invasive, but higher yield sites. Unfortunately, serology is not reliable in making the diagnosis.

Whereas the nontyphoidal salmonellae may grow in animals, and may be transmitted by poultry, eggs, or reptilian pets, *S. typhi* and *S. paratyphi* only grow in humans. Typhoid fever is spread through fecal-oral transmission, but this is usually indirect, through contaminated food or water. Typhoid vaccines are available, and recommended by the Centers for Disease Control before travel to endemic countries, although they are not highly protective as seen in our patient. Three forms, a heat-killed whole-organism vaccine, a live-attenuated oral vaccine, and a capsular polysaccharide vaccine, are available. Typhoid fever is generally treated with fluoroquinolone antibiotics. **Carriage** of the organism can persist for weeks, particularly in patients with gallstones or other anatomic derangements of the gallbladder; carriers can subsequently potentially infect many other people.

Case Conclusion   The patient is given a course of fluoroquinolone treatment, and his fever resolves after 2 days. His case is reported to the Department of Public Health. To minimize the risk of spreading his illness, he is switched to a non-food handling position until follow-up stool cultures are negative for *S. typhi.*

Thumbnail: *Salmonella typhi* and *Salmonella paratyphi*

Type of organism	Aerobic, gram-negative rods
Disease caused	Typhoid fever
Epidemiology	Fecal-oral spread, usually via food or water; a major role is played by asymptomatic carriers; there is no animal reservoir; most typhoid fever in the U.S. is contracted through developing world travel
Diagnosis	Blood culture; stool culture to show carriage; serology is not reliable
Treatment	Fluoroquinolone
Prevention	Typhoid vaccine

Key Points

▶ Most serotypes of *Salmonella* cause gastroenteritis, but *S. typhi* and *S. paratyphi* cause typhoid fever, a more serious, systemic illness

▶ Typhoid fever is spread through fecal-oral transmission

Questions

1. What biochemical feature of *Salmonella* distinguishes it from most of the enteric flora (other Enterobacteriaceae)?
   A. Lactose nonfermenter
   B. Glucose fermenter
   C. Oxidase negative
   D. Nitrate reducer
   E. Failure to produce hydrogen sulfide

2. Which of the following is caused by *Salmonella typhimurium*?
   A. Murine typhus
   B. Epidemic typhus
   C. Scrub typhus
   D. Typhoid fever
   E. Gastroenteritis

HPI: A 36-year-old woman, born in the Philippines, is admitted to the hospital for a work-up of bloody stools. Although this is her first episode of frank blood, she has had episodes of melena over the past 6 months. She notes a 30-pound weight loss over the last 6 months, with occasional fevers and night sweats. She denies cough, hemoptysis, abdominal pain, or orthostasis. She has no family history of cancer.

PE: T 37.9°C BP 120/70 HR 80 RR 14
The patient is a thin woman in no distress. Lungs are clear. There is no abdominal tenderness or palpable masses. A rectal exam shows a small amount of bloody stool, with no palpable masses.

Labs: WBC 12, normal differential. She has a microcytic anemia, with a hematocrit of 29 and a mean corpuscular volume (MCV) of 75. Electrolytes are normal. Amebic serologies are negative.
A chest X-ray shows small calcified upper lobe nodules interpreted as evidence of old granulomatous disease. The patient undergoes colonoscopy. A large 8-cm fungating lesion is seen in her right colon, with an appearance classic for colon cancer. Biopsies are taken and sent to pathology. After the endoscopy, the gastroenterologist tells the patient she likely has cancer. To the gastroenterologist's surprise, the pathologist calls the biopsies inconclusive. Because of her chest X-ray, a purified protein derivative (PPD) tuberculosis is placed, and is positive. The pathologist stains the colon specimens for AFB, but no organisms are seen. Unfortunately, the colonic lesion was not sent for culture. Nonetheless, the patient is started on empiric four-drug TB therapy, with isoniazid, rifampin, pyrazinamide, and ethambutol.

Thought Questions

- Which parts of the body are most commonly affected by tuberculosis?

- Is this patient contagious?

- If four drugs are necessary to treat a case of active tuberculosis, why is only one drug necessary to treat latent tuberculosis infection?

Basic Science Review and Discussion

Mycobacteria are rod-shaped bacteria with a thick waxy coat. The chemical properties of this coat allows them to be detected with an **acid-fast stain**—hence the name acid-fast bacilli (AFB; of note, the acid-fast stain can also stain *Nocardia*). The traditional acid-fast technique is being replaced by a more sensitive fluorescent stain.

Mycobacteria are divided into two groups. The first group is the *Mycobacterium tuberculosis* **complex** (made up of *Mycobacterium tuberculosis*, and the difficult-to-distinguish *Mycobacterium bovis*), which causes tuberculosis, the leading cause of infectious mortality in the world. One third of the world's population is infected with tuberculosis. *M. tuberculosis* is only found in humans, and is acquired by person-to-person contact. A positive culture for *M. tuberculosis* indicates infection that must be treated. The second group is the **nontuberculous mycobacteria,** which by contrast are free-living and acquired from the environment. The nontuberculous mycobacteria usually affect immunocompromised hosts. Their presence in a culture

may reflect disease, but can also be due to colonization or contamination (see Case 21).

M. tuberculosis may be distinguished on culture by its slow rate of growth (taking up to 6 weeks to detect), lack of pigment, and "cording" morphology (the long edges of the bacilli are aligned parallel to each other). *M. tuberculosis* is usually sensitive to the drug isoniazid, whereas many species of nontuberulous mycobacteria are resistant.

Almost all transmission of tuberculosis is due to inhalation of infectious respiratory droplets from an infected patient. The droplets are small, requiring specialized masks to filter them from the air. The droplets may also persist for hours after an infected person has left the room. However, tuberculosis is not easily caught, and transmission usually requires exposure for many hours. Primary infection occurs at the site of inhalation in the lungs, and usually resolves, with the body walling off the bacteria. At a later time, however, the infection can **reactivate,** causing disease. The most frequent site of reactivation is in the lungs, particularly in the apices where the oxygen tension is highest. Tuberculosis can also spread from the lung parenchyma to the pleural space. Tuberculosis can affect almost any part of the body, however. After the lungs, other common sites include the genitourinary system, gastrointestinal tract, meningeal space, lymph nodes, or bone. In some cases, tuberculosis is spread through the bloodstream, creating many tiny foci of infection, referred to as **miliary** tuberculosis. The pathological hallmark of tuberculosis infection is **caseating granuloma** formation at the site of infection.

The **PPD** test can be used to identify people who have ever had primary tuberculosis infection. This test measures cellular immunity against a purified protein derivative of *M. tuberculosis.* The test measures the size of the cell-mediated hypersensitivity response several days after intradermal injection of the PPD. Cut-offs in millimeters for a positive test differ depending on the patient population; in general, patients who are immunocompromised or who have a higher likelihood of reactivation are screened with a lower cut-off, resulting in a more sensitive test. Patients who are anergic due to immunocompromise or overwhelming mycobacterial infection may have false negative tests. Patients who are identified as PPD positive, but have no signs of active infection, are considered to have latent **tuberculosis infection,** and are usually given a course of treatment to kill the remaining tubercle bacilli at the site of primary infection to prevent later reactivation disease. The treatment is usually isoniazid for 6 to 9 months. The long course is necessary because of the slow growth rate of the mycobacteria.

Patients who have active disease are usually diagnosed by AFB smears or cultures from the suspected site of infection. Rarely, patients are treated empirically, and the diagnosis is made by clinical improvement after TB therapy is started. In contrast to latent tuberculosis infection, patients with active tuberculosis have a much larger number of mycobacteria in their bodies, and must be treated with a combination of drugs to avoid the selection of antibiotic-resistant organisms. Usually a patient is treated with four drugs (isoniazid, rifampin, pyrazinamide, and ethambutol) until the susceptibilities of the infecting strain are known. Other drugs exist to treat TB, but are second line because of lower efficacy and difficulties of administration, side effects, or cost. In particular, patients with **multidrug-resistant TB** (defined as

TB resistant to both isoniazid and rifampin) are difficult to treat. Because of the long courses of treatment required for active TB, and the risk of creating resistant strains if partial treatment is given, patients are often given **directly observed therapy** (DOT) if there is any doubt about their ability to adhere to the treatment regimen. Patients with active TB who are in institutional settings (hospitals, nursing homes, or prisons) must be isolated. Epidemiological investigation of all new TB cases, and evaluation of close contacts for disease, are crucial measures in preventing the spread of TB in the community.

The major recent issues in tuberculosis control have been a rise in urban tuberculosis rates coinciding with the HIV epidemic and a rise in multidrug-resistant tuberculosis. These problems have been addressed by increased surveillance and treatment of latent tuberculosis in HIV-positive patients, and by an increase in spending on DOT to improve adherence and prevent the emergence of resistant strains. Recently, most new cases of tuberculosis in the U.S. have been in immigrants who acquired their disease in countries with higher prevalence rates of TB.

A tuberculosis vaccine, **Bacille Calmette-Guérin (BCG),** exists, but is not used in this country. It decreases the incidence of extrapulmonary tuberculosis, especially TB meningitis, but has not been shown to reduce the incidence of pulmonary disease. The vaccination may cause false positive PPDs, but will usually not cause a PPD of greater than 10 mm unless the vaccine has been recently administered. In a patient from a country of high TB prevalence, a positive PPD is more likely to reflect latent tuberculosis infection than represent a false positive test due to the BCG immunization.

Case Conclusion The patient continues on four-drug TB therapy for 1 month, with an improvement in her weight loss and fevers. On repeat endoscopy after 1 month of TB therapy, the colonic lesion has almost completely resolved. The patient finishes a 6-month course of TB therapy.

Thumbnail: *Mycobacterium tuberculosis*

Type of organism	*Mycobacterium;* acid-fast bacillus
Disease caused	Tuberculosis
Epidemiology	Spread person to person through aerosol droplets
Diagnosis	Latent infection is diagnosed through PPD skin testing; active infection is diagnosed via acid-fast smears and mycobacterial cultures from the affected site, usually sputum
Treatment	Latent infection is treated with 6 to 9 months of isoniazid; active infection is usually treated with combination therapy; initially isoniazid, rifampin, pyrazinamide, and ethambutol are given; pyrazinamide and ethambutol can usually be discontinued once antibiotic susceptibilities return

Key Points

- *Mycobacterium tuberculosis* is a slow-growing *Mycobacterium* that is transmitted from person to person via respiratory aerosols
- Most active TB disease results from reactivation of a previous primary infection; the most common site for active TB is the lungs, but infection can be seen at many other sites

- Patients who have been exposed to tuberculosis but have no active disease are said to have latent tuberculosis infection, and are treated to reduce their chances of active tuberculosis in the future
- Active tuberculosis must be treated with multiple drugs to avoid selection for drug-resistant organisms

Questions

1. Which of the following patients is most infectious?
   - A. An 18 year old with tuberculous lymphadenitis of the neck (scrofula)
   - B. A 36 year old with HIV, a negative PPD, lung cavities on chest X-ray, and sputum with a positive AFB smear
   - C. A 46 year old with a positive PPD and no cough
   - D. A 71 year old with a positive PPD, a right upper lobe infiltrate, and sputum that is AFB smear negative but culture positive
   - E. A 24 year old with TB meningitis

2. Which of the following drugs is a first-line agent against tuberculosis?
   - A. Streptomycin
   - B. Pyrazinamide
   - C. Para-aminosalicylic acid (PAS)
   - D. Levofloxacin
   - E. Cycloserine

3. Which toxicity do all of the first-line TB drugs have in common?
   - A. Neuropathy
   - B. Optic neuritis
   - C. Hepatotoxicity
   - D. Serious drug-drug interactions
   - E. Hyperuricemia

4. Which of the following patients needs to be started on multidrug therapy for TB?
   - A. An asymptomatic 9-year-old Philippine immigrant with a positive PPD and a normal chest X-ray
   - B. A 43 year old with a history of tuberculosis treated with three drugs for 6 months, who has calcified granulomas on his chest X-ray
   - C. A 17 year old with a lymph node biopsy growing *Mycobacterium tuberculosis*
   - D. A 51-year-old nurse who was inadvertently exposed to a patient with active pulmonary tuberculosis in an emergency room for 30 minutes
   - E. A 34-year-old man who sat on a bus for 2 hours next to a man with a hacking cough

HPI: MF is a 28-year-old woman who presents to your office with complaints of recurrent boils on her lower extremities. You have seen this patient four times in the past 6 months for recurrent furuncles on both lower extremities. Cultures of these lesions have been negative for bacterial growth. The skin boils seem to have no response to the antibiotics that are commonly used for bacteria that cause skin infections. The lesions seem to resolve spontaneously, but have led to scarring on MF's lower legs. She presents again today with recurrence of the skin boils. MF does not have any fevers or chills. She has never had any problems with skin infections or any other skin conditions prior to 6 months ago. MF receives manicures and pedicures every month and has not changed salons. She has not changed her skin lotion, soap, or detergent. MF shaves her legs with a disposable razor that she changes frequently and she does not use depilatories.

PMH: Intrauterine device infection 3 years ago, requiring removal. MF only takes oral contraceptive pills and has no allergies. Lives with boyfriend and is monogamous. Works at cosmetics counter.

PE: T 37.1°C BP 115/78 HR 70 RR 16
MF has multiple scattered violaceous boils on both her lower extremities. Her lesions are only found below the knee on both legs and several boils have areas of ulceration and bleeding. Multiple scars are visible around the boils on both legs.

Labs: WBC 9.0 with normal neutrophil count. You take cultures of the boil and the lab calls you in 3 days saying that an acid-fast organism is growing on routine bacterial media. The lab subsequently identifies this organism as a mycobacterial species and asks you if MF needs respiratory isolation.

Thought Questions

- How do nontuberculous mycobacteria differ from *Mycobacterium tuberculosis*?

- How are the nontuberculous mycobacteria classified?

- What are the clinical syndromes caused by nontuberculous mycobacteria?

- What are the main species of rapidly growing mycobacteria that cause human disease?

- What are the clinical syndromes caused by rapidly growing mycobacteria?

Basic Science Review and Discussion

Nontuberculous Mycobacteria versus *M. tuberculosis* Nontuberculous mycobacteria (NTM) are defined as mycobacteria species other than the *Mycobacterium tuberculosis* complex (comprised of the species M. *tuberculosis* and *M. bovis*); these species have also been called mycobacteria other than tubercle bacilli (MOTT). Most of the NTM organisms have been isolated from water and soil and are **ubiquitous in the environment.** Hence, even potentially pathogenic isolates of NTM may be found as contaminants or colonizers as well as etiologic agents of infection. Most infections with NTM appear to be acquired by aspiration or inoculation of the organisms from a natural reservoir, and there is little evidence of person-to-person transmission of disease.

As a group, the NTM differ in several respects from the classic tubercle bacilli:

1) NTM present with **varying degrees of acid-fastness.**

2) NTM have a wider temperature range for growth and often grow comfortably at temperatures not found in the human body.

3) **Growth rates tend to be variable:** some species grow in less than 7 days; others have generation times similar to or longer than *M. tuberculosis*.

4) Many of the NTM have colonies that are pigmented yellow to orange.

5) NTM fail to produce progressive disease in guinea pigs, which is the traditional animal model for *M. tuberculosis*.

6) The majority of NTM will produce lesions in mice, however, depending on the route of inoculation.

7) **NTM show a general pattern of resistance to many of the first-line antituberculous agents,** such as rifampin, isoniazid, streptomycin, and ethambutol.

8) Human infections with NTM are frequently associated with pre-existing disease or trauma.

9) Infected persons may or may not show skin hypersensitivity to protein derivatives of these mycobacterial species (analogous to the "PPD" delayed-type hypersensitivity reaction seen with *M. tuberculosis*).

10) NTM generally produce smooth colonies (some rough variants exist) and emulsify readily.

Clinical Syndromes of NTM Dr. Ernst Runyon devised a scheme in the mid-1950s to classify nontuberculous myco-bacteria into four groups based on essentially two criteria: **pigment production and speed of growth.** "Rapid growers" are characterized by the ability to grow rapidly (2 to 7 days) at temperatures ranging from 25°C to 42°C. Colonies of the organisms in this group are generally smooth, but rough variants may occur. The colonies may be pigmented or nonpigmented.

The typical clinical syndromes of NTM, along with their geographic distribution, are presented in Table 21-1.

Syndromes of Rapidly Growing Mycobacteria Rapidly growing mycobacteria are acid-fast rods that resemble diphtheroids on Gram stain. They usually grow as fast as in 1 to 7 days and thrive on most routine laboratory media, as well as special media for isolation of mycobacteria. The ubiquitous rapid growers survive nutritional deprivation and extremes of temperature. They are recovered readily from soil, dust, and water, and have also been isolated from tap water, municipal water supplies, moist areas in hospitals, contaminated biological solutions, aquariums, domestic animals, marine life, and even **contaminated whirlpool footbaths in nail salons.**

Table 21-1 Classification of nontuberclous mycobacteria

Common etiologic species	Geography	Unusual etiologic species
Pulmonary disease		
M. avium-intracellulare	Worldwide	M. simiae, M. chelonae
M. kansasii	U.S., coal mining regions, Europe	M. szulgai, M. fortuitum M. celatum, M. asiaticum
M. abscessus	Worldwide, but mostly U.S.	M. shimodii
M. xenopi	Europe, Canada	M. haemophilum
M. malmoense	UK, northern Europe	M. smegmatis
Lymphadenitis		
M. avium-intracellulare	Worldwide	M. fortuitum
M. scrofulaceum	Worldwide	M. chelonae, M. kansasii
M. malmoense	UK, northern Europe (especially Scandinavia)	M. abscessus M. haemophilum
Skin and soft tissue infection		
M. fortuitum, M. chelonae	Worldwide, mostly U.S.	M. smegmatis
M. abscessus Abscesses, ulcers, sinus tracts		M. haemophilum M. nonchromogenicum
M. marinum Swimming pool granuloma or sporotrichoid presentation	Worldwide	
M. ulcerans Chronic ulcer	Australia, tropics, Africa, SE Asia	
MAC, M. kansasii Hyperimmune reactions	Worldwide or U.S.	
Skeletal (bone, joint, and tendon infections)		
MAC	Worldwide	M. marinum
M. kansasii	Worldwide	M. scrofulaceum
M. fortuitum, M. chelonae	Worldwide, mostly U.S.	
Disseminated infection		
MAC	Worldwide	M. fortuitum
M. kansasii	U.S.	M. xenopi, M. simiae
M. chelonae	U.S.	M. malmoense
M. haemophilum	U.S., Australia	M. genavense M. conspicuum M. marinum

Most of the disease caused by rapid growers is sporadic and community acquired, although nosocomial outbreaks or clustered cases have been reported. For instance, there is a recognized association between rapidly growing mycobacterial wound infections and the procedures of breast augmentation or coronary artery bypass grafting. A recent report[1] described a cluster of cases of lower extremity *Mycobacterium fortuitum* furunculosis in women who received **pedicures** at a certain nail salon in northern California; the whirlpool footbath in this facility was found to be contaminated with *M. fortuitum.* More than 90% of disease caused by rapid growers originates from three species: **M. fortuitum, M. chelonae,** and **M. abscessus.**

Rapid growers are the most common NTM species to cause **skin and subcutaneous tissue infections.** *M. fortuitum, M. chelonae,* and *M. abscessus* are again the three most frequently implicated species. The organisms often form abscesses at the site of puncture wounds (i.e., after stepping on a nail) or after open traumatic injuries or fractures. They can also cause nosocomial skin and soft tissue disease, including infections of long-term intravenous or peritoneal catheters, postinjection abscesses, or surgical wound infections. Incubation periods from the time of injury to clinical infection vary from 1 week to 2 years, but most infections occur within the first month. Infections may resemble pyogenic abscesses with an acute inflammatory reaction and suppuration, or they may progress slowly, with chronic granulomatous inflammation, ulceration, sinus tract formation, and exudates that resemble sporotrichosis. Patients may require **both antibiotic therapy and surgical management** to achieve cure.

Bronchopulmonary infections caused by the rapid growers usually occur following aspiration events. The largest epidemiologic group of patients with lung disease are **elderly (>60 years), Caucasian, female nonsmokers with no predisposing conditions or known lung disease.** Another epidemiologic group of patients susceptible to lung infection with the rapid growers are those with some underlying lung conditions. These patients tend to develop disease at a younger age (<50 years). Predisposing underlying disorders associated with these infections include lung damage produced by prior mycobacterial infection (usually tuberculosis or MAC), gastroesophageal (GE) disorders with chronic vomiting, lipoid pneumonia, cystic fibrosis, and bronchiectasis. Of note, these rapid growers may just colonize respiratory secretions without playing a clinical role in disease.

M. abscessus accounts for approximately 80% of rapidly growing mycobacterial respiratory disease isolates, whereas *M. fortuitum* accounts for approximately 15% of these syndromes. In the small group of patients with GE disorders and chronic vomiting, however, *M. abscessus* and *M. fortuitum* infection occur with equal frequency. The usually presenting symptoms of these pulmonary infections are cough and fatigue, fevers, night sweats, and weight loss (similar to tuberculosis). Chest roentgenograms in these syndromes usually show multilobar, patchy, reticulonodular, or mixed interstitial-alveolar infiltrates with an upper lobe predominance; cavitation occurs in approximately 15% of the cases. High-resolution CT (HRCT) of the lung frequently shows associated cylindrical bronchiectasis and multiple small (<5 mm) nodules. The clinical course is highly variable: in most patients, the course is chronic and inexorably progressive; in others, more fulminant, rapidly progressive disease can occur, especially in association with gastroesophageal disorders. Spontaneous recovery may rarely occur.

Other clinical syndromes of the rapid growers include lymphadenitis, keratitis, endophthalmitis, suppurative arthritis, osteomyelitis, endocarditis (on natural, prosthetic, or porcine valves), aortitis, meningitis, peritonitis, chronic urinary infections, solid pulmonary nodules, bacteremia related to in-dwelling IV catheters, or ventriculoperitoneal (VP) shunts.

Case Conclusion   You tell the lab that respiratory isolation is not necessary for MF and ask for further identification of the mycobacterial organism. The species is identified as *M. fortuitum.* You start MF on ciprofloxacin and doxycycline and notify the local health department to initiate an investigation of the cleanliness of the nail salon frequented by MF.

Thumbnail: Rapidly Growing Mycobacteria

Organisms	*M. fortuitum, M. chelonae, M. abscessus*
Type of organism	Nontuberculous mycobacteria (Runyon group IV)
Diseases caused	Skin and soft tissue infections, pulmonary infections
Epidemiology	Found in soil, dust, and water and can contaminate hospital water supplies; skin and soft tissue infections usually occur secondary to trauma or surgery; pulmonary infections occur in elderly, Caucasian females without underlying risk factors, and younger patients with underlying lung disease
Diagnosis	Culture drainage material, tissue biopsy or sputum; will grow out in 1 to 7 days even on routine bacterial media
Treatment	Take out foreign bodies and debride extensive soft tissue infections; rapid growers resistant to typical TB therapy and usually susceptible to newer macrolides, quinolones, doxycycline, and minocycline, and sulfonamides; IV options for serious infections include amikacin, cefoxitin, and imipenem

Key Points

▶ Nontuberculous mycobacteria (NTM) are ubiquitous in the environment and are classified by their speed of growth and pigment production

▶ The clinically significant rapidly growing mycobacteria are *M. fortuitum, M. chelonae,* and *M. abscessus;* growth occurs in 1 to 7 days and can occur on routine lab media for bacterial cultures

▶ The main clinical syndromes of the rapid growers are skin and soft tissue infections, usually preceded by some sort of trauma or surgery, and pulmonary infections

▶ Rapid growers are usually resistant to typical agents used for TB and may respond to macrolides, fluoroquinolones, tetracyclines, and sulfonamides

Questions

1. The duration of treatment for infections caused by rapidly growing mycobacteria is usually
   A. 7 to 10 days
   B. 10 to 14 days
   C. 14 to 28 days
   D. 1 to 3 months
   E. 4 to 6 months

2. Which drug is currently approved for administration once a week as prophylaxis for MAC in HIV infection?
   A. Rifabutin
   B. Azithromycin
   C. Clarithromycin
   D. Ethambutol
   E. Rifampin

References

1. Winthrop KL, Abrams M, Yakrus M, et al. An outbreak of mycobacterial furunculosis associated with footbaths at a nail salon. N Engl J Med 2002;346:1366–1371.

HPI: An 18-year-old woman is admitted to the hospital for fever and rash. The day of admission she noted a rash that appeared on her palms and soles, and then moved centripetally in towards her torso.

PE: T 39°C BP 90/45 HR 120 RR 14

The patient looks uncomfortable. Exam is notable for neck stiffness. She has a disseminated petechial rash most pronounced over her extremities. Her heart has a 2/6 systolic murmur. Her neurologic exam shows disorientation, but no focal deficits.

Labs: White count is 19. Hematocrit is 40. Platelets are 160. Electrolytes and renal function are normal. RPR (a syphilis test) is nonreactive. A lumbar puncture shows a neutrophilic pleocytosis (10 white cells), elevated protein but normal glucose.

Initially, her doctors consider disseminated *Neisseria meningococcus* infection, as well as possibly endocarditis, and start vancomycin and ceftriaxone. On further questioning, her family reveals that they just returned from a camping trip in North Carolina, where the patient had been bitten by a tick. Doxycycline is added.

Thought Questions

- Many infectious and noninfectious diseases present with fever and rash. How many can you think of?

- Why did this patient receive multiple antibiotics for what was likely a single infection?

- Rickettsiae are obligate intracellular parasites, which makes them difficult to culture. What other pathogens are obligate intracellular parasites?

Basic Science Review and Discussion

Rickettsiae are bacteria which are obligate **intracellular** parasites. Their appearance on Gram stain shows variable coccobacillary morphology.

Most rickettsial diseases are transmitted by **insect** bites. Q fever, which is transmitted through inhalation (or occasionally ingestion), is the exception to this rule, because it is unique among rickettsiae in being able to survive for long periods outside of a host.

Most rickettsial diseases, except for Q fever, feature a **rash.** The etiology of the rash appears to be vasculitis caused by bacterial invasion of the endothelial wall. The clinical appearance of the rash can vary according to the specific rickettsial disease, from the petechial rash of Rocky Mountain spotted fever to the chicken pox-like rash of rickettsialpox. Rickettsialpox and scrub typhus are often accompanied by the formation of an eschar at the site of the mite bite.

Rickettsiae cannot be grown in cell-free media. Because rickettsiae are very difficult to culture at all, diagnosis is usually made **serologically.** When acute and convalescent serum is compared, if there is a 4-fold increase in antibody titer against a rickettsial pathogen in the convalescent phase, the diagnosis is confirmed.

Patients with suspected rickettsial disease are treated with **doxycycline.** Chloramphenicol is also active. Most commonly used β-lactam antibiotics are *not* active against this group of diseases, which is why the diagnosis of rickettsial disease is important not to miss.

Two features that help make a diagnosis of rickettsial disease are a history of an insect bite and presence of a rash. The exception is Q fever, which has no insect vector and does not cause a rash.

Case Conclusion CSF and blood cultures remain negative. The patient makes a full recovery. Several weeks after her hospitalization, her serologic tests for Rocky Mountain spotted fever are performed, comparing acute and convalescent serum. A significant rise in titer confirms the diagnosis of Rocky Mountain spotted fever.

Thumbnail: Rickettsial Diseases

Organism	Spotted fever group			Typhus group			
	Rickettsia rickettsii	**Rickettsia conorii**	**Rickettsia akari**	**Coxiella burnetii**	**Rickettsia prowazekii**	**Rickettsia typhi**	**Rickettsia tsutsugamushi**
Diseases caused	Rocky Mountain spotted fever	Boutonneuse fever, others	Rickettsial pox	Q fever	Epidemic typhus	Murine typhus	Scrub typhus
Epidemiology/ geography	U.S., predominantly East Coast	Africa, India, S. Europe	U.S., Korea, Russia	Worldwide	Asia, Africa, S. America	Worldwide	S.E. Asia, Japan
Vector	Tick	Tick	Mite	None; infection is by inhalation or ingestion of unpasteurized milk	Louse	Flea	Mite
Reservoir	Rodents, dogs	Rodents, dogs	Mice	Cattle, sheep, goats	Humans, flying squirrels	Rodents	Rodents
Diagnosis	Serology	Serology	Serology	Serology	Serology	Serology	Serology
Treatment	Doxycycline	Doxycycline	Doxycycline	Doxycycline	Doxycycline	Doxycycline	Doxycycline

Key Points

▶ Rickettsiae are bacteria that are obligate intracellular parasites

▶ Because rickettsiae cannot be cultured, patients with suspected rickettsial disease need to be treated empirically, usually with doxycycline; the diagnosis may be confirmed retrospectively with serology

▶ Two features that help make a diagnosis of rickettsial disease are a history of an insect bite and presence of a rash; the exception is Q fever, which has no insect vector and does not cause a rash

Questions

1. Which of the following pathogens may be routinely cultured?

   A. *Rickettsiae*
   B. *Chlamydia*
   C. *Mycoplasma*
   D. *Listeria*
   E. *Ehrlichia*

2. Which of the following is a rickettsial disease transmitted by ticks?

   A. Scrub typhus
   B. Q fever
   C. Rickettsialpox
   D. Lyme disease
   E. Rocky Mountain spotted fever

HPI: CB is a 33-year-old woman presenting to the ER complaining of 4 days of headache and nausea and 2 days of fever, shortness of breath, and nonproductive cough. She does not have any other symptoms such as stiff neck, sensitivity to light, pain with urination, vaginal pain, or discharge. She just gave birth 3 months ago to a baby girl. CB's recent history is also significant for a visit to her in-laws' farm in Spain this past month. She just returned 4 days ago. While in Spain, she slept in a room containing three open bags of fresh sheep wool and two sheepskins on the wall. Her husband and baby slept in the same room, but did not get sick.
PMH: Had mild asthma as a child. No allergies or medications.

PE: T 39.0°C HR 110 BP 104/55 RR 24 SaO$_2$ on room air 87%
CB is generally very ill appearing, having a hard time speaking full sentences without labored breathing. Her lung exam has decreased breath sounds in the left lower base with some crackles above that area and crackles in the right upper lung field.

Labs: WBC 5.4 with normal differential. Urine and blood cultures negative. Chest x-ray shows infiltrates in the anterior segment of the right upper lobe and left lower lobe, along with a left-sided pleural effusion.

Thought Questions

- What is this patient's differential diagnosis, especially considering her exposure history?

- What is the microbiology and epidemiology of the suspected agent?

- What are some of its associated clinical syndromes?

- How would you make the diagnosis of this organism?

- What are the best treatment options for this organism?

Basic Science Review and Discussion

Differential Diagnosis The differential diagnosis of CB's **multilobar pneumonia** is broad. More typical community-acquired pathogens include *Streptococcus pneumoniae*, *Haemophilus influenzae,* and *Moraxella catarrhalis*. These pathogens tend to produce an acute respiratory illness with fever, productive cough, and shortness of breath; the typical chest X-ray shows a unilobar or multilobar process. The "atypical" pathogens include *Mycoplasma pneumoniae, Chlamydia pneumoniae,* and *Legionella pneumophila,* which can all present with either diffuse interstitial infiltrates or lobar consolidation on chest radiograph. The "atypical pneumonia" syndromes usually present with a prolonged course of fever, shortness of breath, and a nonproductive cough before coming to medical attention. Less common pathogens of community-acquired pneumonia that present with severe respiratory symptoms include **Staphylococcus aureus** and **gram-negative bacilli, such as Pseudomonas.**

CB's history of **exposure to sheep** widens the differential to include more exotic pathogens such as *Brucella melitensis,* *Bacillus anthracis,* and *Coxiella burnetii* (the agent of Q

fever). Brucellosis does not typically present with pulmonary symptoms, but results in a flu-like syndrome accompanied by fever, weakness, fatigue, malaise, enlarged lymph nodes, and hepatosplenomegaly; chronic *Brucella* infections include osteomyelitis or infective arthritis. *B. anthracis* can present with an extremely severe, often fatal pulmonary process, but usually follows a more massive exposure to sheep's wool than CB experienced; the typical chest x-ray findings of pulmonary anthrax are a widened mediastinum with or without pleural effusions. *Coxiella burnetii* is **extremely infectious and exposure to even a single organism from sheep can lead to one of the syndromes of Q fever,** including an acute pneumonia.

Microbiology *C. burnetii* is a small, highly pleomorphic coccobacillus with a gram-negative cell wall. This organism grows exclusively in eukaryotic cells and was therefore **originally classified in the rickettsial family.** However, *C. burnetii* is most phylogenetically related to the *Legionella* species; both types of organisms are classified in the γ subdivision of *Proteobacteria* on the basis of sequence comparisons in the 16S rRNA-encoding gene. In contrast, the rickettsial species are classified in the α1 subdivision of the *Proteobacteria*.

C. burnetii can only live inside eukaryotic cells within an acidic vacuole (phagolysosomes) at a pH of 4.8. **The microorganism has a spore phase in its life cycle, which explains its ability to withstand harsh environmental conditions.** Spores have been demonstrated to survive for 7 to 10 months on wool at 15°C to 20°C, for more than 1 month on fresh meat in cold storage, and for more than 3 years in skim milk at 4°C to 6°C. *C. burnetii* spores have been isolated from infected tissues stored in formaldehyde for up to 4 to 5 months, although it will eventually be killed by 2% formaldehyde if stored for longer time periods.

C. burnetii has evolved a technique of **"phase variation" that involves alteration of the sugar composition of their lipopolysaccharide layer** depending on the environment. **Virulent and highly infectious isolates are of the phase I type** and are isolated from animals; subculture is required for selection of **the avirulent phase II form** of the organism. These phases are serologically distinguishable and useful in the serodiagnosis of both acute and chronic *C. burnetii* infections.

Epidemiology *C. burnetii* can be harbored in a variety of species and has been identified in arthropods, fish, birds, rodents, marsupials, and livestock. **Worldwide, the most common animal reservoirs are cattle, sheep, and goats,** although there have been urban outbreaks associated with cats, dogs, and rabbits. **Q fever is usually an occupational disease of farmers, veterinarians, abattoir workers, and shepherds,** although, given the very infectious nature of the organism, disease can occur with even minimal exposure to *C. burnetii* spores. Q fever outbreaks have been described among residents living along a road traveled by farm vehicles, for instance, and among **laboratory workers** handling the organism. The infection can also be acquired from ingesting contaminated raw milk. **Reactivation of *Coxiella burnetii* infection occurs in female mammals during pregnancy,** and high concentrations of the infectious agent are found in the placenta of these animals (up to 10^9 bacteria per gram of tissue); there are multiple reports of *C. burnetii* transmission to humans around animal births. *C. burnetii* has also been isolated from the human placenta and human milk, although no cases of transmission through these sources have been documented. Several case reports describe Q fever transmission via blood transfusion, and one case report has described a human-to-human transmission case among members of a household. Essentially, the prevalence of Q fever in humans seems to be highest in places where rickettsiologists live; as diagnosis is made mainly on serology, this disease is thought to be significantly underdiagnosed in regions without Q fever specialists.

Clinical Syndromes *C. burnetii* is an intriguing organism in that the **clinical syndrome of acute Q fever can resemble almost any infectious disease.** The main diagnostic clue that the syndrome could be Q fever is the epidemiological circumstances. The incubation period for the organism is 4 to 39 days with the average time from exposure to onset of clinical symptoms being 20 days. **In addition to the acute clinical syndromes, there are a variety of chronic syndromes** associated with *C. burnetii* that can occur months to years after exposure. Typical clinical syndromes of Q fever (acute and chronic) are outlined in Table 23-1.

Diagnosis The most common diagnostic tool for Q fever is **serology. Antibody against the phase II antigen of the organism predominates in acute Q fever and antibody against the phase I antigen predominates in chronic disease.** Seroconversion is usually detected 7 to 15 days after the onset of clinical symptoms and about 90% of patients have detectable antibodies by the third week. The most commonly used serologic test is indirect immunofluorescence and the following values for antibody titers are required for diagnosis:

> **Acute Q fever**   Anti-phase II IgG $\geq$ 1:200
> Anti-phase II IgM $\geq$ 1:50

Sensitivity 58.4%; specificity 92.2%; negative predictive value 88%–96.6%

> **Chronic Q fever**   Anti-phase I IgG $\geq$ 1:800

Sensitivity 100%; positive predictive value (PPV) 98.6%

(Using anti-phase I IgG $\geq$ 1:1600 enhances PPV to 100%)

C. burnetii can also be cultivated in a shell-vial cell culture system in the laboratory setting. The risk of transmission of this infectious organism to laboratory personnel is extremely high and the agent must be handled only in **special safety facilities.**

Table 23-1 Clinical syndromes of Q fever

Acute clinical syndromes	Chronic clinical syndromes
Self-limited febrile illness (flu-like)	Endocarditis
Isolated fever without other symptoms	Infection of arterial aneurysm or prosthesis
Pneumonia	Osteomyelitis
Hepatitis	Infection during pregnancy
Exanthema associated with fever	Hepatitis
Pericarditis	Pseudotumor of the lung
Myocarditis	?Pulmonary fibrosis
Meningoencephalitis	Immune complex-mediated glomerulonephritis (with endocarditis)
Infections during pregnancy	
Acute glomerulonephritis	

Treatment   The recommended therapy for acute Q fever is **tetracycline compounds,** usually doxycycline, administered for 14 to 21 days. **Second-line therapy is erythromycin with or without rifampin,** for the same time period. **Fluoroquinolones** are also efficacious against *C. burnetii* and should be considered in the treatment of acute Q fever meningoencephalitis, given their superior penetration into the CSF. Chronic Q fever is extremely difficult to treat, and usually involves at least **3 years of treatment** with doxycycline plus or minus a fluoroquinolone or hydroxychloroquine. Treatment may become lifelong and eradication of *C. burnetii* endocarditis often requires valve replacement.

Case Conclusion   CB was admitted and started on levofloxacin and doxycycline. Serologies were sent for *Legionella pneumophila, Mycoplasma pneumoniae,* and *Coxiella burnetii.* CB continued to have fevers and poor oxygenation for the first week of hospitalization, but she improved approximately 10 days into her hospital course. Serum serologies were positive for anti-phase II IgG of *Coxiella burnetii* (≥1:200) and anti-phase II IgM (≥1:50). Anti-phase I antibodies for *C. burnetii* were negative.

Thumbnail: Q fever

Organism	*Coxiella burnetii*
Type of organism	Small, gram-negative, coccobacillus that grows only in eukaryotic cells; no longer classified as rickettsial
Diseases caused	Acute Q fever syndromes (flu-like syndrome, fever, pneumonia, hepatitis, pericarditis, myocarditis, meningoencephalitis, acute glomerulonephritis); chronic Q fever syndromes (endocarditis, osteomyelitis, hepatitis, pseudotumor of the lung)
Epidemiology	Occupational disease of farmers and abattoir workers; exposure to livestock, mostly sheep or cattle
Diagnosis	Serologic; anti-phase II antibodies in acute disease and anti-phase I antibodies in chronic disease
Treatment	Doxycycline for 2 to 3 weeks for acute disease; doxycycline ± quinolone or hydroxychloroquine for at least 3 years in chronic disease

---

Key Points

▶ *C. burnetii,* the agent of Q fever, is no longer classified as a rickettsial organism, although it is an obligate intracellular parasite

▶ Q fever encompasses a variety of acute and clinical syndromes; clue to diagnosis is exposure to animals, especially sheep or livestock

▶ Treatment of choice is doxycycline

Questions

1. Which condition of sheep increases the chance of transmission of *Coxiella burnetii* to other organisms?
   - A. Colic
   - B. Diarrhea
   - C. Parturition
   - D. Vomiting
   - E. Mad cow disease

2. Which pathogen is the agent of "woolsorter's disease"?
   - A. *Coxiella burnetii*
   - B. *Brucella ovis*
   - C. *Brucella melitensis*
   - D. *Bacillus anthracis*
   - E. *Francisella tularensis*

HPI: A 24-year-old man presents to a medical school teaching clinic with complaints of a cough that has lasted 2 weeks, accompanied by fatigue and malaise. The cough is incessant and productive of small amounts of yellow sputum. These symptoms were preceded by several days of rhinitis and a sore throat. He has taken his temperature at home, and it reached a maximum of 100°F.

The patient has no past medical history, and has been taking an over-the-counter decongestant and expectorant.

PE: T 37.3°C BP 120/60 HR 65 RR 14 SaO$_2$ 98% on room air

Physical exam shows a young man in no respiratory distress. There is no conjunctival injection. The oropharynx shows slight erythema. Ear exam shows bullous myringitis of the right tympanic membrane. Lungs are clear to auscultation and percussion. Abdomen is benign, with no hepatosplenomegaly. There is no rash.

Labs: The physician initially suspects viral bronchitis, but decides to check a chest x-ray.

The chest x-ray shows a diffuse interstitial infiltrate, which looks "much worse than the patient."

Although diagnostic testing would usually not be performed in this case, the physician demonstrates some diagnostic tests for the edification of his students. He checks a sputum Gram stain, which shows normal flora and no predominant species. Next, he draws blood into an anticoagulated tube, and places the tube on ice. Within minutes, the red blood cells have clumped together. The clumping reverses with warming.

Thought Questions

- Which infections could cause these symptoms and the findings on chest x-ray?
- What did the blood clumping test show?
- Which antibiotics would be reasonable to prescribe?
- Why was this patient not admitted to the hospital?

Basic Science Review and Discussion

Pneumonia pathogens are often divided into typical and atypical etiologies. **Typical** causes of pneumonia are bacterial: *Streptococcus pneumoniae* (pneumococcus), *Haemophilus influenzae,* and *Moraxella.* **Atypical pneumonia** may be caused by viruses, such as influenza, parainfluenza, and adenovirus, and respiratory syncytial viruses, *Mycoplasma,* or *Chlamydia. Legionella,* often grouped with the atypical agents, is a gram-negative bacterium that usually causes more severe disease than the other atypical agents. *Legionella* is grouped with the other atypical agents, however, because it is an intracellular bacterium that is difficult to diagnose and is treated with similar antibiotics. The clinical distinction between the typical and atypical pneumonias is difficult to make in practice, but classically atypical pneumonia presents as a milder, more subacute illness, sometimes described as "walking pneumonia." Fever is less pronounced, and patients are less likely to die of the illness. Chest X-rays show patchy or interstitial infiltrates (unlike the classic lobar infiltrates of pneumococcal pneumonia) and are often described as "looking worse than the patient." Sputum Gram stains do not reveal the etiologic organism. Because of the milder severity of illness and the difficulty of culturing

Mycoplasma and *Chlamydia,* most diagnoses of atypical pneumonia are made clinically and without cultures. Such patients are usually well enough to be treated as outpatients. Regardless of whether a patient appears to have a "typical" or "atypical" presentation of pneumonia, most patients will be treated with an antibiotic regimen that covers both types of agents. Because the atypical pneumonia agents such as *Chlamydia* and *Legionella* live within mammalian cells, antibiotics with good intracellular penetration such as the macrolides, tetracyclines, and fluoroquinolones are the most effective. β-lactams, although excellent drugs against most typical causes of bacterial pneumonia, do not penetrate mammalian cells. In addition, β-lactams have no activity against *Mycoplasma* which do not have a cell wall.

Mycoplasma pneumoniae is the most frequent cause of atypical pneumonia. The other pathogenic mycoplasma species (*Mycoplasma hominis, Mycoplasma genitalium,* and *Ureaplasma urealyticum*) all infect the genitourinary tract. Mycoplasma are the smallest known free-living organisms. They have no cell wall, which renders them resistant to β-lactam antibiotics, and are invisible on Gram stain. They have no DNA homology with typical bacteria. Unlike viruses, *Mycoplasma* are able to grow in defined, noncellular media; they are extracellular parasites and contain both DNA and RNA.

In addition to pneumonia, *Mycoplasma pneumoniae* infection may also lead to serious skin rashes, such as **erythema multiforme** and **Stevens-Johnson syndrome.** Mycoplasma is also associated with an infection of the tympanic membrane known as **bullous myringitis.** Mycoplasma infection is also associated with immunologic phenomena, most strikingly **cold agglutinins,** described in this case. Cold agglutinins are IgM antibodies directed against the modified

I antigen found on the red blood cells of infected patients. If severe, the cold agglutinins may be associated with Raynaud's phenomenon (spontaneous vasoconstriction of the extremities, associated with cold). The pneumonia of mycoplasma is self-limited without treatment, but treatment shortens the illness and probably reduces spread.

Chlamydia pneumoniae is another major cause of atypical pneumonia. Chlamydia are obligate intracellular parasites distantly related to eubacteria. They have very small genomes for prokaryotes; only *Mycoplasma* genomes are smaller. They cannot synthesize their own energy and must rely on the host cell to supply ATP and GTP. The organisms have a biphasic life cycle. The inert, hardy, extracellular state, known as an elementary body, is stabilized by disulfide cross-linking between membrane proteins. Once taken up into a cell by receptor-mediated endocytosis, the elementary bodies transform into larger reticulate bodies, which are metabolically active and reproduce by binary fission, ultimately giving rise to more elementary bodies. Unlike *C. psittaci*, the agent of psittacosis associated with birds, *C. pneumoniae* has no animal reservoir and is spread from human to human through respiratory secretions. The organism may be present with or without causing disease. Most initial infections occur during school age. Clinical presentations tend to be mild, and similar to *Mycoplasma* pneumonia. Some preliminary research suggests that *Chlamydia* pneumonia infection may be associated with the development of atherosclerosis.

Legionella pneumophila is a gram-negative rod aerobic bacterium, often lumped with the other causes of atypical pneumonia because, like *Chlamydia* and *Mycoplasma,* it is difficult to culture and is resistant to β-lactam antibiotics. *Legionella* can survive for years in water, and is tolerant of chlorine, so it may colonize plumbing or air conditioning systems. *Legionella* may require symbiotic microorganisms for survival in these habitats. Aerosols from these colonized sources, or aspiration of contaminated water, lead to pneumonia. Unlike the other atypical pneumonias, *Legionella* pneumonia tends to be very severe, with almost all patients requiring hospital admission. As with other intracellular pathogens, cell-mediated immunity is the major defense against *Legionella,* and the illness is more severe in patients lacking cell-mediated immunity. *Legionella* may also cause a self-limited febrile illness without pneumonia, known as Pontiac fever.

Unexplained hyponatremia may be a clue to *Legionella* infection. *Legionella* tends to be underdiagnosed, because it will not grow with standard blood or sputum culturing techniques. *Legionella* can be cultured, but requires a special medium made from a charcoal yeast extract at pH 6.9. The organism may be detected with direct fluorescent antibodies, but the test requires a large number of organisms. A urine test for the presence of *Legionella* antigen is a convenient new way to diagnose the illness, although the available test only detects *Legionella pneumophila* serogroup 1 species.

Case Conclusion   The patient is sent home with a 5-day course of azithromycin and instructions to return if he gets worse. His cough resolves several days after finishing the azithromycin course. (Due to its long half-life, azithromycin is still present in the blood days after the patient stops taking the pills.)

Thumbnail: Nonviral Agents of Atypical Pneumonia

Organism	Legionella pneumophila	Mycoplasma pneumoniae	Chlamydia pneumoniae
Diseases caused	Atypical pneumonia or lobar pneumonia, often severe	Atypical pneumonia	Atypical pneumonia; possibly linked to atherosclerosis
Epidemiology	Lives in water and may be spread through plumbing or air conditioning	Endemic	Endemic
Diagnosis	Legionella urinary antigen; legionella culture (special media)	Cold agglutinins; may be detected through serology, culture, or PCR, but usually empirically treated	May be detected through serology, culture or PCR, but usually empirically treated
Treatment	Macrolides, tetracyclines, fluoroquinolones	Macrolides, tetracyclines, fluoroquinolones	Macrolides, tetracyclines, fluoroquinolones

Key Points

▶ The major causes of atypical pneumonia include viral infections such as influenza, parainfluenza, RSV, and adenovirus, *Mycoplasma, Chlamydia,* and *Legionella*

▶ Atypical pneumonia classically presents with prolonged cough and malaise; fevers are less common than in typical pneumonia; although chest X-rays are supposed to show patchy or interstitial infiltrates rather than the lobar infiltrates caused by pneumococcus, the distinction is not reliable

▶ While it can be difficult to distinguish typical and atypical pneumonia agents by their clinical presentation, the distinction is useful because antibiotic therapies differ for the two classes

Questions

1. Which of these antibiotic classes, often used to treat pneumonia, misses atypical agents?
   A. Macrolides
   B. Ketolides
   C. Fluoroquinolones
   D. Tetracyclines
   E. β-lactams

2. Which of the following organisms, if found on a sputum culture, definitely indicates infection?
   A. *Chlamydia pneumoniae*
   B. *Pneumococcus*
   C. *Haemophilus influenzae*
   D. *Legionella pneumophila*
   E. *Moraxella*

3. Which of the following organisms lacks a cell wall?
   A. *Klebsiella pneumoniae*
   B. *Mycoplasma pneumoniae*
   C. *Pneumococcus*
   D. *Moraxella*
   E. *Candida albicans*

4. Which of the following agents of pneumonia is extracellular?
   A. *Chlamydia pneumoniae*
   B. *Mycoplasma pneumoniae*
   C. *Chlamydia psittaci*
   D. *Legionella pneumophila*
   E. Influenza A

HPI: NG is a 22-year-old woman who presents with 24 hours of increasing lower abdominal and pelvic pain. She notes that the pain, which began as a dull ache the prior day, was initially in the middle of her lower abdomen and now is more left sided. She notes no nausea or vomiting, and while she has not taken her temperature, she has felt feverish. PMH: She notes no particular illnesses, no symptoms like this before. She is sexually active, with a new partner for 6 weeks. She uses oral contraceptive pills for contraception and has never been pregnant.

PE: T 38.2°C HR 96 BP 116/72
On abdominal exam, the patient has no peritoneal signs, but is tender in both lower quadrants. On pelvic exam, she has cervical motion tenderness (CMT), with adnexal tenderness particularly on the left.

Labs: WBC 14.5, 77% polys, 9% bands; cervical cultures and DNA studies pending.

Thought Questions

- What are the leading organisms that cause pelvic inflammatory disease (PID)?

- What other diseases do they cause?

- How can each of these organisms be treated?

- What are the most common sequelae from PID?

Basic Science Review and Discussion

The two most common organisms known to cause PID in the U.S. are *Neisseria gonorrhoeae,* known as gonococcus or GC, and *Chlamydia trachomatis* (CT). These two organisms differ in terms of their microbiology; however, they are commonly diagnosed together as the etiology for cervicitis, urethritis, prostatitis, and PID.

N. gonorrhoeae is a gram-negative diplococcus closely related to *N. meningitidis* (meningococcus), which is a common cause of bacterial meningitis. The incidence of gonococcal disease fell in the late 1980s and early 1990s concomitant with the increased awareness regarding sexually transmitted infections (STIs) that accompanied the identification of HIV and its prevention. However, the incidence of gonorrhea has remained relatively stable in the late 1990s and since 2000, with about 100 cases per 100,000 in the U.S.

Gonococcus can cause disease in humans by invading the mucous membranes of the eye, rectum, throat, and commonly the genitourinary (GU) tract. It is thought that the predilection of the gonococcus for these particular sites is based upon the specificity of the organisms pili for these tissues. The pili are 2- to 3-μm appendages that extend from the surface of the bacterium. These pili are composed of pilin proteins, which have enormous variety, particularly at the ends nearest to the host cells (the carboxy terminus).

GC can be diagnosed in several ways, including Gram stain smears (i.e., gram-negative diplococci), culture on modified Thayer-Martin medium grown in a CO_2-enriched atmosphere (organisms are oxidase positive), and via serology using radioimmunoassay and ELISA to specific IgA and IgG antibodies. Because definitive diagnosis can take several days, GC is often treated presumptively in a clinical setting of cervicitis, urethritis, or PID. Because of the high prevalence of penicillinase-producing *N. gonorrhoeae* (PPNG) strains, initial treatment with penicillins is not recommended. Resistance to tetracyclines, spectinomycin, and fluoroquinolones has also been reported. Thus, GC is commonly treated with ceftriaxone or high doses of azithromycin.

Chlamydia species can be considered gram-negative, but they only exist as obligate intracellular parasites. *C. pneumoniae* is a common cause of upper and lower respiratory tract infections worldwide. *C. psittaci* causes psittacosis, an atypical pneumonia contracted after exposure to birds (commonly pigeons, chickens, parrots, etc.). *C. pecorum* is known to infect animals but has not been isolated in humans.

Humans are the natural host for *Chlamydia trachomatis,* which has different serotypes that cause trachoma, an eye infection (serotypes A, B, Ba, and C), infection of the GU tract, neonatal pneumonia (serotypes D-K), and lymphogranuloma venereum (serotypes L1, L2, and L3). *C. trachomatis* is one of the leading causes of blindness worldwide; it is also considered a leading cause of infertility in women due to pelvic infections. Vertical transmission from the mother's genital tract to the newborn can lead to conjunctivitis and pneumonia in the newborn. Lymphogranuloma venereum (LGV) is seen most commonly in tropical areas.

Trachoma was described by the Egyptians almost 4000 years ago. It is a chronic conjunctivitis that leads to scarring of the eye, secondary bacterial infections, and too often, blindness. It can be diagnosed with conjunctival scrapings, which identify cytoplasmic chlamydial inclusions with either fluorescent antibodies or Giemsa staining. Occasionally, *C. trachomatis* can be identified via growth in cycloheximide McCoy cell cultures. Treatment is with tetracyclines, sulfonamides, and macrolides, such as azithromycin.

STIs such as urethritis, cervicitis, chronic salpingitis, and PID in women and epididymitis, prostatitis, and nongonococcal urethritis in men are the most common result of infection with chlamydial serotypes D through K. Unfortunately, many of these infections are asymptomatic, leading to chronic infections that can result in infertility in women and reinfections between untreated partners. Because of the high rate of asymptomatic patients, most women of reproductive age are routinely screened for *C. trachomatis* using the direct fluorescent antibody (DFA) or enzyme-linked immunoassay (EIA) with sensitivities of 80% to 95%. These tests are also used to identify *C. trachomatis* in patients with signs of infection, as are DNA probes of the urine (85% sensitive) and PCR and ligase chain reaction (LCR) amplification tests (95%–99% sensitive). The amplification tests have both a higher sensitivity and specificity than the other tests. When *C. trachomatis* is identified, it can be treated with tetracyclines or azithromycin (the latter should be used in pregnant women). It is important to treat both partners with STIs to prevent reinfection.

LGV, caused by the L1, L2, and L3 serotypes of *C. trachomatis,* is also an STI, but presents initially with a single papule or vesicle and eventually leads to a painful groin adenitis with involvement of the inguinal nodes. The nodes often suppurate and leak pus from tracts to the skin. The disease can become systemic with fever, headaches, arthralgias, nausea, and vomiting, and rarely meningitis or pericarditis. Chronically, the infection can lead to scarring and fibrosis of the lymphatics, which can lead to enlargement (elephantiasis) of the penis or scrotum in males and vulva in females. Diagnosis can be made by identification of the organism from smears of pus using Giemsa stain, or growing the organisms on McCoy cell culture. Serology is also used, with a single antibody titer above 1:64, or the presence of a titer rising over time. LGV is treated with tetracyclines or sulfonamides. In later stages, surgical excision of the lymphatics may be required.

Our patient with PID is likely to have one of these two organisms (GC or *Chlamydia*), possibly with a contribution from other bacterial species. She should consequently be treated for both organisms. Treatment usually involves a second or third generation cephalosporin (ceftriaxone) combined with either doxycycline or azithromycin. In patients suspected to have PID, aggressive treatment is mandated to prevent further transmission, immediate sequelae such as tubo-ovarian abscess (TOA) and perihepatitis known as Fitzhugh-Curtis syndrome, and the long-term sequelae of infertility and ectopic pregnancy.

Case Conclusion   NG is admitted and treated with ceftriaxone and doxycycline. Over the next 2 days her symptoms improve and she is discharged after being afebrile for 48 hours, on a 10-day course of doxycycline.

Thumbnail: PID

Agents causing pelvic inflammatory disease		
Organism	***Neisseria gonorrhoeae***	***Chlamydia trachomatis***
Type of organism	Gram-negative diplococci	Gram-negative bacterium/obligate intracellular parasite
Disease caused	PID, urethritis, cervicitis, proctitis, prostatitis, conjunctivitis	PID, urethritis, cervicitis, prostatitis, conjunctivitis, epididymitis (types D–K), trachoma (types A, B, Ba, and C), lymphogranuloma venereum (types L1, L2, and L3)
Epidemiology	STI, decreased with safe-sex practices, stable at 1/1000	STI, decreased with safe sex practices; vertical transmission to newborns
Diagnosis	Gram stain culture on CO_2-enhanced Thayer Martin media; serology of ELISA for specific IgA and IgG	Identification of inclusion bodies with Giemsa stain; DFA and EIA of genital or urine specimen; DNA probe hybridization; PCR or LCR amplification techniques; serology
Treatment	Third- and second-generation cephalosporins; high-dose azithromycin	Tetracyclines; macrolides: azithromycin, sulfonamides in trachoma and LGV

Key Points

▶ GC and *C. trachomatis* are commonly seen as co-infective agents, so both are commonly treated when patients present with PID

▶ *C. trachomatis* can cause a variety of diseases such as trachoma, LGV, and urogenital infections

▶ The most common long-term sequelae of PID are infertility and ectopic pregnancy

Questions

1. A 19-year-old woman presents with complaints of vaginal discharge and pelvic pain. On physical exam, she has bilateral lower quadrant pain and right upper quadrant pain with no peritoneal signs. On pelvic exam, there are no obvious masses and she has bilateral adnexal tenderness. Her WBC is 15.4. Her most likely diagnosis is:

   A. TOA: tubo-ovarian abscess
   B. TOC: tubo-ovarian complex
   C. Uncomplicated PID
   D. Fitzhugh-Curtis syndrome
   E. Cervicitis

2. A 24-year-old woman presents with pelvic pain, fever, and elevated WBC in her first trimester of pregnancy. She is diagnosed with PID. Which of the following medications should not be used in her treatment?

   A. Second-generation cephalosporin
   B. Third-generation cephalosporin
   C. Doxycycline
   D. Azithromycin
   E. Erythromycin

HPI: A 40-year-old surgeon presents to the ER while vacationing on Nantucket in September. He complains of fever, myalgias, and mild jaundice. He had a splenectomy 14 years ago after a motorcycle accident. He has been vaccinated for hepatitis A and B at work, with documentation of positive titers.

PE: T 38.8°C BP 140/92 HR 118 RR 20
The patient is mildly jaundiced with icteric sclerae. Heart rate is tachycardic with a flow murmur. Lungs are clear. Abdomen has a healed left upper quadrant scar and is tender in the right upper quadrant. He has scattered petechiae on his extremities.

Labs: Hematocrit 33, platelets 20,000. LFTs elevated with AST 198 and ALT 220. Total bilirubin 4.6. The lab technician calls to tell you that she notes intra-erythrocytic inclusions and thinks the patient has malaria.

Thought Questions

■ How was this infection acquired? What other infection(s) may have been transmitted at the same time?

■ Where is this infection found?

■ What risk factors does this patient have for severe clinical disease?

Basic Science Review and Discussion

Babesiosis is a parasitic disease of animals (rodents and cattle) that is transmitted to humans by **hard-bodied (Ixodid) ticks**. *Ixodes dammini* (the deer tick) is the primary vector for *Babesia microti*—this vector can also transmit **Lyme disease** (caused by *Borrelia burgdorferi*) and **human granulocytic ehrlichiosis** (caused by *Ehrlichia equi/phagocytophila*).

The ticks ingest the parasites from infected animals while feeding. The *Babesia* organisms multiply within the gut of the tick and are then **spread into the tick's salivary glands.** The transmission cycle is complete when the ticks inject the vertebrate host during a second feeding (see Figure 26-1).

Trophozoites in the circulation infect red blood cells through a process that probably involves activation of the complement pathway, coating of the parasite with C3b, and attachment to erythrocytes via the C3b receptor. Asexual reproduction of the *Babesia* within host red blood cells produces two to four **merozoites** per cell, with the four daughter parasites attached by cytoplasm, and may lead to the **Maltese cross** form noted on the smear (see Figure 26-2).

Babesia infections in wild and domestic animals are found worldwide, but **human infections are limited to the range of the Ixodes tick**—primarily the **northeast U.S.** (Nantucket and Martha's Vineyard in Massachusetts, Long Island and Shelter Island in New York, and the mainland coast of Connecticut and New York), but cases have been reported in California, Washington State, Missouri, and Wisconsin.

In addition to tick bites, *Babesia* infections have been documented to be spread from human to human via blood transfusions.

Clinical disease with *Babesia* is most often **silent.** Seroprevalence in highly endemic areas is as high as 10% to 20%. In patients with clinical disease, the **incubation period is from 1 to 4 weeks post-tick bite,** although **many patients do not recall a tick bite.** In general, babesiosis may present with fever, malaise, and myalgias. Hepatosplenomegaly and hemolytic anemia may be seen, as well as elevated liver function tests.

Patients who have had a **splenectomy** are at greater risk for severe disease, most likely as a result of higher circulating parasitemia when the spleen is not available to filter infected red blood cells. Other risk factors for more severe infection include older age, AIDS, and IgM or IgA deficiencies.

Diagnosis is firmly established by **visualization of the intra-erythrocytic parasites** on thick and thin smears of blood stained with Giemsa (Figure 26-2). *B. microti* may appear as a small ring form, similar to *P. falciparum.* Serum antibody titers rise over 2 to 4 weeks after infection and wane over 6 to 12 months. Antibody detection tests may be useful in detecting infected individuals with very low-level parasitemia. PCR techniques are also available.

Treatment is not usually necessary in patients with spleens. In splenectomized patients, or in more severe cases, the combination of **quinine and clindamycin** are used, although parasites may persist in the blood for months after treatment. Atovaquone plus azithromycin serves as an alternative treatment regimen. **If parasitemia reaches 10% or greater of erythrocytes, exchange transfusions may be utilized.**

Prevention of disease is achieved by **avoidance of tick bites**—wearing long-sleeved shirts and pants, tucking pant legs into socks, wearing insect repellants (such as DEET), and avoiding wooded or grassy areas during times that ticks are feeding.

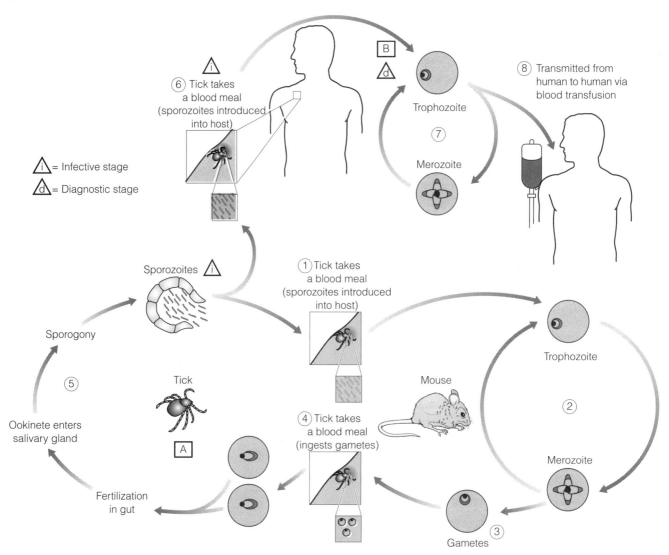

= Infective stage

= Diagnostic stage

⑥ Tick takes a blood meal (sporozoites introduced into host)

B

Trophozoite

⑧ Transmitted from human to human via blood transfusion

⑦

Merozoite

Sporozoites

① Tick takes a blood meal (sporozoites introduced into host)

Trophozoite

Sporogony

Mouse

②

⑤

Tick

Merozoite

Ookinete enters salivary gland

A

④ Tick takes a blood meal (ingests gametes)

③

Fertilization in gut

Gametes

Figure 26-1 *Babesia* life cycle. (Image in public domain on Centers for Disease Control Public Health Image Library.)

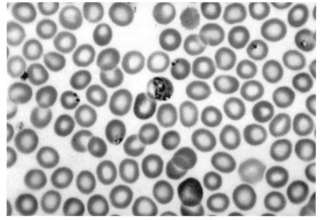

Figure 26-2 Giemsa-stained *Babesia microti* on thin blood smear. (Image in public domain on Centers for Disease Control Public Health Image Library, phil.cdc.gov, courtesy of Dr. Mae Melvin.)

Case Conclusion   When you examine the blood smear in the hematology lab, you note a classic Maltese cross pattern in erythrocytes and diagnose babesiosis. A formal thick and thin smear estimates parasitemia at 25%. The patient is admitted and placed on quinine and clindamycin. After 2 days, his clinical condition worsens and he develops progressive dyspnea. He is treated with exchange transfusions with continued antibiotics. Gradually he improves over several days and eventually returns home with no sequelae.

Thumbnail: *Babesia*

Organism	*Babesia microti*	*Ehrlichia equi/phagocytophila*	*Ehrlichia chaffeensis*
Type of organism	Protozoan (Piroplasm)	Obligate intracellular gram-negative *Rickettsiaceae*	Obligate intracellular gram-negative *Rickettsiaceae*
Type of cell infected	Red blood cell	Granulocytes	Monocytes
Vector	*Ixodes dammini* or *scapularis* ticks	*Ixodes dammini* or *scapularis* ticks	*Amblyomma americanum* or *Dermacentor variabilis* ticks
Diseases caused	Babesiosis	Human granulocytic ehrlichiosis (HGE)	Human monocytic ehrlichiosis (HME)
Epidemiology	Found in northeast; mostly asymptomatic; risk factors for severe infection include splenectomy, AIDS, and old age	Found in upper midwest and northeast; summer seasonality	Found in southcentral and Atlantic states (OK, MI, GA); May–September seasonality
Clinical syndrome	Fever, fatigue, hemolysis, elevated LFTs, thrombocytopenia	Fever, HA, myalgias/arthralgias, leukocytopenia, thrombocytopenia	Fever, HA, chills, rash, elevated LFTs, leukopenia, thrombocytopenia
Diagnosis	Parasites in RBCs on blood smear: "Maltese cross"	Morulae in granulocytes on blood smear; antibody titers	Morulae in monocytes on blood smear; antibody titers
Treatment	Clindamycin + quinine or quinidine; consider exchange transfusion if parasitemia > 10% of erythrocytes	Doxycycline	Doxycycline

Key Points

▶ *Babesia microti* is an intra-erythrocytic parasite that is transmitted by the *Ixodes dammini* tick

▶ Most cases are asymptomatic in the absence of risk factors (splenectomy, AIDS, and old age)

Questions

1. A patient is diagnosed with babesiosis and treated with quinidine and clindamycin. Three weeks after completion of treatment, the patient develops arthritis of her right knee and both wrists. What is the etiology of the arthritis?

   A. Autoimmune arthritis in reaction to *Babesia microti surface proteins*

   B. Deposition of quinine in the joint

   C. Acquisition of *Borrelia* infection at the same time as the *Babesia* infection

   D. Acquisition of *Ehrlichia* infection at the same time as the *Babesia* infection

   E. Relapse of babesiosis due to improper initial treatment

2. Which of the following tick-borne diseases is a virus?

   A. Lyme disease

   B. Rocky Mountain spotted fever

   C. Tularemia

   D. Babesiosis

   E. Colorado tick fever

HPI: A 33-year-old sewer worker in rural Colorado comes to the ER complaining of fever and jaundice. His symptoms began 10 days ago with abrupt onset of fever, chills, headache, and myalgias. He thought he had "the flu" and took acetaminophen and rested. After about a week, his symptoms abated, only to return 3 days later with fever, jaundice, headache, neck pain, and photophobia.
PMH: None. Medications: none.

PE: T 38.6°C BP 130/88 HR 70 RR 22
Skin is jaundiced. Sclerae are icteric, and there is notable conjunctival suffusion. Neck is stiff, with pain on flexion. Abdomen is soft with moderate tenderness in the right upper quadrant.

Labs: WBC 12.2 with 18% neutrophils, no bands; hemoglobin 12.2 mg/dL; platelets 112,000; BUN/creatinine 38/2.1; AST 177; ALT 252; total bilirubin 5.2. Acute hepatitis serologies are negative. Urinalysis shows 2+ WBC, trace blood, and 2+ protein with cellular casts. LP shows 6 RBC/28 WBC (90% lymphocytes), normal glucose, and mildly elevated protein. Cultures of blood, urine, and CSF are pending.

Thought Questions

■ What organisms can be responsible for this constellation of symptoms?

■ What clues from the history are useful in determining the pathogenic organism?

■ What tests may yield a definitive diagnosis in this case?

Basic Science Review and Discussion

Leptospirosis is the clinical syndrome caused by one of the numerous serotypes of the spirochete *Leptospira interrogans*. *Leptospira* are **helical** in shape and are **obligate aerobes.** The organism may be cultured from blood, urine, or CSF samples. The degree of clinical illness depends on the pathogenicity of the infecting strain as well as the general health of the individual infected.

Leptospirosis is the most widespread **zoonosis** in the world, with a high prevalence of infection among numerous species of mammals, including rats, rabbits, dogs, horses, cattle, sheep, and swine. The major mode of transmission is through **contact with animal urine** infected with the virulent organism.

Leptospira reach the environment through animal urine and proliferate in fresh water, damp soil, vegetation, and mud. The occurrence of flooding after heavy rainfall facilitates the spread of the organism from soil into surface waters. Contact with fresh water through white water rafting, kayaking, or adventure racing in areas where leptospirosis is endemic or epidemic is a known risk factor for the disease.

Leptospira from infected water and soil enter the human host through a break in the skin or intact mucosa. Leptospiremia occurs readily and persists throughout the acute illness. Infection of the CSF and kidneys is common. Late

manifestations of the disease may be caused by host immunologic response to the infection.

The clinical syndrome of leptospirosis is a **biphasic illness.** After an incubation period of 7 to 13 days, the first phase, known as the **leptospiremic phase,** is characterized by abrupt onset of fever and chills, frontal headache, and severe myalgias. This phase lasts 4 to 9 days. After a 1- to 3-day period of normal temperatures and mild symptoms, the second phase, known as the **immune phase,** presents with recurrence of fever and earlier symptoms. Meningitic symptoms and jaundice are often more prevalent in this phase.

Weil's syndrome is severe leptospirosis with jaundice, renal failure, hemorrhage, anemia, alterations in consciousness, and continued fever. It is usually seen with the more pathogenic serotypes of *Leptospira*. Other uncommon presentations of leptospirosis include hemorrhagic fever with renal syndrome, atypical pneumonia, aseptic meningoencephalitis, and myocarditis. In contrast to adults, infection in children may be associated with hypertension, pancreatitis, renal calculi, and a desquamative rash on the periphery.

Diagnosis of leptospirosis may be made by either **culture** or **serology.** Culture of the organism may occur from blood or CSF in the first phase of infection or from urine in the second phase of infection. Leptospira grow best on semi-solid media such as Fletcher's or EMJH medium. In the absence of culture-proven leptospirosis, a 4-fold rise in antibody titers during the course and convalescence of illness is diagnostic. Cross-agglutination reactions between serotypes occur, so that determination of the exact serotype of infection cannot be determined serologically.

Many antimicrobial drugs are effective in vitro against *Leptospira interrogans.* Clinical trials have demonstrated a beneficial effect to treatment with penicillin (1.5 million units every 6 hours for 7 days) and doxycycline (100 mg twice daily for 7 days). Resistance to penicillin has not been described. Treatment of leptospirosis (as well as similar organisms such as *Treponema pallidum*) may be accompanied by a characteristic reaction approximately 4 to 6 hours after initiating therapy. This reaction, called a **Jarisch-Herxheimer reaction,** consists of fever, rigors, chills, myalgias, headache, tachycardia, tachypnea, and hypotension. It resolves on its own after a few hours.

The overall mortality of leptospirosis averages 7%. It is higher in older individuals and with certain serotypes of the organism. Death is usually due to hemorrhage or renal failure.

Case Conclusion   This patient is initially placed on ceftriaxone and doxycycline. He begins to feel better by day 2, when urine and CSF cultures turn positive for *Leptospira*. His antibiotics are switched to intravenous penicillin, which he continues for an additional 5 days and he is discharged from the hospital. When he is seen 4 weeks later, his labs have completely normalized and his titers for antibodies to *Leptospira interrogans* have risen from 1:8 while in the hospital to 1:128.

Thumbnail: *Leptospira interrogans*

Organism	*Leptospira interrogans*
Type of organism	Helicoidal, obligate aerobic bacterium
Disease caused	Leptospirosis; Weil's syndrome
Epidemiology	Worldwide distribution; more in the tropics; ubiquitous infection of animals (skunks, opossums, foxes, raccoons, and rats); exposure to animal urine is most common risk factor
Diagnosis	Culture of the organism from blood, CSF, or urine or serology
Treatment	Penicillin or doxycycline

Key Points

▶ Leptospirosis is a zoonotic disease acquired most frequently from contact with animal urine

▶ Leptospirosis is a biphasic illness typified by fever, chills, jaundice, and signs of meningitis; symptoms in the first phase are due to leptospiremia, whereas symptoms in the second phase correlate to the appearance of antibodies to the organism

▶ Weil's syndrome consists of leptospirosis with jaundice, renal failure, bleeding, anemia, and alterations in consciousness

Questions

1. During boot camp in the month of August, six military recruits come down with a syndrome of fever and chills, myalgias, jaundice, and aseptic meningitis. A diagnosis of leptospirosis is made. Which of the following accounts for the outbreak?
   A. The organism is easily spread via the fecal-oral route
   B. The organism is aerosolized in respiratory secretions
   C. Water sources contaminated with animal urine serve as reservoirs of infection
   D. Undercooked pork is a common source of outbreaks
   E. Heat-resistant spores can be passed from person to person in close contact

2. In a patient with leptospirosis, what is the most likely explanation for a sudden temperature spike, chills, myalgias, headache, tachycardia, tachypnea, and relative hypotension approximately 4 to 6 hours following the first dose of penicillin?
   A. Jarisch-Herxheimer reaction
   B. The organism is penicillin resistant
   C. Release of organisms from sequestered areas into the bloodstream
   D. Co-infection with a second organism
   E. Penicillin is the incorrect antibiotic choice

HPI: FS is a 29-year-old man who presents with a red, mildly itchy widespread rash. He denies any new laundry detergents or other causes of contact dermatitis. He has not had any fevers, night sweats, sore throat, or abdominal pain.

PE: On examination, he has a papular erythematous rash over his torso and extremities involving his palms and soles. His mouth shows some white painless mucous patches on his buccal mucosa. Examination of his genitalia shows some new fleshy wart-like lesions.

Further history reveals that 6 weeks ago he had a painless ulcer on his penis, along with some nontender swelling in his groin, presumably lymphadenopathy. The ulcer went away and so the patient did not relate it to the present rash until asked. Upon further questioning, he admits to multiple female sex partners, including prostitutes. He often does not use a condom during vaginal intercourse.

Thought Questions

- What are the major treponemal diseases?

- What is the differential diagnosis of genital ulcerations?

- What are the stages of syphilis, and what are their manifestations?

- How is the diagnosis of syphilis made?

- How is syphilis treated?

- How is he going to explain this to his wife?

Basic Science Review and Discussion

Syphilis is caused by a **spirochete**, *Treponema pallidum* (see Table 28-1). Unique among the spirochetal diseases, it is sexually transmitted. Other spirochetal diseases are **zoonoses** transmitted by insect bites (Lyme disease and relapsing fever) or by exposure to rodent urine (leptospirosis). The other diseases caused by the *Treponema* family are spread through nonsexual contact, and consequently are diseases of childhood. (See Table 28-2.)

Table 28-1 The spirochetes

Genus	Morphology	Diseases
Borrelia	Thick loose coils	Lyme disease (ticks); relapsing fever (lice)
Leptospira	Tight coils, hooked ends	Leptospirosis
Treponema	Slender tight coils	Syphilis; bejel (endemic syphilis); pinta; yaws

Syphilis has several well-defined stages. Although the symptoms of early syphilis (**primary** and **secondary** stages) will resolve without treatment, the infection is still present. Up to one third of patients with untreated **latent** infection will develop the feared complications of **tertiary** syphilis, years after their initial infection. Staging of syphilis is important because it determines proper patient management. See Figure 28-1.

The diagnosis of syphilis can be made by identifying **treponemes** from a patient's lesions. These are usually found by scraping the base of a **chancre** of primary syphilis, but can also be found by scraping the **condyloma lata** lesions of secondary syphilis. In practice, this is rarely done, as treponemes are too narrow to be seen by standard light microscopy and a special **dark-field microscope** is required. *Treponema pallidum* cannot be cultured. Most cases of syphilis are diagnosed by means of serologic tests. The **RPR** and venereal disease research laboratory (**VDRL**) tests are examples of "nontreponemal" tests, which are used for initial screening. These tests are easily performed, but are frequently falsely positive. A second set of confirmatory "**treponemal**" tests, such as the **MHA-TP** or **FTA-ABS**, are used to rule out false positives.

Although other drugs are effective, the mainstay of syphilis treatment is parenteral penicillin. For patients with early syphilis (primary, secondary, or less than 1 year of latent syphilis), a one-time dose of **benzathine penicillin** is given intramuscularly. The benzathine formation ensures that the patient receives the entire dose while providing sustained antibiotic levels that are necessary to kill this slow-growing organism. Patients who have tertiary syphilis or have had latent syphilis for more than 1 year require longer courses of penicillin therapy.

Table 28-2 The treponemal diseases

	Venereal syphilis	Bejel (endemic syphilis)	Yaws	Pinta
Organism	*Treponema pallidum pallidum*	*Treponema pallidum endemicum*	*Treponema pallidum pertenue*	*Treponema carateum*
Transmission	Sexual; congenital	Skin contact	Skin contact	Skin contact
Organ involvement	Skin; bone; heart; CNS	Skin; bone	Skin; bone	Skin

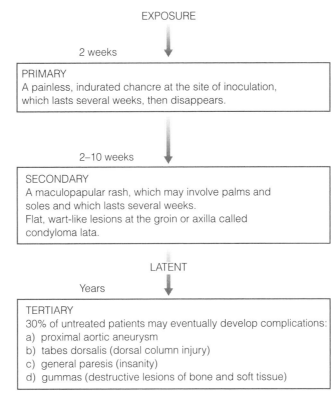

EXPOSURE

2 weeks

PRIMARY
A painless, indurated chancre at the site of inoculation, which lasts several weeks, then disappears.

2–10 weeks

SECONDARY
A maculopapular rash, which may involve palms and soles and which lasts several weeks.
Flat, wart-like lesions at the groin or axilla called condyloma lata.

LATENT

Years

TERTIARY
30% of untreated patients may eventually develop complications:
a) proximal aortic aneurysm
b) tabes dorsalis (dorsal column injury)
c) general paresis (insanity)
d) gummas (destructive lesions of bone and soft tissue)

Figure 28-1 Staging of syphilis.

Case Conclusion　His doctor happens to have a dark-field microscope in the office, and scrapings of the condyloma lata are positive for treponemes. A stat RPR is also performed and is positive. Tests are also sent for gonorrhea, chlamydia, and HIV. The patient is diagnosed with secondary syphilis and is treated with a single intramuscular injection of benzathine penicillin. He is asked to report the names of his recent sexual contacts, and public health workers call these women in for evaluation and treatment.

Thumbnail: Syphilis

Organism	*Treponema pallidum*
Type of organism	Spirochete
Diseases caused	Syphilis; closely related organisms cause bejel, yaws, and pinta
Epidemiology	Sexually transmitted; may also be transmitted transplacentally, causing congenital syphilis
Diagnosis	Characteristic chancre of primary syphilis or rash of secondary syphilis; demonstration of treponemes in lesion by dark-field microscopy; serologies; organism is not culturable
Treatment	Penicillin; no resistance reported; route and duration of therapy depend on stage of disease. Doxycycline is used for penicillin-allergic patients.

Key Points

▸ Syphilis is caused by a spirochete, *Treponema pallidum;* other spirochetal diseases include Lyme disease and leptospirosis

▸ Diagnosis is made on the basis of clinical symptoms suggesting a stage of syphilis, serology, and dark-field microscopy, if available; the organism cannot be cultured

▸ The treatment of choice is penicillin; resistance has not been reported

Questions

1. A patient presents with bony lesions consistent with a treponemal infection. Which of the following lists would be a reasonable differential diagnosis in descending order of probability?

   A. Pinta, syphilis, bejel (endemic syphilis)
   B. Syphilis, yaws, pinta
   C. Bejel (endemic syphilis), yaws, syphilis
   D. Yaws, pinta, syphilis, bejel (endemic syphilis)
   E. Pinta, yaws, bejel (endemic syphilis)

2. A patient is diagnosed with syphilis based on a positive RPR, confirmed by FTA-ABS. His treatment depends on his stage of disease, which is determined by his symptoms. Which of the following is characteristic of secondary syphilis?

   A. Aortic aneurysm
   B. Gummas
   C. Tabes dorsalis
   D. Condyloma lata
   E. Painless chancre

3. When should a patient with syphilis be treated with a drug other than penicillin?

   A. Pregnancy
   B. Penicillin-resistant syphilis is suspected
   C. Neurosyphilis
   D. Patient has a penicillin allergy
   E. Topical treatment of syphilitic chancre in primary syphilis

HPI: LD is a 30-year-old woman who presents with a chief complaint of "I have chronic Lyme disease and need antibiotics." She lives in New York City and complains that she has had chronic fatigue ever since being treated for acute Lyme disease 3 years ago. She had developed a tick bite and a leg rash after camping in Maine at the time and was treated for 3 weeks with oral amoxicillin. Since then, she has noticed progressive fatigue and depression. Her fatigue is so severe that she recently quit her job as a human resources manager and wants to apply for disability insurance. LD also complains of general "all-over" musculoskeletal pain and problems with concentration. She denies any fever, chills, chest pain, joint swelling, shortness of breath, rashes, memory changes, gait changes, abdominal pain, or bowel changes.

PMH: Depression for past year, for which she takes citalopram (Celexa) 20 mg PO once daily. No allergies to medications.

PE: T 36.6°C HR 72 BP 115/75 RR 12
LD is a generally thin, anxious young woman in no acute distress. Physical exam within normal limits; neurologic exam intact; cardiac exam shows regular heart rhythm without any murmurs or rubs; skin exam clear; no joint swelling, warmth, or tenderness.

Labs: WBC 6.5 with normal differential; RPR nonreactive; liver panel, thyroid panel, electrolyte panel, vitamin B_{12}, fasting glucose all within normal limits; ANA and RF negative; *Borrelia burgdorferi* IgG positive; *B. burgdorferi* IgM negative.

Thought Questions

- What is the mode of Lyme disease transmission?

- What is the distribution of Lyme disease?

- What are the stages of Lyme disease?

- How is the diagnosis of Lyme disease made?

- What is the treatment for Lyme disease?

- Would you treat LD for Lyme disease?

Basic Science Review and Discussion

Mode of Transmission and Distribution   **Lyme disease** was first named in 1977 when an outbreak of arthritis was observed in a cluster of children living around Lyme, Connecticut. There are now known to be three distinct foci of Lyme disease in the U.S.: (1) **northeast U.S.,** from southern Maine to Maryland; (2) **upper midwest;** (3) **west coast,** mainly northern California and Oregon. The causative agents of Lyme disease worldwide are three spirochetes called *Borrelia afzelii, Borrelia garinii,* and *Borrelia burgdorferi;* **the latter is the only strain found in the U.S.** By microscopy, *B. burgdorferi* **is a tightly coiled, helical spirochete** of approximately 10 to 25 μm in length.

Lyme disease is transmitted by the **ixodid tick** (Figure 29-1) and is the **most common vector-borne disease in the U.S.,** with an annual incidence of 15,000 cases. The high-risk areas for Lyme disease across the U.S. correspond to the distribution of the *Ixodes* deer ticks: *Ixodes scapularis* (also called *dammini*) accounts for the majority of disease in the

northeast and midwest; *Ixodes pacificus* is responsible for most of the western cases. *B. burgdorferi* is transmitted to humans by *Ixodes* adults or nymphs from their preferred hosts of white-tailed deer or white-tailed mice, respectively. As tick-to-human transmission of *B. burgdorferi* usually requires 1 to 2 days of feeding, **the smaller *Ixodes* nymphs transmit the majority of infections,** as adult ticks are usually noticed and removed from the person's body before transmission can occur. Tick larvae rarely carry *B. burgdorferi* at the time of feeding and are not very important in Lyme transmission. The density of *Ixodes* ticks peaks in June and July and the **yearly Lyme disease outbreak in the U.S. is usually from May 1 to November 30.** Approximately 33% of patients with Lyme disease recall a preceding tick bite.

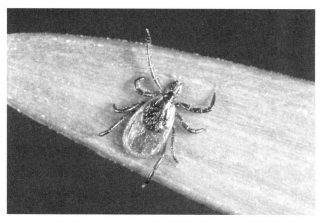

Figure 29-1 Female *Ixodes scapularis* tick. (Image provided by Jim Gathany and is in the public domain on the Centers for Disease Control Public Health Image Library, phil.cdc.gov.)

Stages of Infection There are three main clinical stages of Lyme infection, related to the time since tick exposure.

Stage I Localized infection: this stage occurs 3 to 32 days after tick exposure and usually manifests as a localized skin infection at the tick bite site called *erythema migrans* (EM). EM is seen in 75% to 90% of patients with Lyme disease. The rash usually begins as a red macule or papule at the site of tick engorgement and then expands to approximately 15 cm, with partial central clearing. The lesion is generally flat and the outer borders become erythematous, forming a **"bull's-eye lesion"**; the central portion can turn red, vesicular, or necrotic. The most common sites of the lesion are the thigh, groin, and axilla. Although the rash is often warm, it is rarely painful.

Stage II Disseminated infection: this stage generally occurs 1 to 12 weeks after tick exposure and resembles the **massive spirochetemia phase** of secondary syphilis and the first stage of leptospirosis; the clinical manifestations of all three are protean. Within several days of the onset of the EM lesion, approximately 25% of patients in stage II of Lyme disease develop multiple annular lesions that resemble EM, although they are smaller, lack indurated centers, and have no association with the tick bite site. These skin lesions are usually accompanied by musculoskeletal symptoms, malaise, and fatigue. Other possible signs and symptoms of the disseminated stage of Lyme disease include meningeal irritation, mild encephalopathy, migratory musculoskeletal pain, hepatitis, generalized lymphadenopathy, splenomegaly, pharyngitis, nonproductive cough, and/or testicular swelling. Besides fatigue, the early signs and symptoms of disseminated infection are intermittent and constantly changing.

Several weeks to months following tick exposure, 15% of patients develop a lymphocytic meningitis, usually confirmed by intrathecal IgM, IgG, or IgA antibodies to *B. burgdorferi*. *B. burgdorferi* **meningoencephalitis is often accompanied by cranial nerve palsies**, especially facial palsy, and peripheral radiculoneuropathy. Indeed, **Bell's palsy may be the only manifestation of Lyme meningitis.** In Europe, the most common manifestation of Lyme meningitis is **Bannwarth's syndrome,** which is composed of a headache-free lymphocytic pleocytosis, neuritic pain, and cranial neuritis. This syndrome has also been dubbed tickborne meningopolyneuritis (**Garin-Bujadoux-Bannwarth syndrome**), lymphocytic meningoradiculitis, or chronic lymphocytic meningitis. Approximately 8% of untreated Lyme disease patients develop **cardiac involvement** within weeks to months of tick exposure, usually manifested by a **fluctuating, transient atrioventricular block.**

Stage III Persistent infection: this stage describes persistence of Lyme disease-related symptoms that occur greater than 2 months after tick exposure. There are three main manifestations of stage III Lyme disease:

1) Joint involvement: approximately 60% of untreated patients with Lyme disease will develop frank arthritis within weeks and up to 2 years after the initial tick exposure. The **arthritic syndrome of Lyme is composed of intermittent attacks of asymmetric joint swelling and pain,** primarily in the large joints and especially in the knee. The joints are usually more swollen than painful, and are often warm, but without erythema; **Baker's cysts may form** and rupture in this syndrome. More rarely, patients will experience small joint involvement and symmetric polyarthritis. These attacks of Lyme arthritis can last from weeks to months, with complete periods of remission in between; these arthritic episodes usually decrease with frequency over time. Aspiration of the involved joints reveals a cell count of 500 to 110,000 cells/μL (average 25,000), predominantly neutrophils. Aspirated fluid will also have an elevated protein level, normal glucose level, and elevated C3 and C4 complement levels. The syndrome of **chronic Lyme arthritis** (defined as **continuous** inflammation for over a year) **occurs in 10% of Lyme disease patients** with arthritis and is associated with both the HLA-DRB[401] allele and certain *B. burgdorferi* strains; chronic Lyme arthritis results in synovial destruction accompanied by inflammatory cytokines (such as IL-6 and TNF-α) in the synovial fluid.

2) Neurologic involvement: uncommon late manifestations of Lyme disease **include transverse myelitis, diffuse neuropathy, demyelinating diseases, memory loss, and defects in the seventh and eighth cranial nerves.** Confirmation of Lyme-related neurologic involvement can be made by detecting **IgG antibodies against *B. burgdorferi* in the CSF.**

3) Skin involvement: persistent Lyme infection may result in a chronic skin lesion called *acrodermatitis chronica atrophicans,* denoted by diffuse violaceous infiltrated plaques or nodules that become atrophic on extensor surfaces.

Diagnosis Although *B. burgdorferi* may occasionally be cultured from skin specimens or blood, the **best way to diagnose Lyme disease is by serology.** IgM titers against *Borrelia burgdorferi* reach a peak between the third and sixth week after disease onset and IgG titers are highest months after exposure, during the phase of Lyme arthritis. Most patients with persistent disease and Lyme arthritis have persistently high IgG titers against the organism. As mentioned above, neurologic manifestations of Lyme disease are usually accompanied by intrathecal antibodies to *B. burgdorferi*. PCR for spirochetal DNA is under study and has been successfully tested on joint fluid specimens.

Treatment As with the other spirochetal illnesses, **complete recovery is best achieved if antibiotics are administered**

early in the course of infection. The later sequelae of disseminated Lyme disease or persistent infection can be circumvented by early treatment at the **erythema migrans** stage. Of note, approximately 10% of patients will experience a **Jarisch-Herxheimer-like reaction** (fever, rash, lymphadenopathy, and exacerbation of spirochetal symptoms) during the first 24 hours of antibiotic therapy. The chart below shows the preferred antibiotic regimens for the various symptom stages of Lyme disease. (See Table 29-1.)

In terms of treating our patient, LD, there is evidence that antibiotic treatment is highly effective for the acute and late manifestations of Lyme disease. However, some patients have persistent fatigue, musculoskeletal pain, mood and memory disturbances, or paresthesias after the standard course of antibiotics for Lyme disease. Persistent

symptoms have been reported both in patients who are still seropositive for antibodies against *B. burgdorferi* and in patients who are seronegative. Some case reports and uncontrolled trials showed success with prolonged antibiotic therapy for nonspecific symptoms after treatment of Lyme disease. However, a **recent randomized, placebo-controlled, double-blind trial of antibiotic therapy** in seropositive and seronegative patients who had chronic symptoms after treatment for Lyme disease showed that a **prolonged intravenous and oral antibiotic course for 90 days did not yield any improvement in symptoms over placebo.**[1] By this evidence, LD's symptoms will probably not improve with further antibiotics.

Asymptomatic seropositivity   No treatment necessary.

Table 29-1 Treatment of Lyme disease

Early Lyme disease	Neurologic manifestations	
Primary (localized)	*Bell's-like palsy*	
Amoxicillin (some add probenecid) × 21 days, or	Doxycycline or amoxicillin × 21–28 days	
Doxycycline × 21 days		
	Meningitis	
Secondary (disseminated)	Ceftriaxone IV × 14–28 days	
Cefuroxime axetil × 21 days	Penicillin G IV × 14–28 days	
(Less effective: azithromycin or other macrolides)	Doxycycline IV × 21—28 days	
Carditis	**Arthritis**	
(May need temporary pacing)	Amoxicillin PO × 30–60 days	
Ceftriaxone IV × 14–28 days	Doxycycline PO × 30–60 days	
Penicillin IV × 14–28 days	Ceftriaxone IV × 30 days	
Doxycycline PO × 30 days	Penicillin G IV four times a day × 30 days	
Amoxicillin PO × 30 days		
	Acrodermatitis chronic atrophicans	
Pregnancy	Penicillin VK PO × 30 days	
Localized early disease	Doxycycline × 30 days	
Amoxicillin × 30 days		
Any manifestation of disseminated disease		
Penicillin G IV four times a day × 14–28 days		

Doses for antibiotics Amoxicillin 500 mg PO three times a day; azithromycin 500 mg PO once daily; ceftriaxone (high-dose) 2 g IV once daily; cefuroxime axetil 500 mg PO twice a day; doxycycline 100 mg PO twice a day; penicillin (high-dose) 20 million units IV once daily (divided q4h or q6h); penicillin VK 1 g PO three times a day; probenecid 500 mg PO three times a day.

Case Conclusion   LD was counseled that further antibiotics would not benefit her symptoms. She grew angry in the office, informed you that one of her favorite Internet web sites on Lyme disease recommended further antibiotic therapy, and fired you as her physician.

Thumbnail: Lyme Disease

Organism	*Borrelia burgdorferi*
Type of organism	Tightly coiled, helical spirochete
Diseases caused	Lyme disease; localized infection of *erythema migrans* may be followed by disseminated disease and Lyme meningitis, and then persistent infection, with joint, neurologic, and skin manifestations
Epidemiology	Tick-borne disease from *Ixodes* deer tick; main foci in U.S. are northeast, upper midwest, and west coast, especially in northern California and Oregon
Diagnosis	Serology
Treatment	Oral amoxicillin or doxycycline for acute Lyme; cefuroxime PO for disseminated disease; IV high-dose ceftriaxone or penicillin for meningitis; IV ceftriaxone or penicillin or PO amoxicillin or doxycycline for carditis or arthritis

Key Points

▶ Lyme disease is caused by the tick-borne spirochete, *Borrelia burgdorferi,* in the U.S.

▶ Habitat of the *Ixodes* deer tick determines main regions of exposure in the U.S.: northeast, upper midwest, northern California, and Oregon

▶ Three stages of disease: stage I with localized *erythema migrans;* stage II (disseminated disease) with various, intermittent symptoms and possible meningitis; stage III (persistent infection) with joint, skin, and/or neurologic involvement

▶ Treatment with prolonged PO or IV antibiotics is appropriate for acute and late Lyme, but there is no benefit to prolonged antibiotic therapy for nonspecific symptoms after Lyme therapy

Questions

1. Which of the following diseases are also spread by the *Ixodes* vector?

   A. Human granulocytic ehrlichiosis
   B. Human monocytic ehrlichiosis
   C. Rocky Mountain spotted fever
   D. West Nile virus
   E. Colorado tick fever

2. Which of the following states is a high-risk endemic area for Lyme disease?

   A. Florida
   B. New Jersey
   C. Kentucky
   D. Alabama
   E. Colorado

References

1. Klempner MS, Hu LT, Evans J, et al. Two controlled trials of antibiotic treatment in patients with persistent symptoms and a history of Lyme disease. N Engl J Med 2001;345:85–92.

HPI: HS is a 21-year-old female who presents to your office with complaints of "blisters" in her vulvar area. These lesions appeared in this area with some extension to her inner thighs on the day prior to presentation. She also has had 2 days of low-grade fevers and feels that she has swelling of the lymph nodes in her groin. She denies any abnormal vaginal discharge or bleeding. HS has never experienced these symptoms before. She just became sexually active for the first time approximately 2 months ago with a male partner who told her that he had never had sexual relations before they met. She stopped using condoms with this partner 1 month ago.

PMH: HS has no significant medical history. Just started taking oral contraceptive pills a month ago and has no allergies.

PE: 38.0°C HR 86 BP 118/75 RR 14
Generally anxious, tearful young woman in no acute distress. Genital examination reveals crops of vesicles bilaterally around the inner vulva with sporadic vesicles on both upper inner thighs. Lymph nodes are swollen bilaterally in the inguinal region.

Labs: No blood laboratory tests performed on this visit. A smear of the fluid from the base of one of the vesicles was sent for culture and fluorescent antibody staining.

Thought Questions

■ What are the infectious etiologies of genital ulceration?

■ How would you make the diagnosis of herpes simplex virus (HSV) infection?

■ What are the characteristics of the HSV-1 and HSV-2 viruses?

■ What are some of the clinical syndromes associated with HSV and are there differences between the manifestations of HSV-1 and HSV-2?

■ What is the mechanism of antivirals used in the treatment of HSV infections?

Basic Science Review and Discussion

Differential of Genital Ulcers   In the U.S., the two major infections on the differential of genital ulceration are **herpes** lesions (60%–70%) and primary **syphilis** (10%–20%). The differential is more expansive in nonindustrialized settings and in travelers returning to the U.S. Other agents that cause genital ulceration include the following:

1) **Granuloma inguinale (*Donovanosis*):** this infection is a major cause of genital ulceration in the tropics and is caused by *Calymmatobacterium granulomatis,* an encapsulated pleomorphic gram-negative rod. The primary lesion begins as a small **painless** papule or indurated nodule and then ulcerates to form an exuberant, beefy-red, granulomatous ulcer with rolled edges and with a characteristic satin-like surface that bleeds easily on contact. Interestingly, even large ulcerative lesions are painless. However, spontaneous healing is accompanied

by scar formation, which can produce gross genital deformities. This infection can cause lymphedema; subcutaneous spread of granulomas into the inguinal region can cause groin swellings called **pseudobuboes**. The diagnosis is made by demonstrating typical intracellular *Donovan bodies* in Giemsa-stained smears obtained from lesions, and the treatment is doxycycline for 21 days.

2) **Lymphogranuloma venereum (LGV):** this sexually transmitted disease is caused by **invasive serovars** of *Chlamydia trachomatis* and is mainly found in tropical and subtropical nations of Africa and Asia. The initial manifestation of LGV is a short-lived papular genital lesion followed by massive **painful inguinal lymphadenopathy,** often with systemic symptoms. Diagnosis is made serologically and treatment is doxycycline or erythromycin for 21 days.

3) **Chancroid:** this sexually transmitted infection is caused by *Haemophilus ducreyi,* a small gram-negative rod that is more common in tropical countries. Case 14 discusses this organism in detail. Chancroid infection has been found in the U.S. in association with the use of crack cocaine and selling sex for drugs. This infection is initially manifested by **painful,** nonindurated **(soft) genital ulcers** and local lymphadenitis. The diagnosis is made by culturing the organism from the genital ulcer or a lymph node and treatment is with a single dose of high-dose azithromycin. See Figure 30-1 for a typical chancroid ulcer.

Herpes Simplex Virus 1 and 2 Infections
Properties   There are two serotypes of herpes simplex virus: **types 1 and 2.** All herpes viruses are structurally similar,

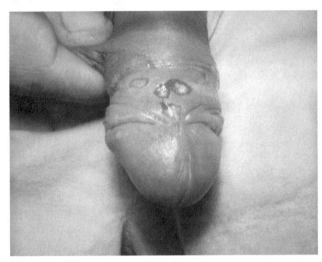

Figure 30-1 Chancroid ulcers of *H. ducreyi* on the penis. (Image in public domain on Centers for Disease Control Public Health Image Library, phil.cdc.gov.)

with an **icosahedral** core surrounded by a **lipoprotein envelope** and a genome composed of **linear double-stranded DNA.** These viruses are large (120–200 nm in diameter) and HSV-1 and -2 are structurally and morphologically indistinguishable. However, the two HSV serotypes can be differentiated by restriction endonuclease patterns of their genomes and type-specific monoclonal antisera.

After entry into the cell, the HSV virions are uncoated and the genome DNA enters the nucleus, where virus mRNA is transcribed by host cell RNA polymerase. Two of the early viral proteins translated are **thymidine kinase** and viral DNA polymerase, which helps replicate the viral genome DNA. Virion assembly occurs in the nucleus, leading to the formation of **intranuclear inclusions.** During **latent** herpes infection, HSV virions are transported to the **dorsal root ganglion** (HSV-1 goes to **trigeminal ganglia** and HSV-2 goes to **lumbar and sacral ganglia**) along peripheral sensory nerves, and multiple copies of HSV DNA are found in the cytoplasm of infected neurons in episomal form.

Transmission and epidemiology HSV-1 infections are transmitted primarily in **saliva** and HSV-2 infections are transmitted mainly by **sexual contact.** Oral-genital contact can lead to HSV-1 infection in the genital area and HSV-2 lesions in the oral cavity in 10% to 20% of cases. **Asymptomatic shedding** of both HSV-1 and HSV-2 can occur and plays an important role in transmission, although these agents are more easily transmitted in the presence of active herpetic lesions. Approximately 80% of the population in the U.S. is infected with HSV-1, with most of these infections occurring during childhood; half of these infections are manifested by recurrent **herpes labialis (cold sores).** Approximately 20% to 25% of the U.S. population is

infected with HSV-2, with 20% of these infections being asymptomatic.

Clinical HSV-1 causes the following conditions:

1) **Gingivostomatitis:** this syndrome is often the manifestation of primary HSV-1 infection and occurs primarily in children. Gingivostomatitis is characterized by fever, irritability, and multiple vesicular lesions in the mouth.

2) **Herpes labialis:** the term describes **fever blisters** or cold sores, which primarily represent recurrent HSV-1 disease.

3) **Keratoconjunctivitis:** a syndrome characterized by corneal ulcers and lesions of the conjunctival epithelium, with recurrences leading to scarring and blindness.

4) **Encephalitis:** HSV-1 is the most common cause of sporadic focal encephalitis in the U.S., with a proclivity for the **temporal lobes.** Symptoms include altered mentation, anosmia, bizarre behavior, and fever; the syndrome has a high mortality rate with neurologic sequelae in those who survive.

5) **Herpetic whitlow:** this condition is a painful infection of the hand involving one or more fingers initiated by viral inoculation of the host through exposure to infected body fluids via a break in the skin. Whitlow is typically seen in **health care workers** after touching a patient's active herpetic lesion.

6) **Disseminated infection:** HSV-1 can cause disseminated conditions in immunocompromised patients such as esophagitis, hepatitis, and pneumonia.

HSV-2 causes the following conditions:

1) **Genital herpes:** this condition is manifested by painful vesicular lesions of the male and female genitalia and the anal area. Lesions are more severe, extensively distributed, and protracted in primary HSV-2 infection than in recurrent disease. Primary HSV-2 infection can also cause fever, inguinal lymphadenopathy, dysuria, urethral discharge, cervicitis, and vaginal discharge. The genital ulcers manifest initially as vesicles, which eventually crust over. Recurrent genital herpes infections are often heralded with a prodrome of localized tingling and are more localized than primary infections, with fewer systemic symptoms.

2) **Neonatal herpes:** the risk of transmission of HSV-2 to the fetus is 33% in the setting of primary HSV-2 infection in the mother, compared with 3% to 5% in the setting of recurrent HSV-2 infection. Hence, cesarean sections are recommended for pregnant women with active HSV-2 lesions to decrease the risk of transmission to the fetus in either situation. Manifestations of neonatal herpes include localized skin, eye, and/or mouth lesions, encephalitis, and disseminated disease.

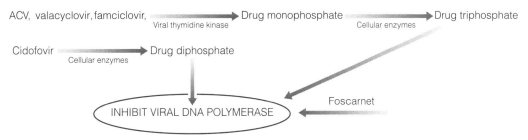

Figure 30-2 Schematizes the mechanisms of action of these antivirals.

3) **Aseptic meningitis:** the syndrome of herpes meningitis is usually caused by HSV-2 rather than HSV-1. The syndrome is usually mild and self-limited without subsequent development of neurologic sequelae.

Diagnosis The most important diagnostic procedure is isolation of the virus from the lesion by growth in cell culture; the typical **cytopathic effect** occurs in 1 to 3 days, after which the virus is identified by **fluorescent antibody staining** of the infected cells. **Tzanck smear** on cells from the base of the vesicle show **multinucleated giant cells** when stained with Giemsa stain. Immunity to HSV-1 and HSV-2 is type specific, and current serologic tests can detect acute infection with either virus by measuring type-specific IgM levels. Diagnosis of encephalitis is best made by PCR analysis of the CSF for HSV-1; the sensitivity of PCR for HSV is 98% and the specificity is 94%.

Treatment The following agents are used to treat HSV-1 and HSV-2 infections: 1) oral agents: acyclovir (ACV; Zovirax); valacyclovir (VACV; Valtrex; prodrug of ACV); famciclovir (FCV;

Famvir). 2) IV agents: acyclovir; foscarnet (Foscavir; for resistant viruses); cidofovir (Vistide; restricted because of renal toxicity); penciclovir (Denavir; investigational; no oral bioavailability).

The above diagram (Figure 30-2) schematizes the mechanism of action of these antivirals.

ACV is phosphorylated by viral thymidine kinase to ACV-monophosphate, which is then phosphorylated to ACV-triphosphate (ACV-TP) by host cell enzymes. ACV-TP inhibits viral DNA polymerase and blocks replicating viral DNA. Most **ACV-resistant** strains have lost the viral thymidine kinase, although drug resistance in HSV can also occur at the level of the viral DNA polymerase. VACV and FCV can be taken less frequently because they are more orally bioavailable than ACV, but all three drugs reduce shedding and hasten time to lesion healing. **Cidofovir** is a nucleotide analog that already exists in the monophosphate form, so that its activation only occurs through cellular enzymes. **Foscarnet** blocks the pyrophosphate binding site of viral DNA polymerase. Both cidofovir and foscarnet can be used against ACV-resistant virus.

Case Conclusion Direct fluorescent antibody (DFA) staining of HS's vesicular lesion was positive for HSV-2. She was treated with acyclovir and she promptly broke up with her boyfriend.

Thumbnail: Herpes Simplex Virus Infections

Organisms	HSV-1 and HSV-2
Type of organism	Large double-stranded DNA virus
Diseases caused	Acute gingivostomatitis, recurrent herpes labialis, keratoconjunctivitis, encephalitis, genital herpes, neonatal herpes, aseptic meningitis, disseminated infection
Epidemiology	80% of the U.S. population is infected with HSV-1, with primary infections occurring predominantly in childhood; 20% to 25% of the U.S. population is HSV-2 infected, with primary infections occurring predominantly in young, sexually active adults
Diagnosis	Direct fluorescent antibody staining in cell culture of fluid scraped from the base of the vesicle
Treatment	Acyclovir, famciclovir, valacyclovir; foscarnet for acyclovir-resistant virus

Key Points

▶ The major causes of genital ulceration in the U.S. are herpes simplex virus infections and primary syphilis (although genital ulcers in the rest of the world can also be caused by *Chlamydia trachomatis, Haemophilus ducreyi,* and *Calymmatobacterium granulomatis*)

▶ HSV-1 is typically spread by saliva and causes oral ulcerations, and HSV-2 is typically spread by sexual contact and causes genital ulcerations, although each virus can cause the converse syndrome

▶ Asymptomatic shedding of virus can occur and is a major source of transmission when active lesions are not visible

▶ Effective antivirals exist for HSV, although drug resistance is emerging

Questions

1. What degree of HSV resistance to acyclovir is seen in the U.S. population?

    A. 0%

    B. 5%

    C. 15%

    D. 50%

    E. Depends on the host

2. Asymptomatic shedding of HSV-2 occurs in what percentage of days out of a year?

    A. 1.2%

    B. 4.3%

    C. 6.7%

    D. 10.2%

    E. 18.5%

HPI: A 41-year-old woman with AIDS and a CD4 count of 20 presents with new onset of diarrhea, up to ten small stools a day. She also has crampy abdominal pain and low-grade fevers. She has been prescribed antiretroviral therapy, but has not been taking it.

PE: T 38°C BP 120/75 HR 95 RR 14
The patient is cachectic and in no acute distress. Her fundoscopic exam is normal. Her oral mucosa is dry with some thrush in the oropharynx. She has a few shotty inguinal nodes but otherwise no lymphadenopathy. Heart and lung exam is normal. Her abdomen has mild left lower quadrant tenderness, but no peritoneal signs. There are no masses or hepatosplenomegaly. Rectal exam shows no masses; stool is brown and guaiac positive.

Labs: White count is 3. Hematocrit is 32. Platelets are 340. She has an elevated BUN of 25, consistent with dehydration. Stool samples are sent for bacterial culture, which is negative for pathogens. A test for *C. difficile* toxin is negative. Stool is also examined for ova and parasites, including cryptosporidium and microsporidium (parasites that can cause diarrhea in advanced AIDS) but none is found. A giardia stool antigen is negative.
A chest X-ray shows no signs of tuberculosis.
The patient is sent for endoscopy, which shows signs of inflammation. Several biopsies are taken. On pathology, characteristic large nuclear inclusion bodies are seen, consistent with cytomegalovirus (CMV) infection. The biopsies ultimately grow out CMV virus.

Thought Questions

- What opportunistic organisms can cause diarrhea in advanced AIDS?
- How will this patient be treated?
- What would be the best strategy for preventing this infection from recurring?

Basic Science Review and Discussion

Cytomegalovirus (CMV) is a member of the **herpes virus family.** The other known herpes viruses are the herpes simplex viruses (HSV-1 and -2), varicella-zoster virus (VZV), Epstein-Barr virus (EBV), and human herpes viruses (HHV-6, -7, and -8). These are all large DNA viruses and CMV is the largest human pathogenic virus. CMV uses its many proteins to down-regulate the host immune response. For example, one CMV protein prevents cellular major histocompatibility (MHC) complexes from being exported to the cell membrane. This prevents T lymphocytes from detecting evidence of viral infection. At the same time, CMV manufactures a "decoy" MHC complex to prevent host natural killer cells (which kill cells *lacking* MHC) from neutralizing the infected cell. CMV is named for the large nuclear inclusion bodies it makes when replicating in infected cells.

CMV infection is common; most people have serologic evidence of prior infection. Lower socioeconomic status is associated with infection; infection prevalence can approach 80% to 90% in urban areas and up to 100% in regions of Africa. Although primary infection is usually asymptomatic, acute CMV can cause a mononucleosis-type

syndrome in immunocompetent hosts. Whereas Epstein-Barr virus is the cause of four out of five cases of mononucleosis, CMV is responsible for the remainder. Compared to EBV, CMV mononucleosis tends to produce more fever, with less adenopathy and splenomegaly. The monospot test for EBV antibodies is negative in CMV mononucleosis. After the acute infection is cleared, the virus is still present in a latent form, and secondary infection can occur when the host's defenses are weakened.

CMV is much more serious in immunosuppressed hosts. If a pregnant woman sustains primary CMV infection, the virus can cause systemic and CNS infection in her fetus, with devastating results. The virus can also be transmitted to neonates at birth. CMV pneumonitis is a major scourge of bone marrow and organ transplant recipients. The more immunosuppressed the patient, the worse the infection can be. Prophylaxis with ganciclovir has been shown to reduce the risk of CMV disease in this population. Blood is screened for CMV antibodies to avoid infecting previously unexposed patients who may undergo bone marrow transplantation in the future. In HIV patients with CD4 counts below 50, CMV can cause retinitis or colitis. Pneumonitis is more rare in this population. HIV patients at risk for retinitis should receive regular eye exams.

All drugs active against CMV are inhibitors of the viral DNA polymerase. CMV lacks a viral thymidine kinase to activate acyclovir, valacyclovir, and famciclovir, so these herpes drugs are not active against CMV. **Ganciclovir** (and its new oral formulation valganciclovir) are the drugs of choice against CMV. In cases of ganciclovir-resistant CMV, other agents, such as foscarnet and cidofovir, may be used. However, these drugs both have serious toxicities, including nephrotoxicity.

Case Conclusion The patient is started on IV ganciclovir, and the diarrhea improves after several weeks of therapy. She is referred to an ophthalmologist for a dilated retinal exam, which is negative for CMV retinitis. Her thrush is treated, and because of her low CD4 count, she is put on prophylaxis for PCP and MAC. After this unpleasant experience, she agrees to take HIV antiretroviral therapy. A year later, her CD4 count is over 300, and her prophylactic medications are discontinued.

Thumbnail: Cytomegalovirus

Organism	Cytomegalovirus
Type of organism	Herpes DNA virus
Diseases caused	Mononucleosis; opportunistic infections in transplant recipients (pneumonitis) and AIDS patients (retinitis and colitis); congenital infection (TORCH)
Epidemiology	Transmission through intimate contact; infected blood transfusions or organ transplants
Diagnosis	CMV culture; CMV antigenemia; CMV PCR
Treatment	Ganciclovir, valganciclovir, cidofovir, foscarnet

Key Points

▶ CMV is a member of the herpes virus family

▶ CMV infection is common and symptoms are visually mild, except in immunocompromised patients (transplant recipients, AIDS patients, and neonates)

▶ All anti-CMV drugs are active against HSV, but many HSV drugs are not active against CMV, because CMV lacks a viral thymidine kinase to activate them

▶ Ganciclovir (or its new oral formulation, valganciclovir) is the drug of choice for CMV, because it has fewer toxicities than the alternatives

Questions

1. Which of the following antiviral drugs is active against CMV?

   A. Acyclovir
   B. Foscarnet
   C. Famciclovir
   D. Lamivudine
   E. Valacyclovir

2. How are asymptomatic HIV patients screened for CMV disease?

   A. Digital rectal exams every month while the absolute neutrophil count is less than 500
   B. Monthly chest X-rays while the HIV viral load is detectable
   C. Quarterly blood cultures for CMV while the CD4 count is less than 100
   D. Eye exams every 6 months while the CD4 count is less than 50
   E. A one-time lumbar puncture when the CD4 count drops below 200

HPI: HV is a 22-year-old man presenting to the ER with 4 days of fever, rash, sore throat, fatigue, muscle pain, joint pain, and swollen lymph nodes. He denies any night sweats, headache, cough, shortness of breath, abdominal pain, nausea, vomiting, diarrhea, or urinary symptoms. No one around him is sick, and he has not started any new medications or had any recent animal exposures or recent travel. HV has sex with men only and recently entered a relationship with a new boyfriend.

PMH: HV had syphilis 4 years ago, which was treated. He does not take any regular medications or have any drug allergies. Condom use is inconsistent.

PE: T 39.2°C BP 120/85 HR 115 RR 12
HV appears acutely ill with a diffuse, erythematous rash over his trunk, back, and upper and lower extremities. His oropharyngeal examination is significant for severe redness in the posterior pharynx and a small ulcer on the inside of his right cheek. Swollen lymph nodes are noted diffusely.

Labs: WBC 3.5 with normal differential.

Thought Questions

- What are the infectious agents that can lead to HV's constellation of symptoms and how would you test for them?

- What are the symptoms of acute HIV infection?

- Why is acute HIV syndrome symptomatic?

- How is acute HIV infection diagnosed?

Basic Science Review and Discussion

Differential Diagnosis Possible infectious etiologies of HV's syndrome include viral syndromes, such as primary EBV or CMV infection, primary HSV infection, acute hepatitis A or B infection, human herpes virus-6 (roseola) infection, acute HIV infection, or rubella. Possible bacterial infections include secondary syphilis, severe (streptococcal) pharyngitis, leptospirosis, meningococcemia, disseminated gonococcal infection, or brucellosis. Protozoal etiologies include acute toxoplasmosis or malaria, although HV has no risk factors for the latter. HV could also be suffering from a severe acute drug reaction (although he reports taking no new medications) or an acute presentation of an autoimmune illness.

Tests to exclude the above-listed infectious causes are cited below (see Table 32-1).

Symptoms of Acute HIV Infection Acute HIV infection can have a number of clinical manifestations, but usually causes a **mononucleosis-like illness** of rapid onset and varying severity. Approximately **80%** of patients manifest some symptoms

Table 32-1 Tests to exclude infectious causes

Infectious agent	Diagnostic test
Bacterial causes	Blood cultures (serology for *Brucella* and throat culture for streptococcal pharyngitis)
Acute EBV infection	Monospot and acute EBV titers
Acute CMV infection	Acute CMV titers
Primary HSV infection	HSV-1 and HSV-2 IgM titers
Acute hepatitis A infection	Hepatitis A IgM and IgG titers
Acute hepatitis B infection	Hepatitis B surface antigen (HepBsAg) Hepatitis B "e" antigen (HepBeAg) Hepatitis B core antibody (HepBcAb) Hepatitis B surface antibody (HepBsAb)
Acute HIV infection	HIV antibody and HIV RNA levels
Syphilis	RPR or VDRL serologic test for syphilis as well as FTA-ABS
Toxoplasmosis	Toxoplasma IgM and IgG titers
Malaria (*Plasmodium* infection)	Thick and thin Giemsa-stained blood smears
Autoimmune disease	Antinuclear antibody (ANA) titer or other specific serologies

Table 32-2 Signs, symptoms, and laboratory abnormalities associated with acute HIV syndrome

Signs, symptoms, laboratory values	Frequency (%)
Fevers	>90%
Fatigue	>90%
Rash	>70%
Headache	32%–70%
Lymphadenopathy	40%–70%
Pharyngitis	50%–70%
Myalgias, arthalgias	50%–70%
Nausea, vomiting, or diarrhea	30%–60%
Night sweats	50%
Oral ulcers	10%–20%
Genital ulcers	5%–15%
Thrombocytopenia	45%
Leukopenia	40%
Elevated hepatic enzymes	21%

during HIV seroconversion. The above table (Table 32-2) shows the frequency of the most common signs, symptoms, and laboratory values associated with primary HIV infection.

Among the most prominent signs and symptoms of acute HIV seroconversion are fever, skin and mucosal lesions, generalized lymphadenopathy, and headache associated with retro-orbital pain. A **maculopapular rash** with primary HIV infection occurs in 30% to 50% or more of patients and is most often nonpruritic, with macular or maculopapular lesions predominantly on the trunk, neck, and face. The

acute seroconversion rash is frequently associated with mucocutaneous oral, genital, and anal ulcers and should resolve spontaneously within 15 days. In most cases, the **acute retroviral syndrome** is self-limited, with a mean duration of 2 to 3 weeks.

Process of HIV Seroconversion HIV seroconversion is marked by the appearance of anti-HIV-specific antibodies in the plasma, which usually occurs 5 to 10 days after the acute retroviral syndrome and 3 to 8 weeks after initial infection. Following exposure to the HIV virus, the sequence of markers to identify HIV infection, in chronological order of appearance in the serum, is as follows: (1) HIV viral RNA; (2) **p24 antigen** (a viral core protein encoded by the HIV *gag* gene); and (3) anti-HIV antibody.

Approximately 2 weeks after the initial infection, **HIV viremia** increases exponentially and then declines to a steady-state level as the host's humoral and cell-mediated immune response controls HIV replication (see Figure 32-1). This time interval, the serologic "**window period,**" is characterized by seronegativity for HIV antibody, detectable p24 antigenemia, detectable HIV RNA levels, and variable CD4 lymphocyte concentrations. The detection of specific antibody to the HIV virus signals the end of the window period and identifies the individual as seropositive. The symptoms of the acute HIV seroconversion syndrome manifest during the stage of massive viremia that follows the initial HIV exposure.

Diagnosis of Acute HIV Infection As can be extrapolated from the figure below, the diagnosis of primary HIV infection is made by the detection of a high HIV RNA level with a negative HIV antibody titer.

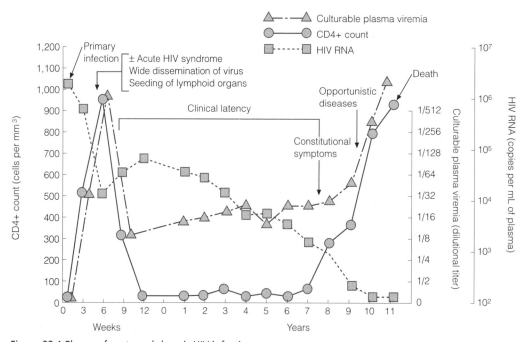

Figure 32-1 Phases of acute and chronic HIV infection.

Case Conclusion The results of HV's laboratory work-up were as follows: blood cultures × 3 negative; monospot and acute EBV titers negative, hepatitis A IgM negative, hepatitis A IgG positive; HepBsAg negative, HepBeAg negative, HepBsAb and HepBcAb both positive, HIV antibody negative, HIV RNA by PCR greater than 100,000 copies/mL; RPR negative, specific fluorescent treponemal antibody absorption test (FTA-ABS) positive; toxoplasma IgM negative, toxoplasma IgG positive; ANA 1:40 with a speckled pattern. These results indicate that HV is undergoing the acute retroviral syndrome of primary HIV infection.

Thumbnail: Acute HIV Seroconversion Syndrome

Organism	Human immunodeficiency virus (HIV)
Type of organism	Retrovirus (single-stranded RNA virus)
Diseases caused	Primary HIV infection; acquired immunodeficiency syndrome (AIDS)
Epidemiology	High-risk groups for acquisition of HIV infection include men who have sex with men (MSM), IV drug users (IVDU), heterosexuals with high-risk sex behaviors (e.g., selling sex for money), individuals who received a blood transfusion prior to 1985 (e.g., hemophiliacs)
Diagnosis	HIV antibody test for chronic HIV infection; high HIV RNA level and negative HIV antibody test for acute HIV infection
Treatment	Therapy for acute HIV infection symptomatic; treatment for acute infection with antiretroviral therapy is controversial; chronic infection should be treated with combination antiretroviral therapy

Key Points

▶ Primary HIV infection manifests with a variety of symptoms in 80% of patients, including fever, rash, fatigue, headaches, lymphadenopathy, pharyngitis, myalgias, gastrointestinal symptoms, and oral or genital ulcers

▶ Syndrome of acute HIV seroconversion corresponds to the phase of massive viremia that occurs approximately 2 weeks after initial infection with HIV

▶ Diagnosis of acute HIV infection is made by detecting high HIV plasma viral load in the face of a negative anti-HIV antibody

▶ Treatment of acute HIV syndrome with antiretroviral therapy is controversial and under study

Questions

1. What is the appropriate *initial* clinical management for this syndrome?

   A. Starting combination antiretroviral therapy immediately

   B. Symptomatic therapy

   C. Prednisone

   D. Cidofovir

   E. High-dose acyclovir

2. The term "retrovirus" refers specifically to the presence of

   A. Reverse transcriptase

   B. *gag* gene complex

   C. Viral envelope

   D. Incorporation of the viral genome into the host genome

   E. Plasmids

HPI: WN is a 58-year-old man who was brought to the ER by his wife because of a 4-day history of fevers, chills, night sweats, and myalgias. WN has also developed significant asymmetric weakness in the right lower leg and left arm. WN does not have a cough, but feels short of breath and is having difficulty swallowing. No changes in speech, no visual changes, abdominal pain, diarrhea, rash, joint pains, or urinary symptoms. Wife notes that WN has seemed confused over the past 2 days. WN has had no recent gastrointestinal or upper respiratory tract infections.

PMH: WN has a history of hypertension and smoking. Takes an antihypertensive medication and has an allergy to sulfa-containing medications, to which he develops a severe rash. Lives with his wife and works as a civil engineer.

PE: 38.6°C HR 112 BP 142/90 RR 18
WN appears in mild respiratory distress with obvious difficulties swallowing. His main physical findings are flaccid paralysis in his left arm and the distal portion of his right leg with loss of reflexes throughout. Sensation is intact throughout. He is alert, but oriented only to self and year. His heart, lung, and abdominal examination are all normal.

Labs: Studies: MRI of the brain was normal and blood and CSF samples were sent for serology.

Thought Questions

- What is the differential of acute flaccid paralysis?
- What is the definition of an arbovirus?
- What are some medically important arboviral infections?
- When was West Nile virus detected in the U.S. and how has it spread since then?

Basic Science Review and Discussion

Differential of Acute Flaccid Paralysis The differential for **acute flaccid paralysis** is limited and includes **paralytic polio virus** infection, enterovirus 71 infection, vaccine-associated paralytic polio infection (VAPP), **Guillain-Barré syndrome,** transverse myelitis, botulism (although *Clostridium botulinum* infection is associated with descending **symmetric** paralysis), and some other causes of encephalitis. **West Nile virus encephalitis** has recently been identified as an infection associated with acute flaccid paralysis.

Arboviruses Arboviruses are arthropod-borne viruses (i.e., spread by mosquitoes and ticks) that include members of the following viral families: **alphaviridae, flaviviridae, bunyaviridae,** and **reoviridae.**

Table 33-1 lists the important known arboviruses.

The life cycle of the arbovirus is based on the ability of these viruses to multiply in both the vertebrate host and the bloodsucking vector. Only the female of the species serves as the vector of viral transmission to the human, because only females require a blood meal for progeny production. Humans are often dead-end hosts for the arbovirus, because viremia is so low in humans that a mosquito or tick cannot ingest enough virus for transmission. In the syndromes of yellow fever and dengue, however, humans have a high-level viremia and the transmitting arthropods are able to acquire the virus through biting humans.

The diseases of arboviruses range in severity from mild to rapidly fatal. The clinical picture of arboviral infections usually fits into one of three categories: (1) **encephalitis;** (2) **hemorrhagic fever;** and (3) fever with myalgia, arthalgias, and nonhemorrhagic rash. Arboviruses have a tendency to cause sudden outbreaks of disease, generally at the interface between human communities and jungle or forest areas where arthropods are found in abundance. (See Table 33-2.)

West Nile Virus
Properties West Nile virus is a member of the **flavivirus** family (single-stranded RNA virus).

Table 33-1 Arboviruses

Viral family	Examples
Alphaviridae	Eastern equine encephalitis, Western equine encephalitis, Venezuelan equine encephalitis
Flaviviridae	Yellow fever virus, Dengue virus, Japanese encephalitis virus, St. Louis encephalitis virus, West Nile virus, tick-borne encephalitis
Bunyaviridae	California encephalitis virus (La Crosse encephalitis)[1]
Reovirus	Colorado tick-borne virus

[1]Hantaviruses are in the bunyavirus family, but they are not considered arboviruses; Hantaviruses are roboviruses (*rodent-*borne viruses).

Table 33-2 Characteristics of important arboviral diseases

Organism	Vector	Animal reservoir	Region
Alphaviridiae			
Eastern equine encephalitis	Swamp mosquito (*Culiseta*)	Wild birds	Atlantic and Gulf states
Western equine encephalitis	*Culex* mosquito	Wild birds	West of Mississippi River
Venezuelan equine encephalitis	Various mosquitoes	Wild birds	South America
Flaviviridae			
St. Louis encephalitis	*Culex* mosquito	Wild birds	Widespread in southern, central, and western states
Japanese encephalitis	*Culex* mosquito	Birds and pigs	Asia, especially southeast Asia
Dengue virus	*Aedes aegypti*	Monkeys/humans	Tropics
Yellow fever	*Aedes aegypti*	Monkeys/humans	Africa/South America
Tick-borne encephalitis; CEE: Central Europe encephalitis; and RSSE: Russian spring summer encephalitis	*Ixodes* tick	Vertebrates	Central Europe
West Nile virus	*Culex* mosquito	Crows and domestic birds; variety of animals	Most eastern and midwestern states
Bunyaviridiae			
California encephalitis virus (La Crosse encephalitis)	*Aedes* mosquito	Small mammals	North-central states
Reoviridae			
Colorado tick fever: *Coltivirus* subfamily	*Dermacentor* tick	Small mammals	Rocky Mountain states

Transmission and epidemiology West Nile virus was first identified as a cause of an encephalitis outbreak in the U.S. eastern seaboard in 1999. The flavivirus had first been identified in a patient in Uganda in 1937, but was not previously recognized in the western hemisphere prior to this outbreak. The virus has spread throughout most of the U.S. and Canada as of the winter of 2002.

West Nile virus (WNV) is primarily an infection of **birds and Culex mosquitoes,** with humans and horses serving as incidental hosts. The incidence of human disease peaks in the late summer and early fall after the emergence of mosquitoes and birds provides an efficient means of geographic distribution of the virus. As of October 2002, there have been 2703 laboratory-positive confirmed human cases of WNV infection and 146 deaths since the beginning of 2001. Besides transmission of infection to humans from mosquito bites, case reports have linked transmission to the **transplantation** of four organs from a single donor during the 2002 outbreak.

Clinical Twenty percent of WNV infections are manifested by a mild, febrile illness, which can include malaise, anorexia, nausea, vomiting, headache, lymphadenopathy, eye pain, and rash. The rash is generally an erythematous macular, papular, or morbilliform eruption involving the neck, trunk, arms, or legs. The incubation period of the infection is thought to range from 3 to 14 days and symptoms of the mild illness usually last 3 to 6 days.

More severe infection manifests as meningitis or encephalitis and develops in approximately 1 out of 150 infections. The neurologic illness develops only rarely in young persons; incidence is higher among persons older than 50 years of age and in immunosuppressed individuals. Encephalitis is more commonly reported than meningitis and is often accompanied by fever, gastrointestinal symptoms, rash, and mental status changes. Other notable features of the syndrome of WNV encephalitis include severe muscle weakness and **flaccid paralysis,** which may serve to distinguish the syndrome of WNV encephalitis from other etiologies. Other neurologic presentations include ataxia and extrapyramidal signs, cranial nerve abnormalities, myelitis, optic neuritis, areflexia, polyradiculitis, and seizures. Case reports from former outbreaks (not in the U.S.) have observed myocarditis, pancreatitis, and fulminant hepatitis with WNV infection.

Case fatality rates range from 4% to 14%, with advanced age being the most important risk factor for death (especially age greater than 70 years). In the New York outbreak of 1999–2000, persons 75 years of age and older were nearly nine times more likely to die than younger persons. Clinical risk factors for death are encephalitis with severe muscle weakness and change in the level of consciousness. Diabetes mellitus and immunosuppression may also be independent risk factors for death. Furthermore, recovery from WNV encephalitis is marked by significant long-term neurologic sequelae.

Diagnosis The most efficient diagnostic method for WNV infection is **detection of IgM antibody** to WNV in the serum or CSF using the IgM antibody capture enzyme-linked immunosorbent assay (MAC-ELISA). Approximately 75% of patients with WNV encephalitis have detectable IgM in serum or CSF during the first 4 days of illness, and nearly all test positive by 7 to 8 days after the onset of illness. IgM antibodies may persist for a year or more after infection. West Nile virus-specific IgM in the CSF is confirmatory for diagnosis of a current WNV infection, but identification of virus-specific IgM in serum indicates only a probable infection and requires con-firmation with acute and convalescent phase antibodies (to identify a change by a factor of four or more in the antibody titer). Patients with recent vaccination against related fla-viviruses (e.g., yellow fever, Japanese encephalitis, dengue) may have positive WNV MAC-ELISA results.

Treatment Treatment is supportive, often involving hospitalization, intravenous fluids, and respiratory support. Ribavirin in high doses and interferon α-2b were found to have some activity against WNV in vitro, but no controlled clinical trials have been performed.

Case Conclusion Our patient developed respiratory paralysis on the second day of admission, requiring intubation for mechanical ventilation. WNV-specific IgM antibodies were positive in WN's CSF on the thirteenth day of hospitalization, confirming the diagnosis of West Nile virus encephalitis. One month after the onset of WN's weakness, he remains in a long-term rehabilitation facility on continued respiratory support.

Thumbnail: West Nile Virus Encephalitis

Organism	West Nile virus
Type of organism	Flavivirus (single-stranded RNA virus)
Diseases caused	Mild febrile illness, meningitis, encephalitis notable for severe muscle weakness, and flaccid paralysis
Epidemiology	The virus was first detected in the U.S. in 1999; since then, WNV has been identified in almost every state; associated with birds and transmitted to humans by the bite of the *Culex* mosquito; transmission has also been linked to the transplantation of four organs from a single donor
Diagnosis	Detection of WNV-specific IgM antibodies in the CSF or a 4-fold rise in antibody titer of IgM in serum acute to convalescent phase samples
Treatment	Supportive

Key Points

▶ The differential for acute flaccid paralysis is limited, including paralytic polio virus infection, transverse myelitis, Guillain-Barré syndrome, and West Nile virus encephalitis

▶ Arboviruses are arthropod-borne viruses (spread by mosquitoes or ticks) and include members of the alphaviridae, flaviviridae, bunyaviridae, and reoviridae families

▶ West Nile virus was first detected in the U.S. in 1999 and is associated with an encephalitic syndrome hallmarked by severe muscle weakness and flaccid paralysis

▶ Definitive diagnosis of WNV encephalitis is made by detection of virus-specific IgM in the CSF

Questions

1. Which of the following measures can be protective against the acquisition of West Nile virus infection?

    A. Mosquito repellant
    B. Not handling dead birds
    C. Testing pets for latent infection
    D. Avoiding zoos
    E. Never keeping pet birds

2. Which of the following host factors is most strongly linked to increased morbidity and mortality of WNV encephalitis?

    A. HIV
    B. Diabetes mellitus
    C. Iatrogenic immunosuppression
    D. Older age
    E. Young age

HPI: A 34-year-old woman comes to the ER because of nausea and jaundice. She has had 4 days of anorexia and malaise. Nausea developed 2 days ago, and this morning she noticed that her eyes were yellow. On questioning, she also notes dark urine and generalized pruritus. She works at a day care center, but does not recall any of the children being ill with similar symptoms. She takes only oral contraceptive pills.

PE: T 36.6°C BP 108/62 HR 88 RR 16
She is notably jaundiced with icteric sclerae and nailbeds. She has mild right upper quadrant tenderness. The remainder of her exam is normal.

Labs: Notable labs include: AST 890; ALT 1202; total bilirubin 5.4; alkaline phosphatase 216. Serologies are sent.

Thought Questions

- What are potential sources for this infection?
- What are potential long-term sequelae of this infection?
- What can be done to prevent infection in people at risk?

Basic Science Review and Discussion

Hepatitis A virus (HAV) is a **nonenveloped, 27- to 30-nm, heat-resistant RNA virus of the Picornavirus (picorna = pico + rna = small RNA) family.** There is only one serotype. **Replication of the virus is limited to the liver,** although virus can be detected in the liver, bile, stool, and blood during active infection. Unlike other hepatitis viruses, HAV will replicate in tissue culture, albeit poorly.

Transmission of HAV occurs almost exclusively from the **fecal-oral route. Person-to-person spread easily occurs** under conditions of poor hygiene and overcrowding. Both large outbreaks and sporadic cases can be traced to contaminated food, water, milk, and shellfish. **Filter-feeding shellfish are an important reservoir for HAV** because they may concentrate large amounts of virus from contaminated water sources during feeding.

Clinically, HAV presents similarly to other types of acute hepatitis with anorexia, nausea, vomiting, and jaundice. The incubation period for HAV ranges from 15 to 45 days, with a mean of 30 days.

Specific diagnosis of HAV is made on the basis of serology. **IgM antibodies to HAV can be detected during the acute illness and are diagnostic of acute infection.** These IgM antibodies persist for several months. During convalescence, IgG titers rise and become the predominant class. Detectable IgG persists indefinitely and indicates immunity to reinfection.

Unlike hepatitis B and C, **there is no carrier state for HAV and no chronic infection occurs,** eliminating the risk of hepatocellular carcinoma that is seen in other chronic viral hepatitides. In general, the prognosis is excellent, with fulminant hepatitis occurring in only 0.1% of cases, more commonly in patients with pre-existing hepatitis C or other forms of liver disease. HAV is most often diagnosed in children and young adults, and many infections are clinically mild or silent.

The disease is **self-limited,** and therapy for acute HAV is supportive, consisting of symptom management and ensuring adequate hydration. Because of its potential importance to public health, any case of acute HAV should be reported to local health officials, and consideration should be given to preventive therapy in exposed, nonimmune contacts.

All preparations of pooled serum immune globulin contain antibodies to HAV. **Postexposure immunoprophylaxis with immune globulin** should be offered within 2 weeks of exposure to household or child care center contacts or those exposed to a common source. Casual contacts and medical personnel do not routinely require immune globulin.

Vaccination against HAV is recommended for at-risk populations (health care workers, child care workers, sexually active gay men, and travelers to endemic areas) and populations in whom disease may be more severe (chronic liver disease, hepatitis C infected).

Case Conclusion The patient was hydrated in the ER and sent home. At follow-up with her primary physician 2 days later, labs from the emergency room demonstrated IgM to hepatitis A virus. She was negative for hepatitis C and showed hepatitis B surface antibody from prior vaccination. Her symptoms continued for 1 week, after which her jaundice slowly resolved. She remained profoundly fatigued for several weeks and was unable to return to work for 5 weeks. Other workers at her day care center, as well as the children and family members of the children, were offered immunoprophylaxis.

Thumbnail: Hepatitis A

Organism	Hepatitis A
Type of organism	Picornavirus: single-stranded RNA virus
Disease caused	Acute hepatitis
Epidemiology	Transmission via fecal-oral route; food-borne outbreaks (shellfish, water, milk) and sexual transmission (oral-anal contact) are common
Diagnosis	HAV IgM antibodies; HAV IgG indicates prior infection or vaccination with subsequent immunity
Treatment	Supportive care; no specific therapy

Key Points

▶ Hepatitis A is the most common cause of acute infectious hepatitis in adults

▶ At-risk populations should be vaccinated

Questions

1. A 41-year-old man presents to the ER with the sudden onset of anorexia, abdominal pain, nausea, and dark urine. He lives with his wife and 2-year-old son who is in day care, neither of whom are ill. He works as a phlebotomist at your hospital and has been successfully immunized for hepatitis B. He drinks one glass of wine daily with dinner and denies IVDU. He takes no medications. On exam he is afebrile with obvious scleral icterus, mild jaundice, and right upper quadrant tenderness. Labs show normal CBC and creatinine, AST 1420, ALT 1824, total bilirubin 4.8, alkaline phosphatase 312. What is the most likely source of his infection?

   A. Tick
   B. Sexual partner
   C. Mother
   D. Occupational exposure
   E. Food

2. A healthy 35-year-old woman is going to a remote village in Mexico for hiking in 2 weeks. She has no history of hepatitis A disease or vaccination. Which of the following strategies for prevention of hepatitis A is appropriate?

   A. Hepatitis A vaccine only
   B. Serum immune globulin only
   C. Both hepatitis A vaccine and serum immune globulin
   D. Give her rimantadine to begin taking immediately if she feels ill
   E. No prevention strategy is necessary, as she is not at risk

HPI: A 35-year-old Taiwanese man presents with fatigue, nausea, and right upper quadrant abdominal pain and bloating over a 2-week period. He has been unable to eat much, and has lost 10 pounds. He does not drink alcohol, and denies recent ingestions such as Tylenol, wild mushrooms, or herbal medications.

PE: T 37.0°C BP 120/75 HR 90 RR 14
The patient has scleral icterus but no jaundice. There are no signs of hepatic failure such as gynecomastia, palmar erythema, testicular atrophy, or asterixis. Abdominal exam shows hepatomegaly with a tender smooth liver edge 8 cm below the costal margin.

Labs: White count is 8.0. Hematocrit is 45. Platelets are 200. Electrolytes and renal function are normal. Liver function tests show albumin 3.8, AST 540, ALT 930, alkaline phosphatase 110, and bilirubin of 3.2. INR is 1.0.
Hepatitis serologies are: **HBsAg** (hepatitis B surface antigen) positive; **HBeAg** (hepatitis B E antigen) positive; **Anti-HBs** (anti-hepatitis B surface antibody) negative; **Anti-HBc** (anti-hepatitis B core antibody) negative. He is HAV (hepatitis A virus) IgG positive. Tests for HCV (hepatitis C virus) and HDV (hepatitis D virus) are negative.
Ultrasound is negative for hepatic masses or blood clots affecting perfusion of the liver.
He is offered a liver biopsy to help stage his hepatitis, but he declines and says he would want treatment "no matter what."

Thought Questions

- What does each test in the hepatitis serology panel tell you about this patient?

- When was this patient likely infected?

- Why do HIV drugs work against hepatitis B virus?

Basic Science Review and Discussion

Hepatitis B is a partially double-stranded DNA virus that infects hepatocytes. Although it is a DNA virus, it replicates through an RNA intermediate, and its polymerase must reverse transcribe the RNA to make new DNA. Therefore, some of the HIV reverse transcriptase inhibitors are also active against HBV.

Hepatitis B can be transmitted through blood or sexual contact. The virus is highly infectious because it reproduces at a very high titer. Its titer and infectivity are approximately 10-fold higher than HCV and 100-fold higher than HIV.

Hepatitis B can cause acute or chronic hepatitis. A useful mnemonic is:

HAV causes Acute hepatitis, HCV causes Chronic, and HBV causes Both.

Rare patients, particularly those with underlying liver disease, may die of fulminant hepatic failure from primary infection with HBV. Most adults make a full recovery. However, neonates or immunocompromised patients infected with HBV are less likely to clear the infection.

These patients risk becoming chronically infected, with HBV integrated into hepatocyte genomes. Neonatal infection leading to chronic infection is most common in Asia. Patients with chronic HBV infection have a greatly increased risk of **cirrhosis.** Interestingly, liver damage in hepatitis B is thought to be due solely to the **host's immune response** to the virus; the virus itself is not harmful to liver cells. Another long-term complication of chronic HBV infection is **hepatocellular carcinoma.** The incidence of this cancer is directly correlated with the duration of chronic HBV infection. Hepatocellular carcinoma can occur independently of cirrhosis, and the virus may increase cancer risk through genetic means—either through disruption of tumor suppressor genes during integration, or possibly through the activity of one of its own genes. See Figure 35-1 and Table 35-1 for a diagram and an explanation of hepatitis B serologic tests.

A recombinant HBV vaccine has been very effective in reducing new cases of hepatitis B. Because it contains only the surface antigen, and not other parts of the virus, people who have been immunized will exhibit anti-HBs, but will not demonstrate anti-HBc, unless they were exposed to the virus in the past.

Treatment for hepatitis B used to be limited to **interferon α-2b,** a very toxic therapy with low rates of success. More recently, new antiviral drugs, particularly **lamivudine, adefovir,** and **tenofovir,** which inhibit the HBV reverse transcriptase, have shown efficacy in reducing viral replication. It is not yet clear whether these drugs should be used sequentially or whether combination therapy modeled after HIV would be better. Compared to HIV, HBV is slower to develop resistance to these drugs. For patients with life-

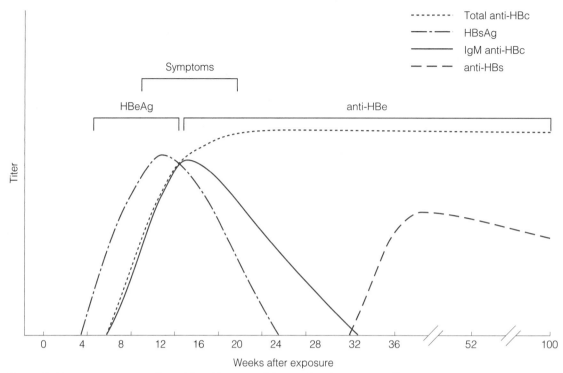

Figure 35-1 Immune response to hepatitis B. (Courtesy of Centers for Disease Control.)

threatening complications of HBV, such as cirrhosis or hepatocellular carcinoma, liver transplantation is an option; recurrence of the HBV infection posttransplant can be prevented by administration of hepatitis B immune globulin.

Patients with multiple hepatitis viral infections have a worse prognosis. All patients with chronic hepatitis should be

immunized against hepatitis A. **Hepatitis D** is a defective single-stranded RNA virus that cannot replicate on its own. However, in patients with concomitant HBV infection, hepatitis D virus is able to replicate and can lead to hepatic decompensation. Hepatitis D is most common in the Mediterranean and is transmitted by blood.

Table 35-1 Interpretation of hepatitis serologies

Results	Interpretation
Anti-HBs +; anti-HBc +	Past infection; now immune
Anti-HBs +; anti-HBc −	Immunization with recombinant HBV vaccine
Anti-HBs −; anti-HBc +	1. Weeks 5–32 in Figure 35-1 after acute infection where anti-HBc has appeared before anti-HBs (months 3–6 in Figure 35-1) 2. Distant infection with waning anti-HBs titer 3. Chronic HBV infection, often seen in HBV patients coinfected with HIV or HCV
HBsAg +	Acute or chronic HBV infection
Anti-HBs −; anti-HBc −; HBsAg −	Never exposed or immunized to HBV
HBeAg +	Active HBV infection at high titer; therefore more infectious

Case Conclusion The patient is started on lamivudine. Within a week, the patient is feeling much better. A repeat HBV viral load shows that the viral DNA has become undetectable. Eighteen months later, the patient develops fatigue, nausea, and right upper quadrant tenderness. An HBV viral load is again detectable. His doctor suspects lamivudine resistance has taken root. Lamivudine is continued to select for "less fit" mutant virus, and tenofovir is added in an attempt to suppress the viral load again.

Thumbnail: Hepatitis B

Organism	Hepatitis B virus
Type of organism	Hepadna virus (DNA)
Disease caused	Acute or chronic hepatitis; hepatocellular carcinoma
Epidemiology	In the U.S., primarily transmitted through blood exposure or sexual contact; primarily transmitted vertically in many Asian countries
Diagnosis	Serology
Treatment	Lamivudine, adefovir, tenofovir, interferon
Prevention	Vaccination

Key Points

▸ HBV is a DNA virus that requires a reverse transcriptase for replication; hence some HIV drugs are active against HBV

▸ HBV can cause acute or chronic hepatitis; mortality stems from acute fulminant liver failure, cirrhosis, or hepatocellular carcinoma

▸ HBV is transmitted through blood exposure, or through sex, similar to HIV

▸ An effective recombinant HBV vaccine is available, although not always accessible in developing nations

Questions

1. Which serologic marker shows immunity to HBV?

   A. Anti-HBe
   B. Anti-HBs
   C. Anti-HBc
   D. HBeAg
   E. HBsAg

2. Which HIV drug is also active against HBV?

   A. ddI
   B. Indinavir
   C. AZT
   D. 3TC (lamivudine)
   E. Nevirapine

HPI: A 34-year-old woman studying chimpanzee behavior in the Ivory Coast found several of the animals were dying. She dissected one several hours after it died and found that it had died of hemorrhage, and had nonclotting blood. She wore household gloves, but no mask or gown during the dissection. Eight days later she developed a fever, headache, and myalgias, which did not respond to empiric malaria treatment. Five days into her illness, she developed vomiting and diarrhea, a rash, and renal failure. Empiric antibacterial antibiotics did not improve her condition either, and she was transported in isolation to Switzerland. There were no clinical signs of bleeding.

PE: 39.0°C BP 110/75 HR 105 RR 14
The patient was lethargic but communicative. Her mucosal membranes had no signs of bleeding. She had no lymphadenopathy. Her lung exam was normal. She had mildly tender and enlarged liver and spleen.

Labs: She had a white count of 3.6, hematocrit of 40, and low platelets of 83. She had a low fibrinogen of 0.8. Her clotting times were normal, however. Liver function tests showed elevated AST of 1380 and ALT of 510, but normal bilirubin.
Serologic tests detected IgM and IgG antibodies against Ebola virus. A new subtype of Ebola virus was isolated from the patient's blood. Ebola virus was also detected in the organs from the dissected chimpanzee. Serologies for anthrax, dengue, chikungunya, and yellow fever, as well as the other viral hemorrhagic fevers (including Crimean-Congo hemorrhagic fever, Marburg, Rift Valley fever, Lassa fever, and Hantavirus) were negative.

Thought Questions

- What are the most common causes of fever in the tropics?

- What about this case made doctors suspect a more unusual etiology?

- How can viruses isolated from different outbreaks be compared to see if they are similar?

Basic Science Review and Discussion

Ebola virus and other causes of hemorrhagic fever have become notorious for the highly lethal illnesses they cause. Up to this point, outbreaks have been relatively rare, with only 1500 known cases of human Ebola virus infection.

Ebola virus is shaped like a thread, hence the name **filovirus**. It is a negative-sense RNA virus. The virus is known to infect humans, primates, and bats, but the ultimate reservoir is unknown.

Ebola virus has been found in several separate outbreaks in Africa, composed of three subtypes. A fourth subtype of Ebola virus has been found in monkeys exported from the Philippines, but does not cause disease in humans. Another filovirus, Marburg virus, has been found in Africa, and in monkeys exported from Africa. There is no serologic cross-reactivity between Ebola and Marburg viruses.

Ebola virus is transmitted through contact with patient body fluids. Many health care workers have become infected when caring for patients. Infectious virions may persist for weeks in the semen of recovered patients. The virus has also been spread through the handling of infected animals.

Clinically, the virus causes sudden onset of fever, weakness, headache, myalgias, and sore throat. This is followed by vomiting and diarrhea, and renal and hepatic failure. The hemorrhagic fever viruses cause DIC, which can lead to internal and external bleeding. Unique among the hemorrhagic fevers, Ebola virus causes a maculopapular rash. The case fatality rate for Ebola virus may exceed 80%.

Diagnosis may be confirmed through serology or culture, but samples may only be handled in laboratories with high-level isolation precautions.

Transfusion of hyperimmune serum from previously infected individuals has been tried as an attempt to treat Ebola infection through passive immunization, but animal studies have not shown any benefit to this practice. Supportive care is important to maintain hydration and blood volume.

To prevent spread of the disease, all patients must be isolated with barrier precautions, and all contacts, including health care workers, should be regularly monitored for signs of fever until 3 weeks after exposure.

Case Conclusion The patient's fever resolved without treatment, and she was discharged from the hospital after 2 weeks, having lost 10% of her body weight. Curiously, her hair fell out 1 month after the illness, but eventually grew back.

Thumbnail: Hemorrhagic Fevers

Organism	Ebola	Marburg	Hantavirus	Crimean-Congo hemorrhagic fever	Lassa virus	South American hemorrhagic fevers (Junin, Machupo, Guanarito)
Type of organism	Filovirus (negative-sense RNA)	Filovirus (negative-sense RNA)	Bunyavirus (negative-sense RNA)	Bunyavirus (negative-sense RNA)	Arenavirus (ambisense RNA)	Arenavirus (ambisense RNA)
Diseases caused	Hemorrhagic fever with rash	Hemorrhagic fever	Fever, shock, and pulmonary edema or renal failure	Hemorrhagic fever; hepatitis	Hemorrhagic fever	Hemorrhagic fever
Epidemiology	Exposure to blood or body fluids; aerosols	Exposure to infected green monkeys	Aerosols from mouse urine	Tick bite or contact with infected animal or human blood	Aerosols from mouse urine	Aerosols from mouse urine
Geography	Central Africa, possibly Philippines	Africa (or animals sent from Africa)	Americas (pulmonary syndrome), Asia, Europe (renal syndrome)	Crimea (former USSR); Africa	West Africa	South America
Diagnosis	Culture; serology	Culture; serology	Serology; PCR	Culture (dangerous); serology; PCR	Culture (throat, blood, urine); serology	Culture; serology
Treatment	Convalescent serum (unproven); supportive care	Unknown	Ribavirin; supportive care	Ribavirin; supportive care	Ribavirin	Convalescent serum; ribavirin

Key Points

▶ Ebola virus and the other causes of hemorrhagic fever are relatively rare, but have a high mortality; they are the prototypical "emerging infectious diseases" that have existed undetected in circumscribed animal reservoirs until ecological changes, due to economic development and increasing travel, lead to infectious outbreaks

▶ Because treatment options are limited, prompt isolation of potential cases is important; body fluid aerosols may infect caregivers

Questions

1. Ribavirin can treat certain hemorrhagic fever viruses as well as severe cases of respiratory syncytial virus. It is also a mainstay of treatment for which of the following?

   A. Hepatitis A
   B. Hepatitis B
   C. Hepatitis C
   D. Hepatitis D
   E. Hepatitis E

2. A previously healthy 28-year-old woman goes camping in New Mexico and develops a fever and severe pulmonary edema requiring intubation. She should be evaluated for:

   A. Lassa virus
   B. Sin Nombre virus
   C. Ebola virus
   D. Junin virus
   E. Machupo virus

HPI: A 16-year-old boy is brought in to the doctor's office one December morning by his mother. For the past 3 days, he has been feeling "terrible," staying in bed all day with fever, headache, fatigue, and severe myalgias. "This is the worst cold I've ever had." He has also had a runny nose and mild nonproductive cough.

The mother's parents live with the family. The grandfather has emphysema, and the grandmother has had a recent myocardial infarction. Their health is tenuous, and the mother is concerned they could catch his illness.

PE: T 38.5°C BP 120/60 HR 65 RR 14 SaO₂ sat 99% on room air

Physical exam shows a young man in no respiratory distress, but looking quite fatigued and uncomfortable. The patient is flushed, but there is no rash. His conjunctivae are injected, and his nose has clear discharge. The oropharynx is red but there is no exudate. The neck is supple, with mild enlargement of anterior cervical lymph nodes. Lungs are clear, and heart exam is regular. Abdomen is benign. There is no edema.

Labs: A nasal wash is sent for a viral DFA panel, which tests for influenza A and B, parainfluenza 1, 2, and 3, adenovirus, and RSV (respiratory syncytial virus). The test is positive for influenza A.

Thought Questions

- Which viruses can cause respiratory symptoms?

- How can a patient with influenza be clinically distinguished from a patient with a cold?

- What measures can be taken to prevent or treat influenza?

- Why is the influenza vaccine required yearly? Who should receive it?

- What are the complications of influenza?

Basic Science Review and Discussion

Influenza is an **orthomyxovirus,** with a segmented negative-sense, single-stranded RNA genome. The virus has a membrane envelope embedded with multiple protein spikes called **hemagglutinin** and **neuraminidase.** These are the major viral antigens, and are used by researchers to distinguish viral strains. The body uses them to drive its immune response, but viral strains with changes in these proteins are able to reinfect people with an immune response to previous strains of virus. The hemagglutinin functions as a viral adhesion molecule, used to bind sialic acid on the host cell surface as a prelude to infection; the neuraminidase is necessary to cleave off sialic acid from already infected cells to allow the virus to spread to new, uninfected cells.

Influenza is an acute illness that is usually much more severe than a cold, presenting with fevers, malaise, myalgias, and fatigue. Usually the illness is self-limited and resolves in about a week. The major complication of influenza is **pneumonia,** which is the primary cause of mortality. Pneumonia is most common in patients with chronic heart or lung disease. The virus itself may cause pneumonia. Viral infec-

tion may also predispose patients to secondary bacterial pneumonia, which usually follows 1 to 2 weeks after the viral infection. Whereas any of the usual bacterial pathogens can cause postviral pneumonia, there is an increased incidence of *S. aureus* pneumonia, which is an unusual lung pathogen in other settings.

Influenza has a pattern of **epidemic** spread, every 1 to 3 years. These epidemics are caused by **antigenic drift** in the virus, moderate changes in the viral coat proteins that allow the virus to infect people who have previously had influenza. Every few decades, an influenza **pandemic** occurs, thought to be due to an **antigenic shift,** where a brand-new subtype of viral coat proteins occurs. The pandemic viruses are always influenza A, and they are thought to be due to recombination of avian and human influenza viruses in swine in Southeast Asia. The new virus usually receives a new designation for its coat proteins. For example, the Spanish pandemic of 1918 was caused by an H1N1 (hemagglutinin type 1, neuraminidase type 1) virus, and was succeeded by the 1968 Hong Kong flu, which was an H2N2 virus. After an antigenic shift, the new virus is able to spread widely because the population has no effective immunity. Such pandemics can be devastating. The 1918 pandemic killed 21 million people, many of them younger individuals.

Influenza may be prevented by vaccinations. Experts survey viruses in human and animal populations to guess in advance which viruses will be circulating the following winter. A vaccine is then manufactured according to these predictions; most years these predictions turn out to be correct and the vaccine is protective. Because of yearly changes in the circulating virus, the vaccine must be administered on a yearly basis, as well.

Two sets of antiviral medications are available for influenza. All must be prescribed within 48 hours of symptom onset in order to have any effect on the course of the illness. The medications may also be used for prophylaxis during influenza outbreaks to prevent illness in those who were not vaccinated. Two drugs, amantadine and rimantadine, act by preventing viral **uncoating.** They are only effective against influenza A. Two newer drugs, the neuraminidase inhibitors oseltamivir and zanamivir, are active against both types of influenza. They inhibit **neuraminidase,** which the virus requires to cleave off sialic acid molecules on the host cell membrane. Without the ability to cleave these receptor molecules off, the virus is trapped on the cell, unable to move to another cell and spread the infection.

Case Conclusion   Because the boy has had symptoms for over 48 hours, it is too late for him to benefit from antiviral medication. He is also at low risk of complications. However, the physician is concerned about the grandparents, in whom influenza could be life threatening. When he hears they did not receive influenza vaccinations this year, he prescribes them prophylactic rimantadine to decrease their chances of contracting the virus. (He chooses rimantadine over amantadine because it is less likely to have CNS side effects in the elderly.)
The grandparents are admonished to have influenza vaccinations every year from now on.

Thumbnail: Respiratory Viruses

Organism	Influenza A and B	Parainfluenza 1, 2, and 3	Respiratory syncytial virus	Adenovirus	Rhinovirus	Coronavirus
Type of organism	Orthomyxovirus (negative-sense, ssRNA virus)	Paramyxovirus (negative-sense, ssRNA virus)	Paramyxovirus (negative-sense, ssRNA virus)	Adenovirus (dsDNA virus)	Picornavirus (positive-sense, ssRNA virus)	Coronavirus (positive-sense, ssRNA virus)
Diseases caused	Influenza	URI, croup, bronchiolitis	Pneumonia, bronchiolitis, tracheobronchitis	Tracheitis, bronchiolitis, pneumonia; subclinical infection common	URI	URI
Epidemiology	Spread by person-to-person contact; pigs serve as a reservoir in which new strains can be generated; annual winter epidemics; regular pandemics every few decades	Person-to-person contact; subtype of outbreaks changes on a yearly pattern	Person-to-person contact; newborns almost universally infected; yearly predictable pattern of outbreaks	Person-to-person contact	Person-to-person contact	Person-to-person contact
Diagnosis	DFA; ELISA; culture	DFA; ELISA; culture; serologies	DFA; ELISA; culture; serologies	DFA; ELISA; culture; serologies	Culture (rarely performed); serology only possible if infecting serotype is known	All rarely performed: culture, antigen detection, RT-PCR
Treatment	Amantadine (A only); rimantadine (A only); oseltamivir; zanamivir	Symptomatic	Ribavirin	Symptomatic	Symptomatic	Symptomatic
Prevention	Immunization; prophylaxis with antiviral agents		Hyperimmune globulin or monoclonal antibody in high-risk infants	Oral vaccine used in the military		

Key Points

▶ Viruses that cause respiratory symptoms include influenza, parainfluenza, RSV, adenovirus, coronavirus, and rhinovirus; influenza tends to cause more systemic symptoms than other causes of viral URIs

▶ Influenza can be prevented with immunization or with prophylactic antiviral medication

▶ The course of illness can be ameliorated if antivirals are administered within 48 hours of onset: Amantadine and rimantadine inhibit viral uncoating, but are only active against influenza A; the neuraminidase inhibitors, oseltamivir and zanamivir, are active against both influenza A and B

Questions

1. Which of the following patients is likely to have influenza?
   A. A 34 year old with 3 days of vomiting and diarrhea
   B. A 12 year old who has trouble paying attention in class because of his nasal congestion and cough
   C. A 25 year old with anorexia, nausea, right upper quadrant abdominal pain, and jaundice
   D. A 21-year-old recent Mexican immigrant with cough, conjunctivitis, runny nose, and a macular erythematous rash
   E. A 29 year old confined to bed with headache, myalgias, fatigue, and high fever

2. Which enzyme is inhibited by zanamivir?
   A. Reverse transcriptase
   B. Hemagglutinin
   C. Protease
   D. Neuraminidase
   E. Dihydrofolate reductase

3. Which of the following is a contraindication to influenza vaccination?
   A. AIDS
   B. Receipt of the vaccine within the previous 5 years
   C. Pregnancy
   D. Allergy to eggs
   E. Severe pulmonary or cardiac disease

4. Which of the following drugs is active against influenza B?
   A. Amantadine
   B. Stavudine
   C. Oseltamivir
   D. Nelfinavir
   E. Rimantadine

HPI: A 22-year-old Honduran woman presents to an urgent care center complaining of a rash and joint pains in the wrists and knees for 2 days. Her rash was preceded by 3 days with a fever, malaise, headache, mild conjunctivitis, mild cough, and lymphadenopathy. Her rash began on her forehead and face and spread downward onto the trunk and extremities. She has had a new sexual partner for the past 3 months and does not use birth control.
PMH: Mild asthma, on albuterol inhaler as needed (PRN).

PE: T 38.2°C BP 110/68 HR 100 RR 22
She has a rash consisting of numerous small, pink, maculopapular lesions on her face, neck, torso, and proximal extremities. Most of the lesions are discrete, but over her chest, they are coalescent. Palms and soles are spared. She has tender adenopathy in the cervical, postauricular, and occipital regions. Her abdomen is mildly tender with a palpable spleen tip. Her uterus is palpable just below her umbilicus. She has mild diffuse swelling and tenderness of her wrists and knees.

Labs: Mild lymphocytosis with a few atypical lymphocytes, otherwise normal. A urine pregnancy test is positive. Viral titers are sent.

Thought Questions

- What risks does this infection pose to the woman? To the fetus?

- What could have been done to prevent this infection?

Basic Science Review and Discussion

Rubella virus is the only member of the genus *Rubivirus,* family Togaviridae. It is a **positive-sense, single-stranded, RNA virus.** It is similar to alphaviridae but has no arthropod vectors; **human beings are essentially the only hosts.**

The initial site of infection of rubella is the **nasopharynx** or respiratory system, and dissemination via the bloodstream follows. **Transplacental transmission** of virus to the fetus can lead to congenital infection.

In the past, most infections occurred in school-age children. Vaccination campaigns initiated in 1969 have changed the epidemiology so that most cases in the U.S. now occur among adults, and often occur in small clusters in places such as university dormitories.

When acquired postnatally, rubella has an incubation period of about 14 days. It is generally a benign exanthem, often preceded with fever, respiratory symptoms, and adenopathy (particularly of the head and neck). **The rash classically starts cranially and spreads downward.** It is pink in color and maculopapular in character. Other symptoms that are commonly seen in rubella include headache, signs of meningitis, thrombocytopenic purpura, and arthralgias. Rubella has been implicated in more chronic forms of arthri-

tis (rheumatoid arthritis and systemic juvenile arthritis), but this is debated.

During an epidemic of rubella in the U.S. from 1964 to 1965, 12.5 million cases were reported, resulting in 11,500 spontaneous abortions, 2100 neonatal deaths, 2000 cases of encephalitis, 11,600 cases of deafness, 3580 cases of blindness, and 1800 cases of mental retardation.

Congenital rubella is the most devastating consequence of infection. The likelihood that a fetus will be infected from a mother with primary rubella during pregnancy depends on the time in gestation, with the **greatest risk being in the first trimester** (up to 85% of fetuses may acquire congenital rubella when the mother is infected in the first trimester). The clinical syndrome of congenital rubella may consist of deafness (especially with infection in the fourth month), eye abnormalities (cataracts, chorioretinitis, or microphthalmia), heart defects (patent ductus arteriosus, ventricular septal defect, or pulmonic stenosis), microcephaly, mental retardation, liver/spleen abnormalities, or bony defects. During the American epidemic of 1964, additional congenital symptoms of thrombocytopenic purpura, hepatosplenomegaly, intrauterine growth retardation, interstitial pneumonia, myocarditis, and metaphyseal bone lesions were identified and led to the term **"expanded rubella syndrome."** Deficiencies in humoral and/or cellular immunity may be seen in children with congenital rubella. Late complications of congenital rubella include mental retardation, diabetes, pneumonitis, and thyroiditis. Neurologic manifestations of congenital infection may not appear for 2 to 4 years after birth, and ongoing viral replication in patients with congenital rubella has been observed at greater than 3 years of age.

For exposures that occur during pregnancy, the mother is considered to be immune if rubella antibodies are present anytime before or within 10 days of exposure; the risk to the fetus in this case is virtually zero.

The clinical diagnosis of rubella is often confused with other diseases that produce exanthems such as measles. Viral culture (usually of nasopharynx or urine) is specific and diagnostic, but not readily available. **The most common mode of diagnosis is a rise in specific IgG antibody titers over the course of illness and convalescence.** Because of the short-lived nature of IgM antibodies and transplacental passage of maternal antibodies, a single demonstration of rubella-specific IgM in a neonate is diagnostic for congenital infection.

There is no specific treatment for rubella infection. The use of immunoglobulin to prevent congenital rubella in exposed pregnant women is ineffective.

The widespread use of **live, attenuated rubella virus vaccine** has greatly reduced the risk of infection. Vaccination is contraindicated in pregnant women and patients with immunosuppression from disease (e.g., cancer, hereditary immune deficiencies) or medications (e.g., steroids, chemotherapy), with the exception of HIV, in which case the vaccine is recommended for asymptomatic HIV-infected adults and children. The presence of rubella antibodies, developed through either vaccination or natural infection, confers long-lasting protection.

Case Conclusion   Titers indicate acute rubella infection. The patient elects not to terminate the pregnancy and gives birth to a child with congenital rubella syndrome. He is determined to have patent ductus arteriosus, mild microcephaly, cataracts, deafness, and mental retardation.

Thumbnail: Rubella Virus

Organism	Rubella virus
Type of organism	Positive-sense, single-stranded RNA virus of the genus *Rubivirus*, family Togaviridae
Diseases caused	Rubella or German measles; congenital rubella syndrome includes heart defects, eye lesions, microcephaly, mental retardation, and deafness
Epidemiology	Historically, infection occurred in school-aged children; since the start of vaccination campaigns in 1969, cases have dramatically declined and are now seen sporadically or in small clusters (e.g., college campuses, hospitals, factories) among adults
Diagnosis	Rise in rubella-specific antibody titers; presence of rubella-specific IgM in neonatal blood is diagnostic of congenital rubella; isolation of virus is uncommon
Treatment	No specific treatment; immunization with live, attenuated rubella virus is protective

---

Key Points

▶ Rubella infection is generally a benign exanthem, with the exception of infection in pregnant women

▶ The main purpose of rubella vaccination is to prevent primary infection in pregnant women

▶ The rash of rubella generally develops head to toe in direction

Questions

1. Which of the following is not an RNA virus?

   A. HIV
   B. Measles virus
   C. Rubella virus
   D. Hepatitis B
   E. Hepatitis C

2. A woman in her first trimester of pregnancy is known to be rubella nonimmune. She is inadvertently exposed to an active case of rubella through a coworker's child. Which of the following is the most appropriate course of action?

   A. Advise termination of the pregnancy, as congenital rubella syndrome will almost certainly occur
   B. Vaccinate the mother for rubella immediately
   C. Simultaneously determine rubella antibody titers on specimens obtained 2 to 4 weeks apart during pregnancy to determine risk to the fetus
   D. Administer IVIg (intravenous immune globulin) to the mother immediately in an effort to protect the fetus
   E. Administer ribavirin to the mother in an effort to protect the fetus

3. Which of the following patients should not be offered a rubella vaccine?

   A. An HIV-infected child
   B. A woman preparing for in vitro fertilization with no detectable rubella antibody
   C. A male nurse applying to work in a prenatal clinic who has no detectable rubella antibody
   D. The husband of a woman in her first trimester of pregnancy; neither parent has detectable rubella antibodies
   E. An asymptomatic HIV-infected adult with no detectable rubella antibodies

HPI: A 19-year-old male military recruit comes to the infirmary with 3 days of sore throat, cough, and watery eyes. He tells you that several other recruits in his barracks have similar symptoms.

PE: T 38.8°C BP 118/82 HR 66 RR 20

His conjunctivae are injected and there is notable lacrimation. Oropharynx is erythematous without exudate. There is shotty anterior and posterior cervical lymphadenopathy. Lungs are clear.

Thought Questions

- What characteristics differentiate various respiratory viruses at the virologic level? At the pathogenesis level? At the clinical level?

- What treatments are available for respiratory viruses?

Basic Science Review and Discussion

Adenoviruses are medium-sized DNA viruses, which have a characteristic **icosahedral** shape. They are mainly pathogens of the eye (conjunctivitis) and respiratory tract; however, in immunocompromised hosts, they may cause widespread and disseminated disease.

The 41 serotypes of human adenoviruses are classified into seven subgroups according to biologic characteristics.

Adenoviruses were the first viruses with demonstrated **oncogenic potential in animals,** but there has been no identified association with tumors in humans.

Adenovirus infections occur most commonly in **infants** and have a **seasonal predilection** from fall to spring. They account for 5% to 10% of all acute respiratory illnesses in children and 2% in adults. In addition to high infection rates in children, certain serotypes of adenovirus have been identified to cause outbreaks among military recruits. By adulthood, nearly 100% of people have serum antibody against multiple serotypes of adenovirus.

The **respiratory tract** is the major portal of entry, although infection may occur through **conjunctival inoculation** and possibly via the **fecal-oral route** as well. The viral life cycle in respiratory tissues may result in a cell lysis or establishment of latent infection, usually in lymphoid tissues.

Immune control of adenoviral infections is due to a complex interaction between monocytes, macrophages, lymphocytes, natural killer cells, and humoral factors, including antibody, complement, interferon, and cytokines. **Cell-mediated immunity** appears to be particularly important to containment and clearance of adenoviral infections, which may explain why individuals with impaired cellular immunity (HIV, transplant, thymic aplasia, and neonates) have a higher risk of disseminated disease.

In children, adenoviral infections typically cause an **upper respiratory illness with prominent rhinitis.** Other manifestations include bronchiolitis, pneumonia, and pharyngoconjunctival fever (a syndrome of fever, conjunctivitis, rhinitis, pharyngitis, and adenopathy, which has been described in outbreaks at summer camps).

The most frequently reported illness in adults is **acute respiratory disease in military recruits** (serotypes 4, 7, and 21). Serotypes of groups B and C are the most common isolates in respiratory infections, often causing pharyngitis, tonsillitis, and nasopharyngitis. Fever is a common feature of adenovirus infections, often reaching 39°C. Adenoviruses are rarely associated with the common cold syndrome in adults.

Ocular disease caused by adenoviruses are commonly characterized as one of three syndromes: **acute follicular conjunctivitis** (hyperemic conjunctivae, increased lacrimation, and a foreign body sensation), **pharyngoconjunctival fever** (sore throat, fever, conjunctivitis, and adenopathy), and **epidemic keratoconjunctivitis** (conjunctivitis with palpebral edema, pain, photophobia, sore throat, and coryza, which may leave corneal opacities, called "shipyard eye" because of its relation to outbreaks among industrial workers).

Adenovirus is associated with a few specific nonrespiratory infections, including acute hemorrhagic cystitis and childhood diarrhea with intussusception.

Other viral respiratory infections may have similar clinical presentations to adenoviruses.

Respiratory syncytial virus (RSV) is the **most common respiratory pathogen** in children, causing both upper respiratory infections and pneumonias mainly in the wintertime. Recurrent disease later in life is associated with a common cold syndrome. In the elderly, more serious infections such as pneumonia can occur. RSV is commonly epidemic and rarely encountered in the summer months. RSV accounts for 2000 deaths per year in the U.S., usually among the very young, the very old, and the immunosuppressed. Rapid diagnosis is available with fluorescent antibody testing of nasal swabs. Aerosolized **ribavirin,** a guanosine analogue, can be used to treat severe RSV infections. RSV immunoglobulin is available for prevention of disease during outbreaks.

Parainfluenza virus is an important cause of **croup** (lower respiratory tract infection with barking cough, hoarseness, and coryza) in children. In adults, it is responsible for common cold syndromes, sometimes involving hoarseness. Treatment is supportive.

Rhinovirus is the **most common cause of the common cold in adults,** isolated in up to 40% of cases. Seasonal peaks occur in fall and in the spring, but infections may occur throughout the year. Treatment is symptomatic and vaccines have been elusive.

Coronavirus infection is similar to rhinovirus infection, most often causing a common cold syndrome. Treatment is symptomatic.

Although diagnosis of acute respiratory infections is usually empiric, relying on epidemiologic and clinical information, **isolation of the infecting agent** is required to establish the diagnosis with certainty. Serum antibody rises may be identified as well.

Treatment of adenoviral infections is purely supportive and symptomatic. Live, attenuated **vaccines** have been developed for use in military recruits, but are not used in civilian populations.

Case Conclusion   The recruit is treated symptomatically with antihistamines and acetaminophen. His symptoms abate and gradually resolve over the next 4 days. A total of 16 recruits are evaluated with similar symptoms. Because of the outbreak, oropharyngeal cultures are obtained from all symptomatic recruits and adenovirus type 7 is cultured from nine individuals. A vaccine program is initiated on base with oral, live, attenuated adenovirus vaccine being administered to all new recruits.

Thumbnail: Common Cold

Organism	Adenoviruses
Type of organism	DNA virus
Diseases caused	Upper respiratory tract infection, pharyngitis, conjunctivitis, rarely pneumonia
Epidemiology	Most frequent in infants and children, also seen in military recruits; outbreaks occur from fall to spring
Diagnosis	Culture of virus from conjunctivae, oropharynx, sputum, urine, or stool
Treatment	Symptomatic and supportive therapy only

Key Points

▶ The clinical syndromes of various respiratory viruses (and *Mycoplasma pneunomiae*) overlap, and empiric diagnosis is often based on epidemiologic and clinical clues

▶ No specific treatment or vaccine is available for the common cold

▶ Most infections are self-limited and resolve completely without sequelae

Questions

1. A 25-year-old medical student develops rhinorrhea, sneezing, nasal congestion, and mild sore throat while on her family medicine rotation in January. She has no fever, headache, or myalgias. Which of the following is the most likely cause of her symptoms?

   A. Rhinovirus
   B. RSV
   C. Enterovirus
   D. Influenza A
   E. *S. pneumoniae*

2. A 23-year-old man presents with acute onset of dysuria, gross hematuria, and suprapubic pain of 2-day duration.

He has no fever. Blood pressure and creatinine are normal. UA shows 3+ hemoglobin, no leukocyte esterase. Microscopic exam of the urine shows numerous RBCs of normal morphology. Routine culture is negative. CT scan of the abdomen is completely normal. His symptoms continue for 3 more days, and then spontaneously subside. What was the cause of his illness?

   A. Kidney stone
   B. *E. coli* UTI
   C. Gonorrhea
   D. Adenovirus
   E. Acute poststreptococcal glomerulonephritis

HPI: A 34-year-old woman is brought to the ER when her roommate returned home to find her lethargic and slightly confused. She had been complaining of a migraine headache and vomiting for 2 days.

PE: T 39.2°C BP 148/92 HR 100 RR 22
She is laying on her back on the gurney with her knees bent. She is groggy but oriented to person, place, and time. Kernig's and Brudzinski's signs are both present. No focal neurologic deficits are present. There is no rash. Electrolytes are normal. LP demonstrates an opening pressure of 83 cm H_2O; 162 WBCs (90% lymphocytes); 23 RBCs; protein 88; glucose 42. Routine cultures are sent.

Thought Questions

■ What are potential causes of meningitis in this young woman?

■ What other diseases are caused by enteroviruses?

■ What explains the variety of clinical syndromes caused by enteroviruses?

Basic Science Review and Discussion

Enteroviruses   Enteroviruses are a group of small, nonenveloped **picornaviruses** with a single, positive RNA strand. Because there are no lipids in their capsid, enteroviruses are **stable** to treatment with ether, ethanol, and various detergents. They are heat stable and can remain viable for several hours on moist surfaces.

Enteroviruses are classified into subgroups (e.g., polio viruses, Coxsackie viruses, and echoviruses) and further into serotypes on the basis of surface proteins; after infection with a specific serotype of enterovirus, an individual remains immune to symptomatic reinfection with the same serotype.

Enteroviruses are **spread via the fecal-oral route.** Epidemics of enterovirus disease, such as polio, usually occur in **late summer months** in more temperate climates. In the tropics, enteroviruses do not demonstrate seasonal variation in disease. There is also a periodicity to the predominant strain isolated from year to year. The majority of infections are **asymptomatic,** and **fecal shedding** from asymptomatic individuals is an important source of spread.

The basic pathogenesis of each of the enteroviruses is the same, regardless of serotype. They enter the body through the **oropharynx** and begin replicating in local tissues, such as the respiratory epithelium and lymphoid tissues. The virus is shed back into oral secretions, and undergoes further rounds of replication in the lumen of the GI tract. It enters the bloodstream through the intestinal wall and travels to specific tissues based on serotype, accounting for

manifestations of specific diseases. Thus, despite their name, enteroviruses do not cause disease of the gastrointestinal tract.

The initial acute tissue damage is caused by lytic effects on the cell, but many of the secondary sequelae are immunologically mediated.

There is widespread overlap among the clinical syndromes of the various enteroviruses, but some of the more common associations are listed below.

Polio virus infections   There are three serotypes of polio virus that cause paralytic human disease. Most infections (90%) are symptomatic. Symptomatic polio is a **biphasic illness.** The first phase, or **minor illness,** consists of fever, malaise, headache, sore throat, and vomiting, which occur within a few days after infection. The **major illness** occurs 3 to 4 days later and consists of symptoms of aseptic meningitis (fever, headache, stiff neck, and vomiting) with or without paralysis. Paralysis begins with muscle stiffness, hyperactivity of muscle reflexes, and fasciculations, and evolves into profound weakness. Poliomyelitis is termed **spinal** if the majority of muscles affected are supplied by nerves from the spinal cord and **bulbar** if the major involvement is in a cranial distribution.

A **postpolio syndrome** of progressive muscle weakness has been noted to occur 20 to 30 years after recovery from an initial syndrome of polio. This syndrome may be progressive and involve both limb and bulbar musculature.

Prevention of polio is possible through vaccination with either **inactivated polio vaccine** (IPV, Salk vaccine) or **oral polio vaccine** (OPV, Sabin vaccine). Both are highly effective vaccines, and the debate over which is preferred continues. IPV consists of injection of an inactivated strain of polio virus and produces 99% to 100% seropositivity after two doses in infants. OPV consists of live, attenuated viruses and produces antibodies in 95% of recipients. Boosters of either vaccine are required to maintain long-lasting protection.

With widespread vaccination, there are no areas of wild polio prevalence in the U.S.; however, polio virus remains widespread throughout the world and imported cases may occur.

Numbered enterovirus infections   The most recently identified enteroviruses are identified by number (numbers 68–71; enterovirus 72 is hepatitis A virus).

Meningitis and meningoencephalitis are the most common manifestations of enterovirus infections. Headache, fever, photophobia, neck stiffness, and nausea are the most common symptoms. Confusion and delirium are common, but localizing sensory and motor deficits are unusual. CSF pleocytosis is initially primarily neutrophilic, but within 48 hours converts to the more familiar lymphocytic predominance. Enteroviral meningitis in adults most often resolves without sequelae, but neurologic deficits and developmental delays may be seen in infants.

Coxsackie virus infections   The clinical manifestations of Coxsackie virus infection vary according to serotype. The main clinical syndromes associated with Coxsackie virus are myocarditis, pharyngitis, oral ulcers (herpangina), epidemic myalgias, pleurodynia (Bornholm disease or "the devil's grippe"), hand-foot-and-mouth disease (vesicular rash with fever), and other febrile illnesses with rashes.

Echoviruses   Echoviruses may cause respiratory infections and are frequently associated with severe neonatal disease with multisystem organ failure. About 60% to 90% of viral meningitis is caused by enterovirus, whereas the rest are caused by arboviruses, HSV, HIV, EBV, or other viruses.

Hepatitis A   Hepatitis A is enterovirus 72. This virus is discussed in detail in Case 34.

Diagnosis of any of the enteroviruses is most readily established by isolation of the virus from throat swabs, stool or rectal swabs, body fluids, and occasionally tissues. Diagnosis is supported by a 4-fold or greater increase in neutralizing antibody titer from paired acute and convalescent serum samples.

There is **no specific antiviral treatment** for any of the enteroviruses. Immune globulins are of no clinical benefit in acute disease. Treatment is entirely supportive and symptomatic. Glucocorticoids are contraindicated.

Case Conclusion   The patient is diagnosed with aseptic meningitis and sent home with acetaminophen-oxycodone hydrochloride (Percocet) for pain and Compazine for nausea. She follows up with her primary care physician 2 days later and is improved. She completely recovers over the next week. Routine bacterial cultures of her CSF are negative and viral cultures grow an echovirus.

Thumbnail: Enteroviruses

Organisms	Polio virus, Coxsackie virus, echovirus, enterovirus
Type of organism	Picornavirus
Diseases caused	Poliomyelitis, meningitis/meningoencephalitis, upper respiratory tract infections and pleurodynia (Bornholm disease), herpangina, acute myocarditis/pericarditis, febrile exanthems, nonspecific febrile illnesses
Epidemiology	Worldwide distribution; epidemics occur in late summer and fall; fecal-oral and direct person-to-person transmission
Diagnosis	Isolation of the virus from bodily fluids (CSF, pleural or pericardial fluids), throat swabs, or stool specimens; 4-fold increase in neutralizing antibody titer in acute and convalescent sera
Treatment	Supportive care; glucocorticoids are contraindicated; vaccine available for polio virus and hepatitis A virus only

Key Points

▶ Enteroviruses cause a number of various illnesses, the most common of which is aseptic meningitis

▶ With no treatment available, vaccination is particularly important in limiting morbidity and mortality from polio virus infections

Questions

1. Which of the following is true about polio virus vaccines?

   A. Inactivated polio vaccine (IPV) is contraindicated in AIDS patients

   B. Oral polio vaccine (OPV) contains serotype 1 virus, whereas IPV contains serotypes 2 and 3 virus

   C. OPV has the advantage of secondary immunization of nonimmune contacts through the shedding of vaccine virus into the intestinal tract

   D. IPV induces both mucosal and humoral antibodies

   E. Booster shots are needed for IPV but not OPV

2. A previously healthy 20-year-old college lacrosse player develops shortness of breath, chest pain, and fatigue several days after an upper respiratory infection. On exam, she is in atrial fibrillation and mild congestive heart failure. Chest x-ray shows an enlarged heart and mild pulmonary edema. Which of the following is the most likely infectious cause of her symptoms?

   A. Pneumococcal pneumonia

   B. Tuberculous pericarditis

   C. *Chlamydia*-induced atherosclerosis and myocardial infarction

   D. Myocarditis due to Coxsackie B virus

   E. Herpes zoster

HPI: AF is a 55-year-old man who had a cadaveric renal transplant a year ago for kidney disease related to his long-standing diabetes mellitus. He is on multiple immunosuppressive medications and has recently needed several courses of steroids to treat rejection of his transplanted organ. AF presents to the office today complaining of 5 days of severe shortness of breath with a cough productive of blood-tinged sputum with black streaks, fevers and chills, severe fatigue, and sharp chest pain with deep breathing or coughing.
PMH: Type II diabetes mellitus and hypertension; medications include insulin injections, atenolol, hydrochlorothiazide, cyclosporine, tacrolimus, and prednisone at a current dose of 6 mg orally every day. No allergies to medications.

HPI: T 38.9°C HR 114 BP 98/62 RR 24 SaO$_2$ 86% on room air
AF is a very ill-appearing, cachectic man, breathing rapidly and having problems speaking secondary to shortness of breath. His lung exam is significant for crackles in the right lung field. Skin is dry without any rashes.

Labs: WBC 14.2 with 82% neutrophils. Sputum Gram stain shows septate hyphae branching at acute angles. Chest X-ray has a cavitary lung lesion in the right upper lobe and peripheral consolidations.

Thought Questions

- What are the possible etiologies of pneumonia in patients on immunosuppressives?

- What is the most likely etiology in this patient?

- What is the microbiology of this organism?

- What is the epidemiology of disease with this organism and what are its syndromes?

- What are its possible treatments?

Basic Science Review and Discussion

Differential   The differential for lower respiratory infections in immunocompromised patients is vast. Although neutropenia is an additional risk factor for many of the fungal or viral pathogens, the use of prednisone or potent immunosuppressive therapy can predispose patients to a number of respiratory infections even without neutropenia. Besides the bacterial agents associated with typical community-acquired and atypical pneumonias, immunocompromised patients are also susceptible to a number of additional pathogens, including **gram-negative bacilli, *Pneumocystis carinii*, *Staphylococcus* species, fungal infections, including the dimorphic fungi and molds, viruses (especially cytomegalovirus), *Nocardia* species, *Rhodococcus equi*, and *Legionella*.** The septate acute-angle branching hyphae in the sputum of this immunosuppressed patient on steroids probably indicates a respiratory tract infection with the dreaded *Aspergillus*.

Microbiology   *Aspergillus* **is a ubiquitous mold** and serves as a saprophytic fungus in soil, its natural ecological niche. *Aspergillus fumigatus* is the usual cause of aspergillosis,

although there are several disease-causing species of *Aspergillus* in humans. *A. fumigatus* is characterized by green conidia, approximately 2.5 to 3 mm in diameter, produced in chains from greenish stalks. A rare isolate of this organism is pigmentless and produces white conidia. The chains of conidia are borne on broad vesicles of approximately 20 to 30 μm in diameter. **Replication is achieved by a process of budding,** and there is no sexual stage. *A. fumigatus* grows relatively rapidly and can reach a colony size of approximately 4 cm within 1 week when grown on special media at 25°C. In nature, *A. fumigatus* is a thermophilic species, with growth occurring at temperatures as high as 55°C and survival maintained at temperatures up to 70°C. *Aspergillus* forms septate, **true hyphae with acute-angle branching at 45°** with clusters of conidia topping the fungal stalks (Figure 41-1). *Aspergillus* cell walls are more or less parallel, in contrast to *Mucor* and *Rhizopus* walls, which are more irregular.

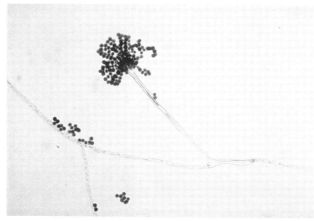

Figure 41-1 Conidia of *Aspergillus fumigatus.* (Image in public domain on Centers for Disease Control Public Health Image Library, phil.cdc.gov.)

Epidemiology Environmental surveys indicate that all humans will inhale at least several hundred *A. fumigatus* conidia per day. As the airborne conidia have a small enough diameter to reach the lung alveoli, **most susceptible patients manifest disease with *A. fumigatus* in the respiratory tract.** However, *Aspergillus* can also **invade the nose and paranasal sinuses, external ear, or traumatized skin,** leading to subsequent infection in these organs. *Aspergillus* can also disseminate to virtually any organ in the severely compromised patient.

The most important determinant in *Aspergillus* infection is the immune status of the host. A 4-fold increase in invasive aspergillosis has been observed in developed countries over the past two decades secondary to increased iatrogenic immunosuppression. The incidence of aspergillosis in certain transplant populations is shown in Table 41-1.

Neutropenia in acute leukemics and bone marrow transplant (BMT) patients is the most important risk factor for aspergillosis, just as the return of bone marrow function is vital to the therapeutic response to antifungals. In solid organ transplant patients, immunosuppression predisposes to infection; **high-dose corticosteroids alone** may predispose to aspergillosis in some patients. Previously normal children with invasive aspergillosis should be evaluated for **chronic granulomatous disease.** Patients in the **late stages of HIV infection** (usually with CD4 counts of less than 50 cells/μL) have an increased susceptibility to invasive aspergillosis, although half of them usually have a secondary predisposing factor, such as leukopenia or corticosteroid therapy. In addition to immunosuppression, **prolonged use of broad-spectrum antibiotics and parenteral nutrition** predispose to this fungal infection. Patient-to-patient spread of *Aspergillus* has not been documented.

Clinical Syndromes *Aspergillus* **can invade tissue planes** or spread hematogenously, leading to a myriad of clinical syndromes. One prominent feature of these infections is **growth of hyphae into and along blood vessels,** leading to hemorrhagic infarction and necrosis of affected tissue. The following organ systems are predominantly infected.

Table 41-1 Incidence of aspergillosis

Iatrogenic procedure	Incidence of invasive aspergillosis
Allogeneic BMT[1]	4%–6%
Autologous BMT	0.7%
Renal transplantation	3.9%
Heart or lung transplant	1.7%
Liver transplant	1.5%

[1]BMT: bone marrow transplant.

Nose and sinus Mucosal invasion by *A. fumigatus* in the nose and sinus can spread rapidly to contiguous structures, causing vascular invasion and necrosis. Infection can ultimately lead to proptosis and monocular blindness.

Eye Minor trauma to the cornea can lead to deep stromal invasion with *Aspergillus* in susceptible patients. Endophthalmitis due to *Aspergillus* can occur hematogenously in immunosuppressed patients or can be a late complication of cataract extraction.

Lungs Four main clinical syndromes:

1) *Allergic bronchopulmonary aspergillosis* **(ABPA):** this disease is defined more as an **allergic response to *Aspergillus* antigens** rather than direct invasion by the organism and usually occurs in immunocompetent asthmatics. The clinical syndrome of ABPA is manifested by **peripheral eosinophilia,** fleeting pulmonary infiltrates from bronchial plugging, an immediate-type skin test response to *Aspergillus* antigens, and **elevation in total serum IgE and anti-*Aspergillus* IgG levels.** Septate hyphae can be seen microscopically in expectorated sputum plugs, with *Aspergillus* growth on culture. **Treatment is usually a combination of high-dose steroids and antifungals.**

2) *Aspergilloma:* this syndrome is described as a "**fungus ball**" in the lungs and is usually caused by growth of *Aspergillus* in a preexisting lung cavity (e.g., from TB, sarcoidosis, histoplasmosis, bronchiectasis, etc.). Aspergillomas can also occur de novo and are marked by severe hemoptysis, intermittent *Aspergillus* in the sputum, and elevated peripheral titers of anti-*Aspergillus* IgG.

3) *Aspergillus pneumonia:* patients with prolonged neutropenia are the highest risk group for acute, rapidly progressing *Aspergillus* pneumonia. This process results in **dense consolidations and cavitations,** with clues to the diagnosis being pleuritic chest pain secondary to extension of the infection to the visceral pleura and hemoptysis from blood vessel invasion.

4) *Pseudomembranous tracheobronchitis:* this condition can be seen in HIV infection or in less severely immunocompromised patients, and is manifested by fever, dyspnea, cough, expectorated sputum plugs, and hemoptysis. Bronchoscopy reveals yellowish plaques or membranes ("**cotton balls**") on a hyperemic tracheobronchial mucosa.

CNS The most common manifestation of CNS aspergillosis is the formation of **brain abscesses** from hematogenous spread of the fungus. **Cerebral infarction** can also occur by occlusion of the cerebral blood vessels by the organism.

Cardiac Cardiac manifestations of *Aspergillus* include endocarditis, myocarditis, and coronary artery embolization by the hyphae.

Other *Aspergillus* can also lead to esophageal or gastrointestinal ulcerations, necrotizing skin ulcers, osteomyelitis, or infection of the kidneys, bone marrow, thyroid gland, adrenal glands, and pancreas.

Diagnosis and Treatment Diagnosis of *Aspergillus* infection is usually made by culturing the organism from the appropriate sample and by viewing septate hyphae with dichotomous 45° angle branching invading tissue under histologic examination. **Blood vessel or tissue invasion by the organism is highly suggestive of true *Aspergillus* infection, rather than colonization.** However, the presence of any *Aspergillus* organisms in the sputum of a highly immunosuppressed patient should be investigated carefully. Serology is helpful in the diagnosis of ABPA or aspergilloma if an increase in anti-*Aspergillus* IgG antibodies is observed.

The mainstay of treatment for invasive *Aspergillus* infections has been intravenous amphotericin B (ampho B), although a recent study suggests that the new triazole, **voriconazole,** is more effective than ampho B for the initial treatment of this infection.[1] As voriconazole is much better tolerated than ampho B and can be given both intravenously and orally, the development of this antifungal may be a major breakthrough in the treatment of invasive aspergillosis. As ABPA was thought to be primarily an allergic response to *Aspergillus* antigen, this condition was initially treated with only high-dose corticosteroids. However, recent data indicates that adding **itraconazole to steroid therapy for ABPA improves treatment response.**[2] Oral itraconazole can be administered for more indolent *Aspergillus* infections, although *Aspergillus* resistance to this agent is emerging. Finally, **surgical resection** of an aspergilloma, an isolated *Aspergillus* pulmonary lesion, or invasive aspergillosis of the brain or sinuses may improve the prognoses of these grim conditions.

Case Conclusion AF had a bronchoscopy for diagnostic purposes and was found to have acute-angle branching septate hyphae with blood vessel invasion on bronchial biopsies. He was started on intravenous voriconazole therapy for invasive pulmonary aspergillosis. AF's respiratory function grew increasingly compromised, requiring intubation upon admission. He suffered respiratory arrest on his third day of hospitalization and expired.

Thumbnail: Aspergillosis

Organism	*Aspergillus fumigatus*
Type of organism	Thermophilic mold; forms septate hyphae that branch at 45° dichotomous angles
Diseases caused	Sinus infections; eye infections; pulmonary infections, including allergic bronchopulmonary aspergillosis, aspergillomas, cavitations, tracheobronchitis, and invasive pneumonias; CNS infections, myocarditis, and endocarditis
Epidemiology	Invasive infection occurs primarily in severely immunocompromised hosts on corticosteroids, immunosuppressive therapy, or with neutropenia
Diagnosis	Culture and demonstrating tissue invasion on biopsy
Treatment	Intravenous or oral voriconazole or intravenous amphotericin B for serious infections; oral itraconazole for indolent infections; steroids and itraconazole for ABPA

Key Points

▶ *A. fumigatus* is a thermophilic mold identified by its septate hyphae that branch at acute angles

▶ Invasive aspergillosis occurs in the severely immunocompromised host and carries a poor prognosis

▶ Intravenous or oral voriconazole will probably replace intravenous amphotericin B as the mainstay of therapy for severe *Aspergillus* infections

Questions

1. Amphotericin B is notable for the following toxicity:

   A. Hepatotoxicity
   B. Renal tubular acidosis
   C. Hyperkalemia
   D. Pulmonary fibrosis
   E. Lupus-like syndrome

2. Mucormycosis can be distinguished from aspergillosis in that *Mucor* branches at angles of

   A. 15°
   B. 30°
   C. 60°
   D. 90°
   E. 150°

References

1. Herbrecht R, Denning DW, Patterson TF, et al. Voriconazole versus amphotericin B for primary therapy of invasive aspergillosis. N Engl J Med 2002;347:408–415.

2. Stevens DA, Schwartz HJ, Lee JY, et al. A randomized trial of itraconazole in allergic bronchopulmonary aspergillosis. N Engl J Med 2000;342:756–762.

HPI: A 37-year-old gay man with long-standing AIDS presents with 10 days of gradually worsening headache, fever, and weakness. He called your office today for an appointment because he began vomiting last night. Despite the fact that he has been compliant with his antiretroviral regimen of didanosine, abacavir, indinavir, and ritonavir, his CD4 count was 74 cells/μL at last check. He also takes TMP-SMZ and weekly azithromycin as well as pravastatin (Pravachol) for hyperlipidemia and atenolol for hypertension.

PE: T 38.6°C BP 148/96 HR 86 RR 12
The patient is groggy, but oriented. Mild meningismus is present. Fundi exam is normal. There are three papular, ulcerated skin lesions, less than 1 cm long, on his upper extremities. Otherwise the exam is normal.

Labs: Opening pressure 280 cm H_2O, WBC 12 (100% lymphocytes), RBC 22, glucose 30, protein 84. Cultures and serology sent.

Thought Questions

- Where did this patient's infection originate?

- How is the causative organism identified?

- What features of this organism add to its virulence?

Basic Science Review and Discussion

Cryptococcus neoformans is a round yeast-like **fungus,** 4 to 6 μm in diameter with a large **polysaccharide capsule. Smooth, creamy white, mucoid colonies** appear within 36 to 72 hours on most simple culture media, including **Sabourand's agar,** at 37°C.

Microscopically, *Cryptococcus* appears as **spherical, budding, encapsulated yeast cells.** The capsule varies in size among different strains, but may be up to twice the width of the individual cell. There are four capsular serotypes (A, B, C, and D), with **serotype A being the most commonly isolated in human disease.** The capsule is composed primarily of glucouroxylomannan (GXM), and the degree of mannosyl substitution of the GXM determines the serotype. Capsular GXM has been shown to inhibit both phagocytosis of the yeast cells and production of antibody.

All *Cryptococcus* species are **nonfermentative, hydrolyze starch, assimilate inositol, and produce urease.** These are the characteristics that distinguish *Cryptococcus* from other medically important yeasts. Additionally, *C. neoformans* produces a **phenoloxidase** that converts catecholamines into dark pigments. This may be important in the virulence of the organism, as mutants lacking phenoloxidase activity may be killed by the epinephrine oxidase system.

Cases of cryptococcal infection occur sporadically worldwide, and the yeast is ubiquitous in soil and **avian fecal material.** Disease may occur in normal hosts but is more commonly seen in patients with some degree of **immuno-suppression** such as AIDS (usually with CD4 counts of less than 200 cell/μL), hematologic malignancies, autoimmune disease, or corticosteroid therapy. Among persons with AIDS, the annual incidence is 2 to 4 cases per 1000.

Infection is acquired by **inhalation** of cells into the lung. Pulmonary infection may be clinically silent and resolve spontaneously, but hematogenous spread to the CNS may lead to a **meningoencephalitis** with scant inflammatory response by the host.

Clinically, patients with cryptococcal meningitis present **subacutely** with headache, fever, nausea, blurred vision, irritability, and gait changes. Because of a mild inflammatory response, nuchal rigidity is often mild. Papilledema is present in only one third of cases. Cerebral edema and/or hydrocephalus may occur in untreated cases, which are invariably fatal.

Lumbar puncture (LP) often reveals a **minimally inflammatory CSF with few lymphocytes.** CSF glucose is low in over half of cases, and protein may be normal to slightly high. **Opening pressure must be carefully measured, as values greater than 250 mm H_2O correlate to poor neurologic outcome and death.** In cases with increased pressure, repeated LPs or continuous CSF drainage must be considered.

Culture of the organism from CSF is the most common means of diagnosis. Blood cultures are often positive, as up to 40% of cases of meningitis involve concurrent fungemia and up to 60% show disseminated infection. The **cryptococcal antigen** (CrAg) test is better than 95% sensitive on either serum or CSF. High titers are often seen, but serum titers are not correlated to clinical or microbiological response on therapy. **India ink** preparation of the CSF often demonstrates the encapsulated yeast cells (see Figure 42-1), but is not frequently used currently due to the widely available CrAg, which has superior sensitivity and specificity.

Isolated pulmonary cryptococcal infection mimics malignancy. Serum CrAg and culture are less reliable, and biopsy

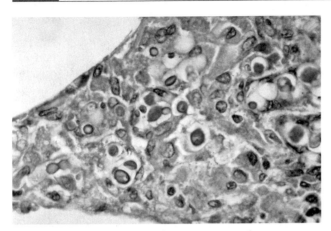

Figure 42-1 Mucicarmine stain of *Cryptococcus neoformans* on histopathology of lung from AIDS patient. (Image in public domain on Centers for Disease Control Public Health Image Library, phil.cdc.gov, courtesy of Dr. Edwin P. Ewing, Jr.)

is often required to make the diagnosis. *Cryptococcus* may also cause ulcerated papular skin lesions, or bone lesions similar to tuberculosis. In these forms of disease, biopsy is the diagnostic tool of choice.

Initial therapy for cryptococcal meningitis in AIDS patients consists of an induction phase with **amphotericin B** with **flucytosine.** The major side effects of amphotericin are renal toxicity with acidosis and elevated creatinine, infusion-associated rigors, hypokalemia, and hypomagnesemia. The major toxicity of flucytosine is bone marrow suppression. After an induction period of 2 weeks or until clinical improvement occurs, suppressive therapy with **fluconazole** is initiated at high doses, and then set at lower doses. Suppressive therapy should continue indefinitely or until a patient is asymptomatic and has a sustained (>6-month) increase in CD4 cells to greater than 100–200 cells/μL while on antiretroviral therapy. Some experts suggest repeating an LP prior to discontinuation of suppressive therapy to ensure clearance of the organism from the CSF.

In patients without AIDS, treatment is with amphotericin alone or in combination with flucytosine. Therapy continues until four weekly CSF cultures (or India ink stains) are negative and CSF glucose is normal. Up to 70% of non-AIDS patients achieve cure. The mortality rate is approxmately 12%.

Case Conclusion   Our patient was admitted to the hospital and started on amphotericin B and flucytosine. Serum and CSF CrAg tests were both positive. Cultures of both CSF and blood grew *C. neoformans.* LP was repeated three more times over the next week with 10 mL of CSF removed each time, in order to control the elevated intracranial pressure. The patient made a gradual recovery and was transferred to a rehabilitation facility 2 weeks later on high-dose fluconazole.

Thumbnail: *Cryptococcus neoformans*

Organism	*Cryptococcus neoformans*
Type of organism	Encapsulated yeast
Diseases caused	Meningoencephalitis; pneumonia; skin and bone lesions
Epidemiology	Common environmental organism in soil worldwide; associated with pigeon droppings; infection via inhalational route; most disease among immunosuppressed patients: AIDS (CD4 counts < 200 cell/μL), hematologic malignancies, autoimmune disease, or corticosteroid therapy
Diagnosis	Culture of CSF or blood; India ink examination of CSF; cryptococcal antigen (CrAg) in serum or CSF; biopsy may be necessary in pulmonary or skin infection
Treatment	Induction therapy with amphotericin B and flucytosine, then high-dose fluconazole, followed by maintenance therapy with lower-dose fluconazole

Key Points

▶ In addition to specific antifungal therapy, control of elevated intracranial pressure is an important determinant of clinical outcome with cryptococcal meningitis

▶ In patients with AIDS and cryptococcal meningitis, long-term suppressive therapy is required until sustained increases in CD4 count on antiretroviral therapy are achieved

Questions

1. A patient with AIDS and cryptococcal meningitis is started on amphotericin B and flucytosine. Which of the following is the major toxicity of flucytosine?
   A. Renal tubular acidosis
   B. Infusion-related fevers and rigors
   C. Hypokalemia
   D. Hypomagnesemia
   E. Pancytopenia

2. Which of the following properties of *Cryptococcus* does not contribute to its virulence?
   A. The capsular polysaccharide inhibits phagocytosis of the yeast
   B. The capsular polysaccharide inhibits antibody production to the yeast
   C. The yeast secretes a toxin that directly kills macrophages
   D. The yeast phenoloxidase enzyme breaks down host catecholamines, which are toxic to the yeast

HPI: A 52-year-old diabetic woman undergoes emergency surgery for a perforated gallbladder, secondary to cholelithiasis. During the surgery, her peritoneum is irrigated with antibiotic solution. She is treated with broad-spectrum antimicrobial therapy with IV piperacillin-tazobactam. Because she cannot be fed, total parenteral nutrition is started through a central intravenous catheter in her right internal jugular vein. She has a persistent fever, and a follow-up CT scan shows the development of several abdominal abscesses. She is brought back to the OR for a repeat laparotomy where the abscesses are drained. Cultures of the abscesses grow *E. coli* and *Enterococcus* sensitive to piperacillin-tazobactam. Three days after the second operation, she develops new fevers, and becomes hypotensive, requiring both epinephrine and phenylephrine to maintain a blood pressure of 110/50. Her diabetes is being managed with an insulin drip.
She has had normal respiratory secretions. She has started to have loose bowel movements over the past 2 days.

PE: T 39°C BP 110/50 on multiple pressors HR 110
Intubated and sedated patient. On a ventilator, requiring increasing support, with a delivered FiO$_2$ of 70% and a positive end-expiratory pressure (PEEP) of 10. The patient has no rashes. Her central line site shows no erythema. Her lung sounds are coarse due to the ventilator. Her heart has a regular rhythm with no murmur. Her abdomen is soft. The abdominal incision shows pink tissue with no exudate or erythema; she is not forming granulation tissue, however. Wound drains are showing minimal output of serosanguinous fluid.

Labs: WBC 18 Hct 31 Platelets 140. Electrolytes are within normal limits.
A chest x-ray shows some bibasilar atelectasis, but no effusions or infiltrates.
A sputum Gram stain shows mixed flora. A stool test for *C. difficile* toxin is negative.
Two out of two blood cultures grow yeast.

Thought Questions

■ What is the difference between yeast and mold?

■ What is the range of infections caused by yeast?

■ Where could this patient's yeast have come from?

■ What options do the doctors have for treating her infection?

■ What are common causes of fever in the ICU?

Basic Science Review and Discussion

Fungi can be divided into **yeast** (e.g., *Candida, Cryptococcus*), which have an oval or round cellular shape, and **molds** (*Aspergillus*), which form long filamentous structures. Some fungi, the **dimorphic fungi** (e.g., *Coccidioides, Blastomyces, Histoplasma*) are able to grow in both forms. Mycologists make many identifications by morphology rather than biochemical testing. *Candida* is an oval budding yeast with pseudohyphae, whereas *Cryptococcus* are round in shape. A **germ tube** test looks for the development of tube-like projections from the *Candida* yeast cells when they are put in a special medium. A positive germ tube test confirms that the yeast is *Candida albicans*. If the test is negative, then the yeast species is determined by chemical tests. The speciation is important because certain yeast species, such as *Candida glabrata* and *Candida krusei* are resistant to fluconazole, a drug frequently used to treat yeast infections. Yeast speciation is often used to choose therapy because the determination of antifungal susceptibilities is time consuming and often not standardized.

Most yeast infections are superficial minor infections, affecting the skin or mucous membranes of the mouth (thrush) or vagina. These infections are more common in patients with impaired cellular immunity, such as diabetics, patients on steroids or other immunosuppressive agents, and AIDS patients. These infections can often be treated with topical azoles or with nystatin.

Systemic yeast infections are uncommon. They tend to occur in seriously compromised hosts, like the patient described in this case. **Risk factors** for infection include recent abdominal surgery (as the gut can be a source of infecting yeast), or in-dwelling central lines (another potential portal of entry). Impaired cell-mediated immunity (from AIDS, diabetes, steroids, and immunosuppression) or neutropenia can also predispose a host to fungal infection. Finally, high blood lipid levels from total parenteral nutrition (TPN), high blood sugar levels from diabetes, and alteration of normal bacterial flora due to administration of broad-spectrum antibiotics can also create favorable circumstances for yeast.

There are several classes of antifungal drugs. The **azoles** (both topical drugs such as miconazole and econazole, and systemic drugs such as fluconazole and voriconazole) act by inhibiting synthesis of **ergosterol,** an analogue of cholesterol that is a required component of fungal membranes but not found in mammalian cell membranes. The **polyenes** (amphotericin and nystatin) act by binding to ergosterol in the fungal cell membrane and creating holes in the membrane, thereby killing the cell. Amphotericin causes both infusion-related toxicity (fever and chills) as well as renal toxicity (decreased glomerular filtration rate [GFR], along with magnesium and potassium wasting). Newer lipid-based forms of amphotericin have been developed in an attempt to reduce the toxicity of this drug. Finally, a new class of drugs, the **echinocandins** (caspofungin) block β-glycan synthesis in the fungal cell wall.

Case Conclusion The patient's central intravenous line is removed, and a temporary line is placed. Another set of blood cultures is drawn before amphotericin B is started. The original cultures are speciated as *Candida albicans,* using the germ tube test; the follow-up blood cultures are negative. The patient tolerates the amphotericin poorly, with her creatinine rising above 2.0 after 3 days of therapy. She is switched to IV fluconazole. A dilated funduscopic exam is done to rule out the complication of *Candida* endophthalmitis, which would necessitate additional local treatment in the eye. Despite treatment of her infections, the patient develops an increasing requirement for vasopressors and for ventilatory support. Several days later, her family decides to withdraw aggressive care, and the patient dies.

Thumbnail: *Candida*

Organism	*Candida albicans*
Type of organism	Yeast (fungus)
Diseases caused	Local infections of perineum, vagina, or oropharynx; line-related bacteremia; hepatosplenic infections
Epidemiology	More prevalent in patients with defects in cellular immunity (AIDS, transplant immunosuppression, steroids)
Diagnosis	Culture
Treatment	Topical treatment of minor infections with azoles or nystatin; systemic treatments of serious infections with fluconazole

Key Points

▶ Fungi can be divided into yeast (e.g., *Candida, Cryptococcus*) and molds (*Aspergillus*); some fungi, the dimorphic fungi (e.g., *Coccidioides, Blastomyces,* and *Histoplasma*) are able to grow in both forms

▶ Most yeast infections are superficial, affecting the skin or mucous membranes of the mouth or vagina

▶ Systemic yeast infections are usually only seen in patients with breaches in their defenses (e.g., in-dwelling lines that provide a route of entry through the skin) or deficiencies in cell-mediated immunity

▶ Minor *Candida* infections are treated topically; serious infections may be treated with azoles, amphotericin, or caspofungin

Questions

1. A physician is obligated to treat yeast grown from which culture site?

   A. Stool
   B. Sputum
   C. Skin
   D. Urine
   E. Blood

2. Which yeast antibiotic has the most toxicity?

   A. Amphotericin B
   B. Miconazole
   C. Nystatin
   D. Econazole
   E. Caspofungin

3. Which of the following drugs acts by blocking yeast cell wall synthesis?

   A. Amphotericin B
   B. Penicillin
   C. Fluconazole
   D. Nystatin
   E. Caspofungin

HPI: A 35-year-old woman who lives in Arizona had a cadaveric renal transplant 8 months ago for end-stage renal disease from rapidly progressive glomerulonephritis. She has been on immunosuppression with FK506 and prednisone. She presents to the hospital with a 3-day history of progressive shortness of breath, productive cough, and fevers.

PE: T 39.0°C HR 125 BP 95/50 RR 25 SaO$_2$ 89% on room air
On exam, she is tired, anxious, and in moderate respiratory distress. She can speak in 2- to 3-word sentences and is using accessory muscles to breathe.

Labs: WBC 18 with a left shift; ABG pH 7.30 pCO$_2$ 45 pO$_2$ 65 on room air
Chest x-ray shows bilateral fluffy infiltrates.
The patient is intubated. Bronchoscopy is done and sputum is sent for culture. Several days later, a mold grows from the culture and is identified as *Coccidioides*.

Thought Questions

- Which infectious agents cause diffuse, bilateral pneumonia?

- What unique types of organisms cause pneumonia in immunocompromised patients?

- What are the endemic fungi and where in the U.S. are they found?

- Aside from culture, how can the diagnosis of coccidioidomycosis be made?

- Besides giving the patient antifungal agents, what else can be done to improve her ability to fight off this life-threatening infection?

- Why are the lab workers angry at the patient's doctors when they find *Coccidioides* growing in the cultures and had not been warned about the possibility of this organism?

Basic Science Review and Discussion

In a normal host, diffuse pneumonia is usually caused by so-called **atypical agents** such as *Mycoplasma, Chlamydia,* or *Legionella.* Respiratory viruses, such as the influenza A and B viruses, parainfluenza viruses, and adenovirus, can also potentially produce this picture. The **endemic fungal infections** such as **coccidioidomycosis, blastomycosis,** and **histoplasmosis** can all cause diffuse infiltrates. *S. pneumoniae* classically causes lobar infiltrates, although studies have shown that it is difficult to distinguish the causative agent of a pneumonia by radiographic appearance alone.

In the host with compromised **cell-mediated immunity,** such as this transplant patient or a patient with AIDS, the differential diagnosis grows larger and includes *P. carinii* pneumonia (PCP), and disseminated viral infections including varicella-zoster virus (VZV) and cytomegalovirus (CMV).

Fungal Infections The endemic fungi have many characteristics in common. All are found in the soil in restricted geographic areas. Infection with these organisms is unlikely if the patient has not spent time in or near these areas. Infections are more common in children and people who have recently moved to the endemic area. The infections are usually contracted by breathing in fungi from the soil, although skin can occasionally be inoculated directly. These organisms can cause a wide range of infections. Most patients develop self-limited respiratory symptoms with fever, cough, and pleuritic chest pain. Other patients, such as the immunocompromised, pregnant women, and certain ethnic groups (African Americans, Native Americans, and Filipinos) can develop life-threatening disseminated infections. One feared site of disseminated infection is to the meninges; other common sites include bones, joints, and skin and subcutaneous tissues.

Diagnosis Diagnosis of *Coccidioides* can occasionally be made by direct culture of sputum or other body fluids. Unlike other fungi, such as *C. albicans,* which can be either a colonizer or a pathogen depending on the situation, the presence of *Coccidioides* or any endemic fungus in a patient sample is generally regarded as evidence of infection with that fungus. The endemic fungi, unlike most nonpathogenic fungi, have two forms: they grow as **yeasts** at body temperature and as **molds** at room temperature. This trait can be used to help identify them in the laboratory. The **dimorphic** character can also explain their success as pathogens; the mold form is easily spread through the air to new victims, and the yeast form survives well in the body. Classically, *Coccidioides* is diagnosed by finding a **spherule,** which is a round cyst filled with small endospores, either on a pathologic sample or by inducing it to form on special medium. Today, however, biochemical and molecular techniques are more likely to be used for speciation.

Most of the time, *Coccidioides* is diagnosed through serologic means rather than culture. There are two approaches to serologic diagnosis. One test, called **complement fixation,** allows the lab to measure the amount of anti-*Coccidioides* antibody the patient has. If the antibody titer is high, this suggests active, severe infection. The antibody titer should decrease with effective treatment. Patients who do not have active disease will have a negative complement fixation test. A second test, called **immunodiffusion,** measures IgM and IgG antibodies to *Coccidioides* to distinguish between recent and chronic infection, respectively. A 4-fold rise in serum IgG titers from acute to convalescent serum can diagnose coccidioidomycosis in retrospect. A skin test, called **coccidioidin,** is not used to diagnose acutely ill patients, but rather to determine whether a patient has ever been exposed to *Coccidoides* in the past. It measures a cell-mediated immune response, similar to a PPD test for tuberculosis. It is primarily used for public health surveys.

Treatment and Prognosis In an immunocompetent patient, *Coccidioides* pneumonia is a self-limited illness that does not require any treatment. Our patient is immunocompromised, with respiratory failure, however, and she requires antifungal treatment. This patient was treated with **amphotericin B,** a systemic antifungal agent of the **polyene** class, which binds to **ergosterol** in the fungal membranes and disrupts cell membrane integrity. This drug is highly toxic with infusion-related side effects of fevers and rigors, as well as nephrotoxicity, including decreased glomerular filtration rate (GFR) and magnesium and potassium wasting. The

drug is still commonly used for severe fungal infections as clinicians have the most experience with it. Another class of drugs, the **azole** class, prevents synthesis of ergosterol by interfering with P450 enzyme function. Members of this class, such as fluconazole or itraconazole, are often prescribed for serious fungal infections as well.

In an immunocompromised patient, consideration must also be given to improving the patient's immune function if possible. For example, a patient with deficient **humoral** immunity may be given γ-globulin to boost his antibody response. A patient with HIV may be started on antiretroviral therapy to allow his immune system to recover and fight off an opportunistic infection. In this case, the patient's immunosuppression was iatrogenic, and her immunosuppressant medicines were curtailed and eventually held. This risked losing her transplanted kidney to rejection, but it was a necessary risk in the face of life-threatening infection.

As a final note, it is dangerous for laboratory workers to handle any of the endemic fungi, particularly in their mold state, without taking adequate precautions to avoid infection through the respiratory route. Other unusual organisms that can easily infect laboratory workers from routine culture plates in the laboratory include *Brucella, Coxiella burnetti,* and *Francisella tularensis.* Whereas *Mycobacterium tuberculosis* has the potential to infect laboratory workers, routine precautions with AFB cultures usually prevent this from happening.

Case Conclusion The patient was treated with amphotericin B in a liposomal formulation to avoid harming her transplanted kidney. Her immunosuppressants, FK506 and prednisone, were held. Unfortunately, her infection progressed, and involved her eyes, pericardium, skin, and gastrointestinal tract. Despite stopping her immunosuppressants and trying several new antifungal agents such as caspofungin and voriconazole, the patient died of overwhelming infection.

Thumbnail: The Endemic Mycoses

Organism	*Coccidioides immitis*	*Blastomyces dermatitidis*	*Histoplasma capsulatum*
Type of organism	Dimorphic fungus	Dimorphic fungus	Dimorphic fungus
Diseases caused	Self-limited pneumonia; skin nodules; lung cavities; osteomyelitis; meningitis; disseminated disease	Rarely self-limited; cutaneous pneumonia; meningitis; disseminated disease	Self-limited pneumonia; pulmonary mediastinitis; pericarditis meningitis; disseminated disease
Epidemiology/ geography	Arizona; Central Valley of California	Mississippi, Ohio, and Missouri valleys	Tennessee, Ohio, and Mississippi valleys
Soil types	Dry alkaline soil at low elevations; rodent burrows	Decomposing wood	Bat or bird excrement
Diagnosis	Culture; serology (complement fixation and immunodiffusion); may form spherules with endospores at 37°	Culture	Culture; histoplasma urinary antigen
Treatment	Azoles; amphotericin	Itraconazole; amphotericin	Itraconazole; amphotericin

Key Points

▶ Making the diagnosis of endemic fungal infection requires taking a careful travel history

▶ These organisms are not always easy to culture, and if suspected, serology and antigen tests are often used to make the diagnosis

▶ These fungi are dangerous to laboratory personnel and the lab should be warned if they are suspected

▶ The three major endemic fungi are dimorphic, and exist as yeast at body temperature and as molds at room temperature

Questions

1. A healthy 21-year-old woman moves to the Central Valley region of California, and develops signs of an acute pneumonia with fevers, shortness of breath, and cough. Her doctor diagnoses *Coccidioides* pneumonia. What is the recommended treatment for her pneumonia?

   A. Levofloxacin
   B. Fluconazole
   C. Terbinafine
   D. Amphotericin B
   E. None of the above

2. A 34-year-old man has a skin nodule removed. Which morphologic finding on pathology confirms the diagnosis of *Coccidioides*:

   A. Morula
   B. Spherule
   C. Round encapsulated yeast
   D. Acutely branching septate hyphae
   E. Gram-positive cocci in clusters

3. A 25-year-old hiker returns from a hiking trip outside Tucson, Arizona. He notes a large painful nodule on his arm. The nodule is cultured and is found to grow a dimorphic fungus, but final identification is pending. Which is most likely?

   A. *Histoplasma capsulatum*
   B. *Blastomyces dermatitidis*
   C. *Sporothrix schenckii*
   D. *Coccidioides immitis*
   E. *Penicillium marneffei*

HPI: PF is a 23-year-old woman who presents to the emergency department with a chief complaint of fever. She describes fevers, chills, a severe headache, mild abdominal pain, and nausea for the past 3 days. PF had just returned from 6 weeks in Nepal 5 days ago, where she was helping to set up a women's clinic in a rural village over the summer. She took chloroquine prophylaxis for malaria when she was there, was immunized for hepatitis A before she went, and always drank boiled water. She did not have any sexual exposures, nor was she in contact with any animals in Nepal. She does not have any cough, shortness of breath, diarrhea, constipation, or urinary symptoms.

PMH: History of *Chlamydia* STD when she was 19; bacterial pneumonia as a child, requiring hospitalization. Takes a multivitamin every day and stopped her chloroquine 5 days ago when she got back. No allergies. Not currently sexually active.

PE: 38.9°C HR 115 BP 105/80 RR 18
PF was flushed but in no acute distress. Her lungs were clear and her heart rate was regular, although rapid. Abdominal examination revealed mild diffuse tenderness to palpation with an enlarged spleen. No rashes.

Labs: WBC 4.8 with hematocrit count 35.0, platelet count 140,000/μL. Renal and liver function normal.

Thought Questions

- What is the differential diagnosis for fever in a traveler?

- What are PF's risk factors for developing malaria?

- What is the life cycle of the *Plasmodia* species?

- What are the pathogenesis and clinical manifestations of malaria?

- What are prophylactic and treatment options for malaria?

Basic Science Review and Discussion

Fever in a Traveler The differential for fever in a traveler depends on the location and activities during travel (insect contact, sexual exposures, animal exposures, food or water exposures, etc.; see Table 45-1).

Table 45-1 Fever in a traveler

Vector-borne:
Malaria, dengue, Lassa fever, typhus, rickettsial diseases, trypanosomiasis, yellow fever
Animal contacts:
Rabies, Q fever, tularemia, brucellosis, echinococcus
Infected person contact:
Hemorrhagic fevers, enteric fevers, meningococcal infection, tuberculosis, sexually transmitted diseases
Food/water borne:
Enteric infections, trichinosis, tapeworms (cestodes), salmonellosis (nontyphoid and typhoid), shigellosis, campylobacter, hepatitis A, enterovirus, aeromonas, plesimonas, toxin-mediated illnesses (staphylococcal, *Bacillus cereus*), *Listeria, E. coli*

Malaria

Epidemiology **Malaria is one of the most common infectious diseases globally,** with 200 to 300 million cases worldwide and 1 to 2 million deaths per year. Malaria is caused by infection with any of four species of the *Plasmodium* protozoa (i.e., ***Plasmodium falciparum, P. vivax, P. ovale,*** and ***P. malariae***) and is spread to humans by the **female *Anopheles* mosquito. Approximately 500 to 600 cases of imported malaria** in civilians are seen in the U.S. every year, mostly from travelers to Africa, South America, and Asia.

The CDC performed an analysis of malaria surveillance data on all reported cases in the U.S. with an onset of illness between August 1, 2000, and December 31, 2000. Two hundred forty-six cases of imported malaria in civilians were seen during that time period; 91.1% of them had prior information regarding the use of chemoprophylaxis to help prevent malaria infection, but 53.6% of these did not take any chemoprophylaxis and 10.7% did not take appropriate prophylaxis, leaving only one third on adequate malaria chemoprophylaxis. As elucidated in the **chemoprophylaxis** section below, our patient PF was taking an ineffective regimen for malaria for her region of travel.

Life cycle and pathogenesis *Plasmodia* species are spread by *Anopheles* mosquitoes. The lifecycle of the protozoal organisms is summarized below.

Stages of the life cycle:

1) Female *Anopheles* mosquito bites human (intermediate host), injecting **sporozoite** form of the *Plasmodium* protozoa from mosquito saliva into the bloodstream.

2) **Sporozoites** travel to the liver where they mature and undergo asexual reproduction (**exoerythrocytic schizogony**) to produce **schizonts** within the hepatocytes.

3) A massive number of **merozoites** are released from the **schizonts** within the liver, producing symptomatic infection as they invade and destroy red blood cells (RBCs).

4) In *P. vivax* and *P. ovale* infection, some parasites remain dormant in the liver as **hypnozoites**, which can cause **relapsing malaria** with these two species.

5) **Merozoites** invade RBCs, where **erythrocytic schizogony** occurs: cell division (asexual reproduction) produces *Plasmodia* **ring forms** (an immature form with the same appearance in all four species), **trophozoites**, and **schizonts**, which contain more merozoites.

6) The schizont-containing RBC eventually bursts, releasing **merozoites** into the bloodstream where they invade new RBCs and the process is continued.

7) After several generations of **erythrocytic schizogony**, some of the **merozoites** develop into male and female **gametocytes** within RBCs, which are subsequently ingested by a mosquito when she takes a blood meal.

Diagnosis   The diagnosis of malaria is made by viewing one of the **intra-erythrocytic parasite stages (including gametocyte forms) on thick or thin blood smears** from the patient. *P. falciparum* has a characteristic banana-shaped gametocyte. Figure 45-1 shows the ring forms of *Plasmodia falciparum*. The ring forms of each species are indistinguishable, but the appearance of multiple ring forms within the same erythrocyte almost always indicates infection with the rapidly replicating *P. falciparum*.

Pathogenesis and clinical manifestations   Of all the species, *P. falciparum* **results in the most severe clinical manifesta-**

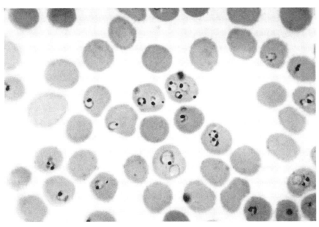

Figure 45-1 Blood smear depicting ring forms of *P. falciparum* inside erythrocytes. The term "ring" is derived from the morphologic appearance of this stage, which includes chromatin (red) and cytoplasm (blue), often arranged in a ring shape around a central vacuole; biologically, the ring is a young trophozoite. (Image in public domain on Centers for Disease Control Public Health Image Library, phil.cdc.gov.)

tions, because *P. falciparum* can invade RBCs in all stages of maturation and lead to profound degrees of parasitemia (up to 10^6 organisms/mL*). P. vivax* and *P. ovale* can only invade immature RBCs (reticulocytes) and *P. malariae* can only invade older RBCs, limiting the degree of parasitemia to fewer than 10,000 organisms/mL. **The immune response to malaria is not protective,** as there are multiple circulating parasitic stages, as well as antigenic variability among strains and between species. Hence, malaria can be contracted multiple times within a lifetime, although partial immunity conferring limited protection does occur. Disease manifestations are mediated by cytokine production and **obstruction of the microvasculature by peripheral sequestration of the parasitized RBC,** a phenomenon directly proportional to the degree of parasitemia.

The dominant clinical manifestation of malarial infection is **fever** (the oft-quoted cyclical pattern of fevers in malarial illnesses is not sensitive for diagnosis); 98% of imported malaria cases present with fever. Other symptoms include chills, headache, nausea, myalgias, arthralgias, malaise, vomiting, abdominal pain, anorexia, diarrhea, cough, and **dark urine.** Physical findings usually involve a temperature above 38.0°C and may include **splenomegaly** (due to splenic sequestration of infected RBCs), abdominal pain, hepatomegaly, jaundice, or scleral icterus (due to hemolysis of parasitized erythrocytes). Obstruction of the microvasculature by diseased RBCs can cause illness in almost any organ system:

- **Cerebral malaria:** can lead to coma and carries a substantial mortality rate. **Hypoglycemia** contributes to the cerebral manifestations of malaria: hypoglycemia can be caused by glucose consumption by massive parasitemia, poor glycogen stores in an ill patient, or the release of insulin by pancreatic β-cell elicited by quinidine or quinine treatment.

- **Renal malaria:** can see an immune complex-mediated nephrotic syndrome or an acute tubular necrosis caused by the massive amounts of free hemoglobin in the bloodstream from hemolysis (the dark urine from hemoglobinuria has led to the nickname of **blackwater fever** for malaria).

- **Pulmonary:** malaria can cause a **noncardiogenic pulmonary edema,** likely from the protozoal production of cytokines such as tumor necrosis factor-α.

- **Hematologic:** will usually see **anemia** from hemolysis of diseased RBCs and subsequent splenic enlargement (a late complication of *P. vivax* and *P. ovale* infection is splenic rupture); thrombocytopenia is observed in two thirds of patients with malaria.

- **Gastrointestinal:** most likely diarrhea from ischemic compromise of the bowel secondary to microvascular obstruction.

Chemoprophylaxis Prevention of imported cases of malaria in developing world travelers relies on an adequate knowledge of effective chemoprophylactic regimens for malaria by both physicians and patients. Effective regimens include:

- **Chloroquine:** used to be the drug of choice for chemoprophylaxis, but **chloroquine resistance in *P. falciparum* (and in *P. vivax* to a lesser extent) is burgeoning in Southeast Asia, South America, and Africa (chloroquine resistance is now found in *P. vivax*). Chloroquine prophylaxis is only effective for travelers to malaria-risk areas in Mexico, Haiti, the Dominican Republic, and certain countries in Central America, the Middle East, and Eastern Europe. The regimen is 500 mg orally per week for 1 week prior to travel, during travel, and 4 weeks afterward. Hence, PF failed malaria chemoprophylaxis because there was bound to be chloroquine-resistant *P. falciparum* in Nepal. Furthermore, she did not take the prophylactic medication for the prescribed dosing interval following travel.

- **Mefloquine:** used in chloroquine-resistant areas. Dose is 250 mg orally per week for 1 week prior to travel, during travel, and 4 weeks afterward. **Neurologic symptoms** such as dizziness, confusion, concentration difficulties, anxiety, and even psychosis can occur.

- **Doxycycline:** used in chloroquine-resistant areas. Dose is 100 mg orally every day for the same dosing interval as mefloquine. **Photosensitivity is a common problem** with this medication.

- **Malarone:** new antimalarial combination drug composed of **atovaquone and proguanil** (Malarone). Adult dosage is 1 tablet (250 mg atovaquone/100 mg proguanil) orally every day. Take first dose 1 to 3 days before travel, during travel, and 7 days after travel. **Contraindicated in severe renal impairment, pregnant women, breast-feeding women, and infants less than 24 pounds.** Common side effects are abdominal pain, nausea, vomiting, and headache.

- **Hydroxychloroquine sulfate (Plaquenil):** dose is 400 mg orally every week for the same dosing interval as mefloquine.

Finally, **insect control and pyrethrin-impregnated mosquito bed nets** are essential preventive measures for travelers to regions with high exposure to mosquitoes.

Case Conclusion PF's thick and thin blood smears revealed multiple RBCs with ring forms of the *Plasmodia* parasite. No other parasitic stage was observed and she was presumed to have chloroquine-resistant *P. falciparum* malaria. Quinine sulfate 650 mg orally every 8 hours for 3 days followed by a single dose of pyrimethamine (for eradication of the liver form of the parasite if *P. vivax* or *P. ovale* was present) was administered. PF defervesced and started to plan her upcoming Uganda trip by asking about mefloquine prophylaxis for malaria.

Thumbnail: Malaria

Organisms	*Plasmodium falciparum, Plasmodium vivax, Plasmodium ovale,* and *Plasmodium malariae*
Type of organism	Sporozoans (category of protozoan)
Diseases caused	Malaria, including manifestations of fever, neurologic compromise, anemia, hemoglobinemia, and hemoglobinuria (dark urine)
Epidemiology	200 to 300 million cases yearly in developing areas of the world harboring the *Anopheles* mosquito, including areas in South America, Africa, and Asia; approximately 500 imported cases of malaria per year in the U.S.
Diagnosis	Observation of intra-erythrocytic parasite on thick and thin blood smears
Treatment	Chemoprophylaxis prior to travel; treatment is usually with quinine, although atovaquone-proguanil or mefloquine can be used for treatment; an agent such as primaquine, pyrimethamine, or doxycycline should be administered after the quinine to kill hypnozoites in the liver from *P. vivax* or *P. ovale*

Key Points

▶ Cases of imported malaria in the U.S. often reflect inadequate chemoprophylaxis: mefloquine, doxycycline, hydroxychloroquine sulfate, or atovaquone-proguanil should be used for travel in areas where chloroquine-resistant *P. falciparum* has been reported

▶ Malaria is caused by four species (*P. falciparum, P. malaria, P. vivax,* and *P. ovale*), with *P. falciparum* causing the highest morbidity and mortality and *P. vivax/P. ovale* causing chronic relapses from establishment of an intrahepatic parasitic stage

▶ Diagnosis is made by seeing intra-erythrocytic parasites on thick and thin blood smears

Questions

1. Which of the following enzyme levels in the host should be checked prior to initiating primaquine therapy to eradicate the intrahepatic parasitic stage?

   A. Dihydrofolate reductase
   B. Phenylalanine hydroxylase
   C. Glucose 6-phosphate dehydrogenase
   D. Insulin
   E. Pepsinogen

2. Although PF was thought to only have *P. falciparum* infection, her likelihood of having another *Plasmodia* species in addition to *falciparum* is

   A. 100%
   B. 75%
   C. 50%
   D. 20%
   E. 5%

HPI: A 27-year-old woman presents to an urgent care center because of 6 days of increasing abdominal pain, bloating, and nonbloody diarrhea with four or five loose bowel movements per day. She has had mild nausea, but no vomiting and has been passing increased amounts of flatus. She has had no fever. Two weeks before the onset of diarrhea, she went on a 3-day camping and rafting trip with her girlfriend, who is experiencing similar symptoms. Meds: Multivitamin with iron.

PE: T 36.6°C BP 108/72 HR 110 RR 18

Abdomen is mildly distended with no guarding. Her abdomen is diffusely tender. Rectal exam demonstrates pale-colored stool, which tests negative for occult blood. Pelvic exam is normal.

Thought Questions

- What diagnostic tests are appropriate to send?
- Describe the life cycle of this organism.
- How does this organism cause diarrhea?
- How could this infection have been prevented?

Basic Science Review and Discussion

Giardia lamblia is a common **protozoal parasite** in the intestinal tract of humans and other mammals. Infection occurs following the **ingestion of cysts,** which can contaminate fresh water sources such as lakes, rivers, streams, and municipal water systems or can be spread via the fecal-oral route, through oral-anal sexual practices, or commonly at day care centers. Beavers are often implicated as an intermediate host, giving rise to the name "**beaver fever**" for giardiasis.

In the proximal small intestine, the organism excysts, releasing **trophozoites,** which may reproduce to large numbers by binary fission. The trophozoites attach to the mucosal epithelium of the small intestine by means of a **ventral sucking disk.** In response to environmental stresses such as changes in bile salt concentration, pH, or osmolality, the trophozoites may form the hearty cysts that are more commonly seen in stool. The cysts may remain viable for months in fresh water, but do not tolerate heating or desiccation. Viable cysts may be removed from fresh water by heating or filtration. Ingestion of as few as ten cysts may cause disease. (See Figure 46-1 for a diagram of the life cycle of *Giardia.*)

Infection with *Giardia* is found in both developed and developing countries. *Giardia* is the most common source of infection identified in **water-borne outbreaks** of diarrheal disease in the U.S. In developing countries, cumulative rates of infection approach 100% by 2 years of age, and prevalences of 30% or higher can be seen in adults.

The clinical presentation of *Giardia* infection may range from asymptomatic carriers to fulminant diarrhea. The diarrhea may be acute or chronic, often persisting for months before diagnosis is made. In acute giardiasis, symptoms usually begin after an incubation period of 1 to 3 weeks, with a minimum of 5 days. Prominent symptoms include diarrhea, bloating, abdominal pain, nausea and vomiting, flatus, and belching. The diarrhea of giardiasis is without blood or mucus, such that the presence of blood or mucus should call the diagnosis into question. The exact mechanism by which *Giardia* causes diarrhea is unclear, and histology of the small bowel in acute infection is often normal. In chronic infection, intestinal villi may be flattened and varying amounts of inflammation may be seen in the lamina propria.

Giardiasis often presents with a more subacute or chronic diarrhea, possibly with intermittent or recurrent symptoms. In its most severe form, the disease can be associated with malabsorption, weight loss, growth retardation in children, dehydration, and rarely, death.

Diagnosis is suspected by ascertaining a history of exposure to possibly infected fresh water sources or common fecal-oral sources of infection. On examination of the stool, both cysts and trophozoites may be seen (Figure 46-2). Cysts are oval in shape, 7 to 10 μm by 11 to 14 μm. Immature cysts contain two nuclei; mature cysts contain four. Trophozoites appear as pear-shaped, flattened organisms with two prominent nuclei and four pairs of flagella (two ventral, one lateral, and one caudal). The trophozoite is motile by a rolling motion and measures 4 to 8 μm by 10 to 15 μm. **ELISA for *Giardia* antigens in stool** is a sensitive and specific method of detection and is gradually replacing microscopic stool examination, which has a high false negative rate.

Treatment for giardiasis is with metronidazole 250 mg three times a day for 5 days. Mepacrine dichlorohydrate (Quinacrine; 100 mg twice a day for 5 days) is equally effective. In cases of treatment failure with the above regimens, retreatment can occur with a different drug or a longer course of the same drug, and in very refractory cases, combined treatment with both agents has been effective. Tinidazole, which is not available in the U.S., is more effec-

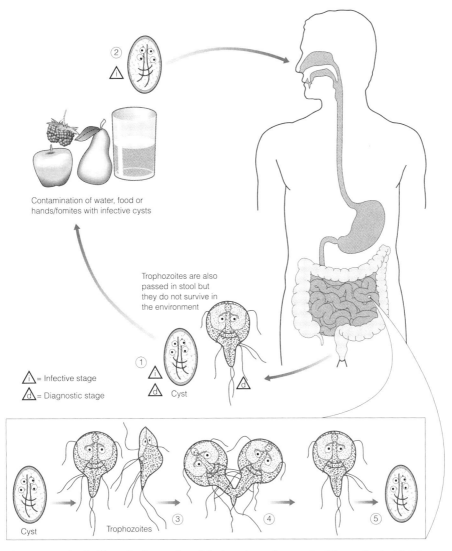

Contamination of water, food or hands/fomites with infective cysts

Trophozoites are also passed in stool but they do not survive in the environment

△i = Infective stage

△d = Diagnostic stage

① Cyst

Cyst   Trophozoites   ③   ④   ⑤

Figure 46-1 *Giardia* life cycle. (Image in public domain on Centers for Disease Control Public Health Image Library, phil.cdc.gov.)

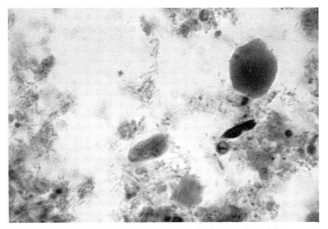

Figure 46-2 *Giardia* cyst on trichrome stain. (Image in public domain on Centers for Disease Control Public Health Image Library, phil.cdc.gov.)

tive than either metronidazole or mepacrine dichlorohydrate. Paromomycin can be used in symptomatic pregnant women.

Prevention of disease is the best treatment. Cooking food adequately and boiling or filtering potentially contaminated water prevents infection.

Case Conclusion Examination of stool specimens demonstrated trophozoites and cysts of *Giardia lamblia*. Giardia antigen test on the stool was also positive. Our patient was prescribed metronidazole 250 mg three times a day for 5 days. Her girlfriend was also treated. Their diarrhea resolved quickly.

Thumbnail: *Giardia lamblia*

Organism	*Giardia lamblia*
Type of organism	Protozoan
Disease caused	Diarrhea; disease may range from asymptomatic to fulminant diarrhea and malabsorption
Epidemiology	Infections are common in both the developed and developing world; associated with contaminated fresh water sources such as streams, lakes, rivers, and municipal water systems; spread commonly through fecal-oral route, in day care centers, and with oral-anal sexual contact
Diagnosis	Identification of cysts or trophozoites in the stool; *Giardia* antigen tests on stool
Treatment	Metronidazole 250 mg three times a day for 5 days

Key Points

▶ Giardiasis is a protozoal infection of the small intestine that causes acute or chronic, nonbloody diarrhea; abdominal pain, bloating, or nausea may be more or less prominent features of illness

▶ Diagnosis is made by observing cysts or trophozoites in the stool or by assays of the stool for *Giardia* antigen

Questions

1. Which of the following is the most sensitive method for making the diagnosis of *Giardia*?

   A. Stool culture
   B. Identification of *Giardia lamblia* cysts in a stool specimen
   C. Identification of *Giardia lamblia* trophozoites in a stool specimen
   D. Serology for *Giardia lamblia*
   E. ELISA for *Giardia* antigens in stool

2. Which of the following is not a characteristic of the trophozoite stage of *Giardia*?

   A. They divide by binary fission
   B. They are motile with four pairs of flagella
   C. They are the infectious form of the organism
   D. They contain two nuclei
   E. They attach to small intestinal mucosal epithelium via a ventral sucking disk

HPI: A 32-year-old female intravenous drug user presents to the ER with 1 week of progressive shortness of breath, dry cough, and low-grade fever. She is homeless and has been staying in shelters. She has also experienced a 20-pound weight loss over the past 6 months. She takes no medications and has not seen a doctor in several years.

PE: T 38.8°C BP 110/92 HR 122 RR 26 SaO_2 89% on room air
She is a thin, chronically ill-appearing woman in obvious respiratory distress. Oral exam reveals thrush. She has diffusely enlarged lymph nodes throughout her neck, axilla, and groin. Lung exam reveals only faint rales at the base. A spleen tip is palpable on abdominal exam.

Labs: WBC 1.2; hemoglobin 11.2; platelets 124,000; AST/ALT normal; LDH 333; arterial blood gas shows PO_2 48, PCO_2 46, pH 7.44.
Chest x-ray demonstrates bilateral diffuse perihilar infiltrates in a "butterfly" pattern.

Thought Questions

- What are the most common characteristics of patients who get PCP?

- How is PCP diagnosed?

- How do the clinical clues to the diagnosis of PCP relate to the organism's pathogenesis?

Basic Science Review and Discussion

Pneumocystis carinii pneumonia (PCP) was recently renamed *Pneumocystis jiroveci* pneumonia (PcP). This disease is seen almost exclusively in immunocompromised patients: AIDS, organ transplantation, chronic corticosteroid administration, and premature malnourished infants. The taxonomy of *Pneumocystis* is somewhat controversial. It has some characteristics of a protozoan, but is most commonly classified as a **fungus** on the basis of ribosomal RNA sequences, mitochondrial proteins, and major enzymes (dihydrofolate reductase and thymidine synthase).

The major structural forms of the organism are the **trophozoite** (1–4 μm with a thin wall) and the **cyst** (4–6 μm with a thick wall and up to eight intracystic bodies). An intermediate stage, called the precyst, may also be seen. All stages may be simultaneously present in an infected individual. The exact method of replication of the organism is not known, but likely involves asexual replication by the trophozoite and sexual replication by the cyst, which leads to release of the intracystic bodies.

It is generally thought that clinical disease results from reactivation of latent infection in the setting of **impaired host cellular immunity,** whether by immunosuppressive drugs (corticosteroids) or by progressive immunologic dysfunction, such as in patients with AIDS.

In the lung, the organism attaches firmly to **alveolar type I pneumocytes.** The organisms gradually replicate to fill the alveoli, impairing oxygen exchange. Changes that occur within the alveolus include **increased capillary-alveolar permeability and alterations in the composition of pulmonary surfactants,** resulting in the filling of alveoli with foamy, vacuolated exudates. In severe disease, interstitial edema, fibrosis, and hyaline membrane formation may be seen. Host immune responses consist of **hypertrophy of alveolar type II pneumocytes and a mild mononuclear cell interstitial infiltrate.**

Clinically, patients with PCP present with **dyspnea, fever, and nonproductive cough** over a period of several days to weeks. Physical findings include tachypnea, tachycardia, cyanosis, and **hypoxia.** Auscultation of the lungs may sound relatively normal. Arterial blood gases demonstrate hypoxemia, an increased alveolar-arterial O_2 gradient ($AaDO_2$), and respiratory alkalosis. WBC counts may be variable, being primarily determined by the underlying cause of immunosuppression. Elevations of lactate dehydrogenase (LDH) reflect general lung damage and are not specific to *Pneumocystis* disease.

Chest x-ray patterns in PCP are highly variable, and almost any picture is possible. The classic radiographic finding is **bilateral diffuse perihilar infiltrates,** but other features, including nodules, cavities, and even lobar infiltrates have been reported. Peripheral pneumatoceles may burst, causing pneumothoraces. Patients on aerosolized pentamidine as prophylaxis for PCP may present with primarily upper lobe infiltrates.

Because much of the pulmonary symptomatology is due to host inflammatory response, PCP may become clinically apparent in patients on chronic immunosuppressant medication during a taper of corticosteroids.

Extrapulmonary disease is rare, but can be seen in patients with advanced immunosuppression. Sites of disseminated involvement include the lymph nodes, liver, spleen, skin, bone marrow, and thyroid gland.

Pneumocystis **cannot be cultured, so diagnosis is typically made by staining of the organism on induced sputum or bronchial alveolar lavage fluid** (Figure 47-1). Wright-Giemsa, methenamine silver, or toluidine blue stains are most commonly used. Both cysts and trophozoites are commonly seen. In immunosuppressed patients, organism burden may be very high. Techniques of molecular identification and PCR of oral secretions are under investigation as diagnostic tools.

Treatment for PCP is most often with high-dose **TMP-SMZ,** which acts by inhibiting dihydrofolate reductase. Intravenous pentamidine is equally effective, although it is associated with hypoglycemia and pancreatitis. The mode of action of pentamidine against *Pneumocystis* is unclear. Other drugs with activity against PCP include dapsone, trimetrexate, clindamycin plus primaquine, and atovaquone.

In vitro resistance of *Pneumocystis* to TMP-SMZ has been described, but its clinical significance remains unclear.

Because of the contributions of host inflammatory response to lung damage in PCP, administration of adjuvant corticosteroids is indicated in moderate to severe PCP (indications for steroids include a $PaO_2 < 70$ mm Hg or $AaDO_2 > 35$ mm Hg on room air).

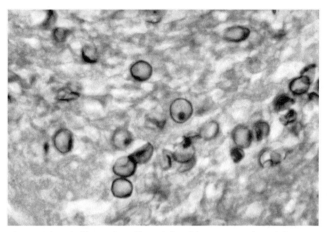

Figure 47-1 Methenamine silver stain of *Pneumocystis* cysts from histopathology specimen of lung from AIDS patient. (Image in public domain on Centers for Disease Control Public Health Image Library, phil.cdc.gov, courtesy of Dr. Edwin P. Ewing, Jr.)

Patients at high risk for PCP (chronic high-dose corticosteroids, organ transplant recipients on significant immunosuppression, and AIDS patients with CD4 counts less than 200 cells/μL or a history prior PCP at any CD4 count) are candidates for prophylactic PCP therapy. The drugs most commonly used for this purpose are TMP-SMZ, dapsone, or aerosolized pentamidine.

Case Conclusion The patient was intubated and admitted to the ICU. She was started on intravenous TMP-SMZ and solumedrol. Bronchoalveolar lavage demonstrated *Pneumocystis carinii* trophozoites and cysts. A diagnosis of HIV infection was established serologically. After a prolonged course, she eventually recovered and was discharged to a drug recovery program, to begin care for her HIV disease.

Thumbnail: *Pneumocystis carinii*

Organism	*Pneumocystis carinii (jiroveci)*
Type of organism	Debated; has characteristics of a protozoan, but analysis of rRNA, mitochondrial proteins, and major enzymes classifies it as a fungus
Diseases caused	Pneumonia (PCP); rarely extrapulmonary disease
Epidemiology	Worldwide distribution among humans and a variety of animals; possible human-to-human transmission
Diagnosis	Staining of induced sputum or bronchoalveolar lavage fluid with methenamine silver, toluidine blue, or Wright-Giemsa stain
Treatment	Trimethoprim-methoxazole (TMP-SMZ), intravenous pentamidine, dapsone, trimetrexate, clindamycin and primaquine, and atovaquone; corticosteroids are indicated in moderate to severe disease ($PaO_2 < 70$ mm Hg or $AaDO_2 > 35$ mm Hg on room air)

Key Points

▶ PCP occurs primarily in hosts with impaired cell-mediated immunity

▶ Hypoxia, which is a common clinical feature of PCP, arises from filling of the alveoli with foamy exudates and changes in surfactant as well as interstitial edema and inflammatory infiltrate

Questions

1. Which of the following is true regarding *Pneumocystis* in HIV-infected patients:

    A. PCP only occurs at CD4 counts less than 200 cells/μL

    B. Primary and secondary PCP prophylaxis may be stopped when antiretroviral treatment results in an increase in CD4 count to greater than 200 cells/μL for at least 3 months

    C. *Pneumocystis* infection occurs only in the lungs and mediastinal lymph nodes

    D. Respiratory isolation is required for all HIV-infected patients in whom PCP is suspected

2. In which clinical scenario would PCP be least likely?

    A. An elderly patient with temporal arteritis on prednisone 60 mg a day

    B. A patient with HIV, on antiretroviral therapy with a CD4 count of 110 cells/μL

    C. A patient with chronic granulomatous disease (CGD)

    D. A premature infant in the ICU

HPI: A 27-year-old woman presents to the city health clinic because of 1 week of vaginal itching and foul-smelling discharge. She is sexually active with several male partners and does not use condoms or other forms of birth control. She has tried over-the-counter vaginal fungal cream without improvement.

PE: Pelvic exam shows moderate erythema of the vaginal and vulvar epithelium with profuse foul-smelling yellow discharge.

Labs: Examination of the discharge demonstrates a pH of 7.0 with a fishy odor when potassium hydroxide (KOH) is placed on the slide. Under the microscope, moderate leukocytes are present along with motile pear-shaped organisms. Pregnancy testing is negative.

Thought Questions

- What is the most effective method of rapid diagnosis of vaginitis?

- What characteristics allow the differentiation of various causes of vaginitis?

Basic Science Review and Discussion

Trichomonas vaginalis is a **pear-shaped, actively motile protozoan,** 7 by 10 μm in size. In women, the organism primarily infects vaginal epithelium and less commonly the endocervix. In men, it infects the urethra and prostate. It replicates by **binary fission** and there is no cyst stage. (See Figure 48-1.)

The majority (50%–90%) of infected men are **asymptomatic,** whereas only 20% to 50% of women are symptomatic. The most common complaints in women are **vaginal itching, dysuria or urinary frequency, and dyspareunia.** These symptoms are accompanied by a notable yellow-colored, **malodorous vaginal discharge.**

Physical examination demonstrates an erythematous, inflamed vaginal and vulvar epithelium. Petechial lesions seen on the cervix during colposcopy give a characteristic **"strawberry cervix"** appearance. The **pH of vaginal fluid is usually 5.0 or greater** (normal vaginal pH is 3.8–4.4), a characteristic that is important in the pathogenesis of the organism, which does not survive more acidic environments. An **amine, or "fishy" odor** can be detected with the addition of KOH to a sample of vaginal fluid.

Diagnosis may be quickly established by **microscopic examination of wet mounts** of vaginal or prostatic secretions. Pear-shaped organisms may be directly visualized and demonstrate characteristic **jerking movements.** Sensitivity of wet-mount diagnosis is only 50% to 60%. Culture is not readily available and takes 3 to 7 days. Dried smears of exudates may be stained with Papanicolau, Giemsa, or acridine-orange to demonstrate organisms if immediate microscopy is not available. Direct immunofluorescent staining is also available but rarely used.

Differential diagnosis of vaginitis includes **bacterial vaginosis (BV)** and **vulvovaginal candidiasis.** See the Thumbnail section for a comparison of these conditions. Testing for other sexually transmitted diseases, such as gonorrhea, chlamydia, syphilis, and HIV, should be considered when trichomoniasis is confirmed.

Metronidazole is the drug of choice for the treatment of trichomoniasis. It can be dosed as a single 2-g oral dose, or 500 mg twice a day for 7 days. Vaginal metronidazole gel, which is effective in treating BV, is less effective in trichomoniasis. Metronidazole is not recommended in the first trimester of pregnancy. Acidic douching to restore the normal pH of the vaginal canal may be helpful, as can daily clotrimazole vaginal suppositories. Partners should be evaluated and treated as well.

Case Conclusion The woman is treated with a single 2-g dose of metronidazole. She undergoes HIV and STD counseling and testing, all of which are negative.

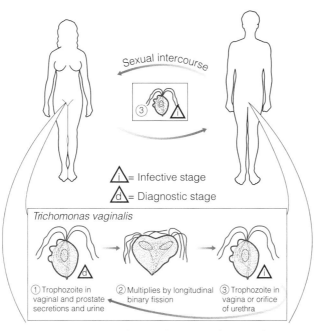

Figure 48-1 *Trichomonas* life cycle. (Courtesy of Centers for Disease Control.)

Thumbnail: Agents Causing Vaginitis

Organism	*Trichomonas vaginalis*	*Gardnerella vaginalis*	*Candida* spp.
Type of organism	Protozoan	Bacteria	Yeast
Diseases caused	Trichomonal vaginitis	Bacterial vaginosis (BV)	Vulvovaginal candidiasis
Epidemiology	Sexually transmitted; 3 to 4 million infections per year in women in the U.S.	Occurs with various anaerobic bacteria and mycoplasma	Associated with antibiotic use, diabetes, and HIV infection
Diagnosis	Motile trichomonads seen on wet mount; pH > 5.0; fishy smell with KOH; profuse yellow discharge	"Clue cells" seen on wet mount; pH 4.5; scant, thin discharge	Yeast forms seen on KOH prep; pH < 4.5; no fishy smell; scant white discharge
Treatment	Metronidazole 2-g single-dose orally; treat partners	Clindamycin or metronidazole cream/gel; oral metronidazole for 7 days; no need to treat partners	Intravaginal antifungal creams; fluconazole 150-mg single-dose orally; treat partner only if candidal dermatitis is present

Key Points

▶ Diagnosis of trichomoniasis can be made by visualizing the motile protozoans on wet mount of vaginal secretions

▶ Diagnosis of trichomoniasis requires thorough evaluation, testing, and counseling for other sexually transmitted diseases

Questions

1. Which of the following is the best method of making the diagnosis of trichomoniasis in men?

   A. Culture of a midstream urine specimen
   B. Microscopic examination of urethral discharge following prostate massage
   C. Serology
   D. Testicular ultrasound
   E. Visualization of clue cells on a urethral swab

2. A 19-year-old college freshman complains of intense vaginal itching and burning. Examination shows scant discharge and erythematous vaginal epithelium. There are scattered white plaques loosely adherent to the vaginal mucosa. Vaginal pH is 3.9. Which of the following is true about her condition?

   A. She most likely acquired the infection from a sexual partner
   B. She will likely have a positive RPR
   C. The most common sequelae of this infection are pelvic inflammatory disease (PID) and infertility
   D. This condition is associated with recent antibiotic use
   E. This infection is associated with cervical cancer

HPI: A 42-year-old female intravenous drug user with known AIDS presents to the urgent care clinic after being lost to follow-up for 8 months. When last seen, her CD4 count was 190 cells/μL and her HIV RNA viral load was 32,000 copies/μL. She had been prescribed zidovudine, lamivudine, indinavir, and TMP-SMZ at that time, but she admits to not taking any medications for the last 5 months. She presents now because of increased confusion, low-grade fevers, and headache over the last several days, with the new development of right leg weakness over the last day. A review of her hospital record indicates she was seen in the ER 3 days ago because of a seizure. Lumbar puncture was performed at that time and showed 6 WBC (100% lymphocytes), mildly elevated protein, and a normal glucose; cryptococcal antigen was negative, as were VDRL and routine cultures. She was monitored overnight, put on a rapid benzodiazepine taper for alcohol withdrawal, and discharged 2 days later with a diagnosis of alcohol withdrawal seizures.

PE: T 37.8° BP 112/92 HR 110 RR 22
She is alert, but oriented only to person and year. There is no papilledema. Kernig's and Brudzinski's signs are absent. She has a left temporal homonomous hemianopsia, and is unable to abduct her right eye. Her strength is three out of five in her right lower extremity, but normal elsewhere. She is mildly ataxic.
Emergent head CT demonstrates multiple ring enhancing lesions in both hemispheres, including the left basal ganglia and brain stem.

Thought Questions

- What are the different clinical presentations of toxoplasmosis in immunocompetent and immunocompromised hosts?

- What are the different modes of transmission of *Toxoplasma*?

- What is the life cycle of the organism?

Basic Science Review and Discussion

Toxoplasma gondii is an **obligate intracellular parasite** that causes infection of the central nervous susytem (CNS) and eyes, heart, lungs, and lymph nodes. *Toxoplasma* also causes congenital infection.

Cats are the only definitive hosts for *Toxoplasma* and acquire the parasite by eating infected meat. The sexual lifestyle in the cat occurs in the epithelial cells of the intestine and results in the production of **oocysts,** which are passed in the stool. Mature oocysts sporulate in the presence of air to produce eight **sporozoite** progeny. If these mature oocytes are ingested by an intermediate host (such as a human changing cat litter), infection results in **trophozoite** replication in many tissues. Alternatively, human infection may occur from ingestion of **cysts** (containing **bradyzoites**) from improperly cooked meat, especially lamb and pork (sheep and pigs are other examples of intermediate hosts). In humans, cysts may form, primarily in the CNS and muscle (including cardiac muscle) tissue. (See Figure 49-1.)

Acute toxoplasmosis in immunocompetent hosts is usually asymptomatic, making diagnosis difficult. This is particularly important in pregnant women, in whom acute infection will lead to transplacental infection of the fetus in one third of cases.

Ocular infection with *Toxoplasma gondii* is the cause of 35% of cases of chorioretinitis in the U.S. and Europe. Most ocular involvement is a result of congenital infection and may cause blurred vision, scotoma, photophobia, and eye pain. Ophthalmologic examination shows yellow-white, cotton-like patches with hyperemic margins, which may be unilateral or bilateral. Sequelae of glaucoma and cataracts are common.

In the immunocompromised person, such as a person with AIDS and a CD4+ cell count below 100 cells/μL, toxoplasmosis typically causes **encephalitis.** CNS disease is usually a result of reactivation of latent infection, but may be due to acquisition of parasites from exogenous sources. The presentation of cerebral toxoplasmosis includes altered mental status, fever, seizures, headaches, and focal neurologic findings. Symptoms may occur rapidly or subacutely.

The areas of the brain most commonly involved are the brain stem, basal ganglia, pituitary gland, and corticomedullary junction. **Multifocal, ring-enhancing lesions** are usually seen on CT scan or MRI of the brain. While suggestive, these findings are not pathognomonic of toxoplasmosis, and CNS lymphoma is often a consideration. Single lesions are uncommon in toxoplasmosis, and if only one lesion is seen, a brain biopsy is often necessary for diagnosis.

Although **brain biopsy** is the definitive method of diagnosis, a combination of **clinical presentation, positive serology, and supportive radiology have an 80% positive predictive value in making the diagnosis.** Treatment is usually initi-

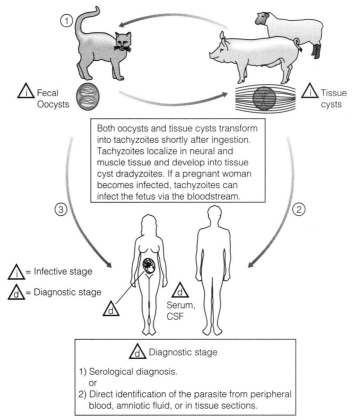

Both oocysts and tissue cysts transform into tachyzoites shortly after ingestion. Tachyzoites localize in neural and muscle tissue and develop into tissue cyst dradyzoites. If a pregnant woman becomes infected, tachyzoites can infect the fetus via the bloodstream.

Fecal Oocysts

Tissue cysts

△i = Infective stage
△d = Diagnostic stage

Serum, CSF

△d Diagnostic stage

1) Serological diagnosis.
   or
2) Direct identification of the parasite from peripheral blood, amniotic fluid, or in tissue sections.

Figure 49-1 *Toxoplasma* life cycle. (Courtesy of Centers for Disease Control.)

ated in such cases, and clinical improvement is seen in 90% of patients by day 7 and radiologic improvement is usually seen by day 21; if such clinical or radiologic improvement is not seen, a brain biopsy is indicated. In congenital infection, rise in IgM antibodies after 1 week of life is diagnostic. Parasites may be isolated from the peritoneal fluid of mice injected with infected body fluids.

There is no treatment necessary for acute infections in most cases among immunocompetent hosts. First-line treatment of toxoplasma encephalitis in the immunocompromised host is **pyrimethamine and sulfadiazine.** Both pyrimethamine and sulfadiazine inhibit the enzyme dihydrofolate reduc-

tase, and leucovorin is necessary to prevent bone marrow suppression in the host. An alternate regimen is clindamycin with pyrimethamine. Spiramycin reduces maternal-fetal transmission. Untreated cerebral toxoplasmosis is uniformly fatal.

Prophylaxis for toxoplasmosis in AIDS patients with CD4+ counts below 100 cells/μL is most effective with TMP-SMZ, but dapsone, atovaquone, azithromycin, and clarithromycin may all be used in combination with pyrimethamine. Additionally, avoiding cat feces, not eating undercooked meat, and washing hands as well as fruits and vegetables are other methods of preventing infection.

Case Conclusion   Our patient is admitted to the hospital with a presumptive diagnosis of *Toxoplasma* encephalitis and started on sulfadiazine and pyrimethamine. On hospital day 2, a *Toxoplasma* antibody serology returns as positive. Over the next 4 days her symptoms improve, and she regains strength in her right lower extremity. On hospital day 7, she leaves against medical advice and does not keep follow-up appointments in the HIV clinic.

Thumbnail: *Toxoplasmosis*

Organism	***Toxoplasma gondii***
Type of organism	Obligate intracellular parasite
Diseases caused	Cervical adenopathy or chorioretinitis in immunocompetent hosts; cerebral toxoplasmosis in immunocompromised hosts (AIDS with CD4 counts less than 100 cells/μL; lymphoproliferative disorders); congenital infection with hydrocephalus, microcephaly, mental retardation, chorioretinitis, and occasionally, fetal death
Epidemiology	Seroprevalence in the U.S. increases at about 1% per year; transmission is primarily transplacental or oral, where it is associated with ingestion of oocysts from cat feces or contaminated soil, or ingestion of bradyzoites from undercooked meat
Diagnosis	Brain biopsy; isolation of organism after injection of infected body fluids into the peritoneum of mice; serum IgG and IgM antibody titers are helpful in determining infection; characteristic radiologic findings on head CT or MRI of the brain
Treatment	Sulfadiazine plus pyrimethamine (with leucovorin); alternatives include clindamycin and spiramycin (in pregnancy); adjuvant glucocorticoids with eye involvement

Key Points

▶ Acute toxoplasmosis is usually asymptomatic and not serious—except in pregnant women

▶ *Toxoplasma* encephalitis in immunocompromised hosts may present with focal or nonfocal findings

▶ TMP-SMZ is a very effective prophylaxis in AIDS patients at risk for toxoplasmosis due to low CD4+ counts

Questions

1. *Toxoplasma gondii* is most closely related to which of the following parasites?

   A. *Trypanosoma cruzi*
   B. *Plasmodium falciparum*
   C. *Giardia lamblia*
   D. *Naegleria fowleri*
   E. *Trichomonas vaginalis*

2. In the U.S., *Toxoplasma gondii* is most often transmitted by which of the following?

   A. Dog feces
   B. Cat feces
   C. Inadequately cooked fish
   D. Ticks
   E. Cat scratches

HPI: A 45-year-old migrant farm worker from Mexico presents to the ER following a generalized tonic-clonic seizure, which stopped spontaneously prior to his arrival in the ER. He has no history of seizures and takes no medications.

PE: He is postictal (mildly disoriented and amnesic for the event), but exam is otherwise normal, including neurologic exam. Head CT demonstrates multiple calcified cystic lesions.

Thought Questions

- What are the two distinct clinical diseases produced by this organism?

- How does the organism's life cycle affect the clinical presentation of disease?

- What epidemiological clues hint at the diagnosis?

Basic Science Review and Discussion

Cestodes, or **tapeworms,** are segmented worms. Each ribbon-shaped adult tapeworm is composed of a conjoined chain (**strobila**) of segments (**proglottids**). The worm attaches to the intestinal mucosa by means of sucking cups or grooves located on the head (**scolex**). Behind the scolex, proglottids emerge from a short germinal center (neck). Maturation of proglottids proceeds toward the posterior of the worm, being progressively termed immature, mature, and gravid. Each proglottid contains both male and female sex organs.

Gravid proglottids, full of eggs, may detach from the strobila and pass in the stool. Eggs may survive in the environment for several months. After ingestion by an **intermediate host,** an egg develops into a **larval oncosphere,** which penetrates the intestinal mucosa, migrates to various organs, and develops into an encapsulated **cysticercus** (single scolex), **coenerus** (multiple scolices), or **hydatid** (cyst with daughter cysts, each containing several scolices), depending on the species. If a cyst is ingested by the **definitive host,** the scolex may mature into an adult intestinal tapeworm, and the cycle repeats. **Autoinfection** is possible with *Taenia solium*. (See Figure 50-1.)

When humans function as the definitive host, the adult tapeworms live in the gastrointestinal tract (as in infections with *Taenia saginata, Diphyllobothrium, Hymenolepis,* and *Dipylidium caninum*). When humans function as the intermediate host, the larval-stage parasites are present in various tissues (as in infections with *Echinococcus, Spargana,* and *Spirometra*). In the case of *Taenia solium,* humans may act as either the intermediate or definitive host.

Adult tapeworms may live up to 25 years in the intestine, be up to 10 m in length, and contain over 3000 proglottids, each of which may produce up to 50,000 eggs. Adult tapeworms do not contain a digestive tract, but absorb most of their nutrients directly through the body wall (**tegument**).

Despite their impressive size, clinical infection is often asymptomatic. Occasionally, vague gastrointestinal symptoms or malabsorption may be present. Often, the first indication of clinical infection is passing proglottids in the stool.

There are many varieties of intestinal cestodes, which come from various intermediate hosts and have various appearances. Diagnosis of the infecting organism depends on examination of a scolex or proglottid, as the eggs often appear morphologically similar. Serologic tests are not helpful, and eosinophilia is the only laboratory abnormality that may be seen.

Treatment is with **praziquantel** or **niclosamide.** Proper cooking of beef and pork and proper disposal of fecal material are key preventive measures.

When tissue infection with the larval form of *Taenia solium* occurs, the disease is termed **cysticercosis.** The cysts have a predilection for **brain and muscle tissue;** less common sites of infection include the retina, heart, liver, lungs, and kidneys. Multiple lesions are usually present.

Cysts in the brain may present with headache, nausea, focal neurologic symptoms, and seizures. Cerebral imaging studies are helpful in making the diagnosis. CT scan demonstrates multiple parenchymal lesions of varying number and size, which may be either cystic or solid and are often calcified (indicating a dead, degenerated lesion). MRI is more sensitive at identifying lesions, whereas CT is better at picking up calcification.

Cysts in the muscle are often asymptomatic and may be detected on plain films obtained for other reasons. Lesions in the retina may produce visual symptoms, and cysts in the heart muscle may lead to conduction abnormalities.

Treatment of neurocysticercosis involves either **praziquantel** or **albendazole.** Dying cysts may invoke an inflammatory response, in which case glucocorticoid therapy may be of benefit. Surgical intervention may be necessary for lesions causing mass effect or intractable seizures. Asymptomatic patients require no therapy.

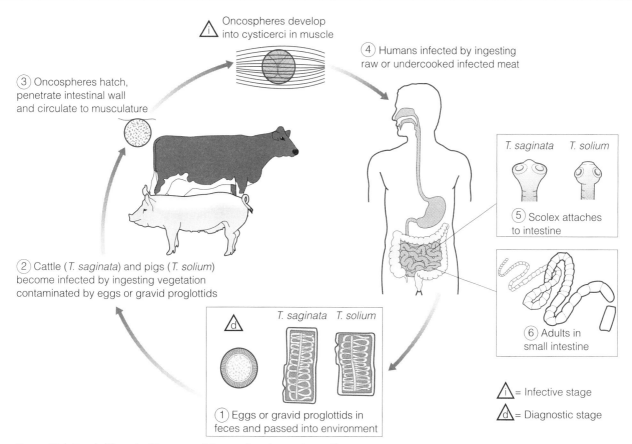

Figure 50-1 *Taenia* life cycle. (Courtesy of Centers for Disease Control.)

Case Conclusion   The patient is started on dilantin for his seizure. An MRI is characteristic of cysticercosis—multiple lesions are seen and a high-intensity rim is visible around the cysts on T-2 weighted images. He is started on praziquantel and prednisone. He is discharged home to continue therapy. He has no more seizures, and a repeat CT scan 4 months later shows slight decrease in size of the lesions.

Thumbnail: *Taenia solium*

Organism	*Taenia solium*
Type of organism	Cestode (tapeworm)
Diseases caused	Adult tapeworms in the intestine; larval form in tissues (brain, muscle) is called cysticercosis
Epidemiology	Humans are only definitive host; intermediate hosts are pigs, less commonly deer, camels, dogs, cats, and sheep; present worldwide, most commonly in Mexico, South America, Africa, Southeast Asia, and Eastern Europe; acquired from ingesting undercooked infected pork (intestinal form) or eggs from fecal contamination of food (cysticercosis)
Diagnosis	Intestinal infection diagnosed by demonstrating eggs or proglottids in stool; definitive diagnosis of cysticercosis requires examination of the larval form in affected tissue; presumptive diagnosis can be made in the proper clinical setting with CT or MRI imaging and/or serology
Treatment	Niclosamide or praziquantel for intestinal infection; cysticercosis may be treated with combinations of chemotherapy (praziquantel and albendazole) and/or surgery

Key Points

▶ Examination of a mature proglottid or scolex is required to distinguish *T. solium* (the pork tapeworm) from *T. saginata* (the beef tapeworm), as the eggs are identical

▶ Treatment of neurocysticercosis may elicit an inflammatory response by dying cysticerci, requiring glucocorticoids for treatment

Questions

1. A 67-year-old woman from Norway is diagnosed with megaloblastic anemia. On further evaluation, she is noted to have a mild eosinophilia and a stool specimen demonstrates thin-shelled ovoid eggs, 45 by 70 μm, with an operculum (lid) at one end. What is her infection?

   A. *Taenia solium*
   B. *Taenia saginata*
   C. *Echinococcus granulosis*
   D. *Hymenolepis nana*
   E. *Diphyllobothrium latum*

2. Which cestode may cause expanding hepatic cysts?

   A. *Taenia saginata*
   B. *Schistosoma mansoni*
   C. *Echinococcus multilocularis*
   D. *Onchocerca volvulus*
   E. *Hymenolepis nana*

HPI: A 56-year-old man from Panama with a 50 pack year smoking history was recently admitted for an exacerbation of chronic obstructive pulmonary disease (COPD). He was treated with high-dose intravenous steroids, and then discharged on a slow taper of oral steroids. He returns 1 week later because of increased shortness of breath.
PMH: Intermittent diarrhea over the past decade.

PE: T 38.0°C BP 140/90 HR 130 RR 34
The patient is in severe respiratory distress. He is using accessory muscles of respiration, and can only speak one word at a time. He is not oriented to place or date. Lung exam features diffuse rales and rhonchi. Heart exam has no murmur. There is severe abdominal tenderness but no peritoneal signs.

Labs: WBC 22, differential significant for 30% eosinophils. A blood gas shows a pH of 7.30, pCO_2 55, and PO_2 of 60 on room air.
A sputum Gram stain showed many white cells but minimal bacteria. Sputum cultures were negative. One of two blood cultures grew *E. coli*.
The patient was taken to the intensive care unit and intubated, and IV steroids were redosed. An initial diagnosis of nosocomial bacterial pneumonia was made, but the patient deteriorated on broad-spectrum antibiotics. Given the patient's immigrant origin and the **eosinophilia**, a parasitic diagnosis was entertained. Stool samples were sent for microscopic examination for ova and parasites. The patient's sputum was resubmitted, this time for a microscopic examination under lower power for parasites, rather than the usual high-power examination for bacteria. Nematodes were seen both in stool and sputum, and the diagnosis of *Strongyloides* hyperinfection was made.

Thought Questions

- How do the routes *Strongyloides* takes through the body explain this patient's symptoms?

- What was the origin of this patient's bacteremia?

Basic Science Review and Discussion

The parasitic worms, or **helminths**, are divided into two phyla, the roundworms (**nematodes**), discussed here, and the flatworms (**cestodes** and **trematodes**), discussed in other cases.

The nematodes are among the most common pathogens on earth. *Ascaris* and hookworms each infect more than one quarter of the world's population. Most nematode infections are spread through **ingestion** or **contact** with the nematode, but the following tissue nematode infections are spread through **insect vectors**: *Onchocerca volvulus,* Loa Loa, and the various agents of elephantiasis. Some nematodes are not primarily human parasites, but can be contracted by humans as dead-end hosts. Examples are aniskiasis (a fish parasite), hookworms (cat or dog parasites), and *Angiostrongyloides* (a rat parasite).

Nematodes can cause disease in several ways. Several worm species cause blockage of the lymphatic system because of the persistence of large numbers of larvae (microfilariae), which in severe cases can cause elephantiasis. Other nema-

todes can cause skin problems ranging from dermatitis (cutaneous larva migrans, *Onchocerca volvulus*) and subcutaneous swellings (Loa Loa) to the ulcers and superinfection that can result from infection with the large Guinea worm. Various organs may be damaged by larval migration through the affected tissue, including the brain (angiostrongyloidiasis), muscles (*Trichinella*), liver (visceral larva migrans), and the eye (*Onchocerca volvulus*). Most intestinal nematodes are well adapted to living with a human host, and do not cause disease, except in heavy infestations. Hookworms can cause anemia, and the large *Ascaris* worms can cause intestinal obstruction.

The patient in this case suffered from *Strongyloides* **hyperinfection.** *Strongyloides* is usually not symptomatic in chronically infected immunocompetent hosts. However, when a patient with established intestinal strongyloidiasis is immunosuppressed with high-dose steroids, the dreaded complication of hyperinfection can occur. In *Strongyloides* hyperinfection, the immunosuppressed host is reinfected by larvae in the colon that then pass through the bloodstream to the lungs. In the alveoli, they pass from the blood to the airway and then migrate up to the pharynx where they are swallowed back down into the gastrointestinal tract. The worms are able to multiply in an uncontrolled fashion, and can cause pulmonary disease, as well as sepsis due to breaches in the integrity of the intestinal mucosa. The outcome is usually fatal, so it is important to diagnose and treat strongyloidiasis before steroids are given, if at all possible.

Thumbnail: Nematode Infections

Gastrointestinal Nematodes

Organism	*Strongyloides stercoralis*	*Ascaris lumbricoides*	*Ancylostoma duodenale; Necator americanus*	*Enterobius vermicularis*	*Anisakis*	*Trichuris trichiura*
Type of organism	Microscopic nematode	Large nematode	Hookworm	Pinworm	Nematode	Whipworm
Diseases caused	Small intestine; hyperinfection	Small intestine; intestinal, biliary obstruction, or pulmonary infiltrates	Small intestine; iron deficiency, anemia, and malnutrition	Cecum; pruritus ani	Anisakiasis; larvae burrow in stomach, intestine	Large intestine; bloody diarrhea; growth retardation
Epidemiology/ geography	Worldwide	Worldwide	Worldwide	Worldwide	Japan, Hawaii, California	Worldwide
Route of infection	Larvae penetrate skin	Ingestion of eggs	Larvae penetrate skin	Anal-oral; often spread through family	Consumption of raw marine fish	Ingestion of eggs
Diagnosis	Larvae in feces or duodenal fluid	Eggs in feces	Eggs in feces	Worms captured on adhesive tape on anus at night	Endoscopy	Eggs in feces
Treatment	Thiabendazole; albendazole	Mebendazole; pyrantel pamoate	Mebendazole	Mebendazole; albendazole; pyrantel pamoate	Endoscopy or surgery	Mebendazole

Tissue Nematodes

Organism	*Angiostrongylus cantonensis*	*Ancylostoma braziliense and others*	*Toxocara canis and others*	*Trichinella*	*Dracunculus medinensis*	*Loa Loa*	*Onchocerca volvulus*	*Brugia malayi; Brugia timori; Wuchereria bancrofti*
Type of organism	Rat lungworm	Dog hook-worm	Dog and cat roundworms	Pig roundworm	Nematode	Nematode	Nematode	Nematode
Diseases caused	Eosinophilic meningoen-cephalitis	Cutaneous larva migrans; dermatitis	Visceral larva migrans; eosinophilia; liver and other organ involvement	Trichinosis; eosinophilia, periorbital edema, myositis, fever	Guinea worm; ulcer with protruding worm; secondary infections	Loiasis; transient subcuta-neous swellings	River blindness; dermatitis; choriore-tinitis	Lymphatic filariasis (elephanti-asis); chronic lymphadenopa-thy; lymph-edema; hydrocele
Epidemiology/ geography	Pacific	Worldwide	Worldwide	Worldwide	Africa, Asia	West Africa	Africa, Central and South America	Africa, Asia
Route of infection	Consumption of raw crustaceans, snails, slugs, infested lettuce	Skin contact with eggs in dog and cat stool	Ingestion of eggs from animal stool	Ingestion of larvae from under-cooked pork and other meats	Ingestion of fresh water containing infected crustaceans	Deer fly (Chrysops) bite	Black fly bite	Mosquito bite
Diagnosis	Suggested by eosinophilia in CSF	Clinical	Biopsy; ELISA; serology	Serology; biopsy	Examination of worm	Microfilariae on blood smear	Biopsy; Mazzotti reaction to diethylcar-bamazine	Microfilariae on blood smear
Treatment	Mebendazole	Thiabendazole albendazole; ivermectin	Usually none	Symptomatic only	Removal of worm by winding around stick	Ivermectin; albendazole; diethylcar-bamazine	Surgery; ivermectin	Surgery

Strongyloides is unusual because only a few helminth species are actually able to multiply in a human host. Therefore, the worm burden in most types of infection is due to the number of worms contracted at the time of infection. In addition to *Strongyloides, Trichinella* can also reproduce in an infected host. However, the new *Trichinella* progeny are unable to mature past the larval stage. These encysted larvae can cause life-threatening immune reactions. Other parasites may repeatedly infect the same host. One example is pinworm. Although the worm has a lifespan of days, infections may persist because of repeated infection by a child transferring worms from the anus back to the mouth.

Case Conclusion The patient was treated with albendazole, but because of overwhelming infection and his poor baseline pulmonary status, he did poorly. He required increasing ventilatory support, and died 2 days later.

Key Points

▶ Eosinophilia can be an important clue to helminthic infections

▶ Patients with *Strongyloides* can develop the life-threatening hyperinfection syndrome if immunosuppressed with high-dose steroids

Questions

1. Which of the following nematode infections is spread by an insect vector?
   A. *Ascaris lumbricoides*
   B. Pinworm
   C. River blindness
   D. Hookworm
   E. Guinea worm

2. The proscription against eating pork in the Old Testament may have been a preventive measure against which infection?
   A. Strongyloidiasis
   B. Anisakiasis
   C. Trichinosis
   D. Elephantiasis
   E. Pinworm

HPI: A 52-year-old man who recently emigrated from Uganda sees a doctor for the first time, complaining of fatigue. Over the past 2 years, he has noted burning and gross blood towards the end of his urination. Upon further questioning, he says he used to take daily swims in a pond near his home in Uganda.

PE: Exam shows an enlarged liver.

Labs: Laboratories were significant for a white count of 20 with 25% eosinophils, anemia with a hematocrit of 34, and an elevated creatinine of 1.5. A urine sample is grossly bloody. Ultrasound of the kidneys shows enlargement of the right kidney. Urine shows large numbers of *Schistosoma haematobium* ova.

Thought Questions

- What is unique about the route of transmission of schistosomiasis compared to other trematodes?

- Why can an infected immigrant to the U.S. not spread schistosomiasis to other people?

Basic Science Review and Discussion

The trematodes are one of the three types of **helminths,** or worms, that cause human disease. The **trematodes,** or **flukes,** are flat nonsegmented worms. The other two types are **nematodes,** which are round, and **cestodes,** which are segmented tapeworms.

More than 200 million people are infected with schistosomiasis. Each of five species has a fresh water **snail** as an obligate intermediate host. The habitat of each snail determines the geographical distribution of disease.

Adult worms in the human host produce eggs that are excreted in the host's urine or feces. The eggs hatch in fresh water, releasing **miracidia,** which infect the snail intermediate host. The miracidia multiply asexually inside the snail, and emerge as **cercariae,** the forms that infect humans by penetrating through the skin of the unwary wader or bather. Once through the skin, the cercariae transform into **schistosomula.** The schistosomula initially migrate to the lungs and liver. After 6 weeks, they mature to the adult stage and migrate to their ultimate locations in the venous system. *Schistosoma haematobium* primarily affects the veins surrounding the urinary **bladder,** while the other schistosome species target the **mesenteric veins.** The adult worms may live up to decades in their final location. See Figure 52-1.

Schistosomiasis infection can cause disease at several stages of the life cycle. Exposure to parasites in the water may cause an acute dermatitis called **swimmer's itch.** When the adults begin to lay eggs, an acute illness may ensue, **Katayama fever,** which features fever, headache, cough, and lymphadenopathy. Egg deposition in the portal venous system may lead to portal hypertension,

hepatosplenomegaly, and potentially lethal complications. Other sequelae are caused by chronic inflammation of the target organs where the adult worms live. *Schistosoma haematobium* can cause obstruction of the urinary system. *Schistosoma mansoni, S. japonicum,* and *S. mekongi* can cause intestinal granulomatous lesions leading to gastrointestinal bleeding and iron deficiency anemia. The multiple stages of parasite migration through the body stimulate a brisk eosinophilia in many patients with schistosomiasis.

In contrast to schistosomiasis, the other trematodes all cause infection through ingestion—in most cases, of undercooked fish or seafood. Like schistosomiasis, these flukes have a snail intermediate host, but the cercariae of these species pass from the snail to a second intermediate host (fish, crustaceans, or aquatic plants), which are then ingested. Most of these species have a predilection for the gastrointestinal tract: either the intestine or the liver. *Clonorchis sinensis* and *Opisthorchis* are notable for causing chronic inflammation of the biliary tract, which can result in biliary obstruction requiring surgery. Patients with these biliary flukes have an increased incidence of cholangiocarcinoma.

Paragonimus westermani is unique among ingested flukes in that adult worms travel beyond the gastrointestinal tract to infect the lungs or brain.

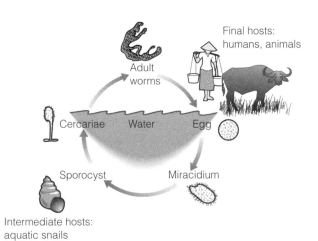

Figure 52-1 The schistosome life cycle. (Courtesy of Centers for Disease Control.)

Case Conclusion The parasitic infection is cured with two doses of **praziquantel** in 1 day. Our patient undergoes cystoscopy to evaluate the bladder, which shows numerous papillomatous irregularities. A right ureteral stent is placed to relieve the hydronephrosis of his right kidney.

Thumbnail: Schistosomes

Blood Flukes

Organism	*Schistosoma haematobium*	*Schistosoma japonicum*	*Schistosoma mansoni*	*Schistosoma mekongi*
Type of organism	Trematode; blood fluke	Trematode; blood fluke	Trematode; blood fluke	Trematode; blood fluke
Diseases caused	Veins of urinary bladder, colon, liver	Veins of intestine, liver	Veins of colon, liver	Veins of intestine, liver
Geography/ epidemiology	Africa, Middle East	China, Philippines, Japan	Africa, Middle East, South America, the Caribbean	Mekong Delta of Thailand
Route of infection	Larvae penetrate skin in snail-infested water	Larvae penetrate skin in snail-infested water	Larvae penetrate skin in snail-infested water	Larvae penetrate skin in snail-infested water
Diagnosis	Ova in urine or feces	Ova in feces	Ova in feces	Ova in feces
Treatment	Praziquantel	Praziquantel	Praziquantel; oxamniquine	Praziquantel

Other Flukes

Organism	*Clonorchis sinensis*	*Fasciola hepatica*	*Fasciolopsis buski*	*Heterophyes heterophyes*	*Metagonimus yokogawai*	*Opisthorchis felineus/viverrini*	*Paragonimus westermani*
Type of organism	Chinese liver fluke	Sheep liver fluke (humans are incidental hosts)	Giant intestinal fluke	Intestinal fish fluke	Intestinal fish fluke	Southeast Asian liver fluke	Lung fluke
Diseases caused	Bile duct obstruction; cholangio-carcinoma	Migration through liver parenchyma to bile ducts	Small intestine	Small intestine	Small intestine	Bile duct	Paragonimiasis (lung, brain cysts)
Geography/ epidemiology	East Asia	Worldwide, especially in sheep-raising areas	East and Southeast Asia	East Asia, Middle East	East Asia, Middle East, Russia, Balkans, Spain	Eastern Europe, Russia, Thailand	Asia, North central Africa, South America
Route of infection	Eating under-cooked fish	Eating contaminated watercress or other aquatic plants	Eating contaminated water plants	Eating uncooked fish	Eating uncooked fish	Eating uncooked fish	Eating raw crabs and other freshwater crustaceans
Diagnosis	Ova in feces	Ova in feces or bile	Ova or parasites in stool	Ova in stool	Ova in stool	Ova in stool	Microscopy of sputum or feces; serology
Treatment	Praziquantel; albendazole	Bithionol; triclabendazole	Praziquantel	Praziquantel	Praziquantel	Praziquantel	Praziquantel; bithionol

Key Points

▶ The trematodes fall in two major categories: (1) the schistosoma blood flukes, acquired through the skin, and (2) the liver, intestinal, and lung flukes, acquired through ingestion

▶ All trematodes have an aquatic snail as an intermediate host

▶ The treatment of choice for most trematode (and cestode) infections is praziquantel

Questions

1. A 43-year-old man from Asia presents with multiple lung nodules. Which of the following flukes may be responsible?
   A. *Clonorchis sinensis*
   B. *Opisthorchis viverrini*
   C. *Paragonimus westermani*
   D. *Fasciolopsis buski*
   E. *Schistosoma mansoni*

2. Praziquantel is the drug of choice for almost all trematode infections. Its mechanism of action is:
   A. Stimulates the neuromuscular junction
   B. Opens calcium channels
   C. Affects folate synthesis
   D. Disrupts microtubule function
   E. Forms free radicals

HPI: A 54-year-old woman who grew up in rural Brazil presents to a gastroenterologist complaining of odynophagia and dysphagia, with frequent episodes of regurgitating undigested food about 20 minutes after eating. The symptoms have gotten progressively worse over the past year. Aside from two hospitalizations for right middle lobe pneumonia over the past year, her health has been good. She denies any chest pain, dyspnea, edema, or palpitations. She has had no problems with abdominal pain or constipation. She denies any changes in her skin, Raynaud's phenomenon, or any history of autoimmune disease. She does not smoke or drink.

PE: T 37.5°C BP 120/70 HR 80 RR 14
The patient is a thin woman in no acute distress.
She has no lymphadenopathy. Her lungs are clear, and her heart has a regular rhythm, with no gallops. Her abdomen is soft and nontender. She has no edema. Her skin and nailbeds are normal.
A barium swallow shows an enormously dilated esophagus with constriction at the lower esophageal sphincter. There is minimal passage of contrast into the stomach on follow-up films.
An ECG shows normal sinus rhythm, with normal-sized heart chambers, and an echocardiogram confirms the normal heart size.
A serologic test for *Trypanosoma cruzi* is positive.

Thought Questions

- How could the patient's episodes of pneumonia be connected to the rest of her symptoms?

- What kind of cardiac problems was she evaluated for, and why?

Basic Science Review and Discussion

Trypanosomes are protozoan parasites; two species are human pathogens, transmitted by insect bites. *Trypanosoma cruzi* is found in Latin America and causes **Chagas disease.** *Trypanosoma brucei* is found in Africa and causes **African sleeping sickness.** *Trypanosoma cruzi* has both intracellular and extracellular phases in its life cycle, whereas *Trypanosoma brucei* is an exclusively extracellular parasite.

Trypanosoma cruzi is transmitted from a mammalian reservoir to humans by triatomine insects, known as kissing bugs. Kissing bugs tend to infest poorer dwellings in rural areas. The insect takes up the parasite while feeding on a blood meal from an infected mammal. The parasites multiply in the bug's gastrointestinal tract. When the insect bites a human host, the parasites are then transmitted in the bug's feces onto the skin. If these feces contaminate mucous membranes or breaks in the skin, the parasites are able to enter the bloodstream and establish a new infection. Chagas disease can also be transmitted through blood transfusions, and the blood supply in Latin America is routinely screened for this dieseaes.

The acute phase of Chagas disease is often subclinical. A skin lesion, or **chagoma,** may form at the parasite's site of entry through the skin. If the parasite enters through the conjuctiva, then local swelling around the eye can occur. These local symptoms are followed by systemic symptoms including fever, anorexia, malaise, hepatosplenomegaly, and generalized lymphadenopathy. These symptoms resolve within weeks, although the parasitic infection persists.

Less than one third of patients with chronic trypanosomal infection will eventually develop the symptoms of chronic Chagas disease, and this chronic phase may occur years to decades after the initial infection. Chagas disease causes **cardiomyopathy,** which can result in heart failure, arrhythmias, and thromboembolic disease. Chagas disease can also affect gastrointestinal motility. In the esophagus, **achalasia** can occur, resulting in dysphagia and odynophagia, megaesophagus, and predispose the patient to aspiration. In the colon, poor motility can cause abdominal pain and constipation, megacolon, and lead to acute colonic obstruction, volvulus, or perforation. The course of Chagas disease is greatly exacerbated by immunosuppression.

The diagnosis of Chagas disease requires a history of exposure, through immigration, travel, or possibly blood transfusion. Acute Chagas disease is diagnosed by detecting parasites in the blood through microscopic examination or PCR. Traditionally, the yield of blood examinations was improved by a technique called **xenodiagnosis:** uninfected kissing bugs are deliberately allowed to sample the patient's blood, and then the bugs themselves are examined for evidence of the parasite. Chronic Chagas disease is usually diagnosed through serology.

Chagas disease may be treated with the drugs nifurtimox or benznidazole. Whereas these drugs can eliminate the parasite from up to 70% of acutely infected patients, the benefit in chronic infection is much smaller—the goal is to slow the progression of chronic sequelae. The sequelae of Chagas disease are usually treated symptomatically: car-

diomyopathy is treated with heart failure medications and pacemakers if necessary, esophageal disease may require lower esophageal sphincter dilation or surgery, and colonic disease may eventually require surgery as well.

Case Conclusion The patient begins a course of nifurtimox, but stops it early because of abdominal pain and insomnia. She then tries benznidazole, but develops a rash. She decides not to try any more antiparasitic treatments, as the benefits of these drugs are limited at this chronic stage of disease.

She undergoes a balloon dilation of her lower esophageal sphincter, which gives her relief for several months, but her symptoms recur and she needs two more repeat dilations. Finally, she undergoes surgery, wide esophagocardiomyectomy of the anterior gastroesophageal resection, with a valvuloplasty to prevent reflux, and her symptoms are relieved.

Thumbnail: Trypanosomal Diseases

Organism	*Trypanosoma cruzi*	*Trypanosoma brucei gambiense* (W. Africa); *Trypanosoma brucei rhodesiense* (E. Africa)
Type of organism	Trypanosome	Trypanosome
Diseases caused	Chagas disease	African sleeping sickness
Epidemiology/geography	Kissing bug bite; Latin America	Tsetse fly bite; Africa
Diagnosis	Acute: blood smears; xenodiagnosis chronic: serology	Demonstration of parasite in blood, CSF, bone marrow, lymphatic tissue or skin lesions
Treatment	Nifurtimox; benznidazole	Stage I (hemolymphatic): suramin; stage II (meningoencephalitic): difluoromethylornithine (W. Africa) or melarsoprol (E. Africa)

Key Points

▶ Trypanosomes cause two distinct illnesses in distinct geographical areas: Chagas disease in Latin America, and sleeping sickness in Africa

▶ The chronic sequelae of Chagas disease are cardiomyopathy, achalasia, and colonic dysmotility; antiparasitic therapy at the acute stage of infection can prevent these sequelae, but once the sequelae have developed, antiparasitic therapy may slow their progression but will not reverse them

---

Questions

1. Which of the following is a chronic sequela of Chagas disease?

   A. Cardiomyopathy
   B. Lytic lesions of the bone
   C. Lymphedema
   D. Malabsorption
   E. Alopecia

2. Which of the following is an exclusively extracellular protozoan parasite?

   A. *Plasmodium falciparum*
   B. *Babesia microti*
   C. *Leishmania donovani*
   D. *Trypanosoma brucei*
   E. *Pneumocystis carinii*

Case 1
1. B
2. C
3. E
4. D

Case 2
1. D
2. C

Case 3
1. B
2. D

Case 4
1. D
2. A

Case 5
1. B
2. A

Case 6
1. C
2. D

Case 7
1. C
2. B
3. D

Case 8
1. E
2. A

Case 9
1. C
2. B

Case 10
1. C
2. E

Case 11
1. E
2. D

Case 12
1. B
2. C

Case 13
1. C
2. A

Case 14
1. E
2. B

Case 15
1. D
2. B
3. C

Case 16
1. D
2. E

Case 17
1. E
2. B
3. A

Case 18
1. A
2. B

Case 19
1. A
2. E

Case 20
1. B
2. B
3. C
4. C

Case 21
1. E
2. B

Case 22
1. D
2. E

Case 23
1. C
2. D

Case 24
1. E
2. D
3. B
4. B

Case 25
1. D
2. C

Case 26
1. C
2. E

Case 27
1. C
2. A

Case 28
1. C
2. D
3. D

Case 29
1. A
2. B

Case 30
1. E
2. B

Case 31
1. B
2. D

Case 32
1. B
2. A

Case 33
1. A
2. D

Case 34
1. E
2. C

Case 35
1. B
2. D

Case 36
1. C
2. B

Case 37
1. E
2. D
3. D
4. C

Case 38
1. D
2. C
3. D

Case 39
1. A
2. D

Case 40
1. C
2. D

Case 41
1. B
2. D

Case 42
1. E
2. C

Case 43
1. E
2. A
3. E

Case 44
1. E
2. B
3. C

Case 45
1. C
2. E

Case 46
1. E
2. C

Case 47
1. B
2. C

Case 48
1. B
2. D

Case 49
1. B
2. B

Case 50
1. E
2. C

Case 51
1. C
2. C

Case 52
1. C
2. B

Case 53
1. A
2. D

Part II

Immunology

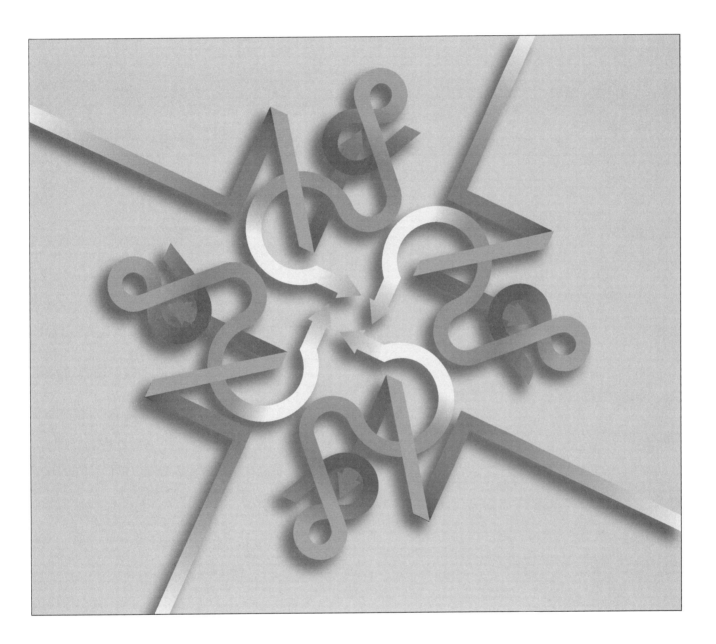

> **HPI:** IL is a 45-year-old diabetic man **who had a kidney transplant** 2 weeks ago. IL now presents with **shortness of breath, severe hypertension, rapid weight gain,** and **oliguria** (decreased urine production). He has gained 10 pounds over the last 2 days and his blood pressure has increased from 130/85 to the 190s/100s. He has also had a progressive decline in urine output to 500 mL/day. He reports increased shortness of breath with new onset of **orthopnea.** The patient is taking **cyclophosphamide for immunosuppression.**
>
> **PE:** T 38.0°C HR 85 BP **190/105** RR 22 SaO$_2$ 96% on room air
> On exam, he is in mild respiratory distress. His exam is significant for diffusely **increased skin turgor, bibasilar crackles** to the midchest, a **cardiac flow murmur,** a **distended abdomen** with left lower quadrant tenderness to palpation, and significant lower extremity **pitting edema.**
>
> **Labs:** He has a normal CBC but an elevated potassium. His serum **creatinine is elevated** at 5.0. UA reveals **3+ protein** and WBC. Blood cultures are negative.

Thought Questions

- What is cell-mediated immunity and how does it defend against invading pathogens and foreign cells?

- What is the major histocompatibility complex and its involvement in antigen presentation? What are cytokines and how are they involved?

- How does tolerance to self-antigen develop among T-lymphocytes?

- How are foreign cells recognized and eliminated? What implication does this have on allogeneic transplant rejection?

- What is the pathogenesis of the different forms of transplant rejection and their clinical manifestations? How is transplant rejection medically suppressed?

Basic Science Review and Discussion

Cell-mediated immunity, an arm of the adaptive immune system, is involved in the surveillance of not only the extracellular but also the **intracellular compartment** for the elimination of pathogens. Its mediators not only help B-cells produce antibodies to neutralize extracellular pathogens but also eliminate intracellular pathogens by killing cells that harbor these pathogens. Targets of cellular immunity include mycobacteria, fungi, and cells viewed as defective or foreign, such as tumor cells and transplanted cells. Like the humoral immune system, the cellular immune system must be capable of (1) **specific recognition** of its targets, (2) processing and **presenting antigen** to effector cells involved in the immune response, (3) activating the most appropriate components of the immune response to optimize **pathogen elimination,** and (4) **establishing memory** of these pathogens for more rapid elimination upon re-exposure.

T-Lymphocyte Development T-lymphocytes are the primary effectors of cellular immunity. They arise from lymphoid progenitors in the bone marrow that mature and eventually migrate to the thymus where they undergo further development. On the next page is a diagram of T-cell development and the key receptors present in each stage. (See Figure 54-1.)

Antigen recognition in T-cells is mediated by the **T-cell receptor (TCR).** TCR is similar to the B-cell receptor in that it consists of two subunits, α and β, homologous to immunoglobulin heavy and light chains. The α-chain genes include multiple alleles for the V, J, and C regions. The β-chain genes include multiple alleles for the V, D, J, and C regions. The final TCR product consists of recombinations of these alleles within each region of the α- or β-chains. This rearrangement during development allows for the production of an almost infinite array of antigen-recognizing TCRs using relatively few genes.

Following migration to the thymus, T-cells undergo a process whereby they develop **the ability to distinguish self from nonself.** Within the thymus, T-cells are exposed to thymic epithelial cells and antigen-presenting cells (macrophages and dendritic cells) that expose them to the majority of self-peptides. Immature T-cells that recognize self-antigen are destroyed by **negative selection.** Those that successfully recognize MHC-I or MHC-II receptors, and not self antigens, undergo **positive selection.** Those that fail to recognize MHC at all die of attrition.

CD4+ T-cells become **T-helper cells,** which become restricted to recognizing antigen complexed to **class II MHC.** These cells support T- and B-cells in orchestrating the adaptive immune response. **CD8+ T-cells** become **cytotoxic T-cells,** restricted to recognizing antigen bound to **class I MHC** and to the lysis of virus-infected, tumor, or foreign cells. CD4+ and CD8+ T cells are released from the thymus into the bloodstream to mediate cellular immunity.

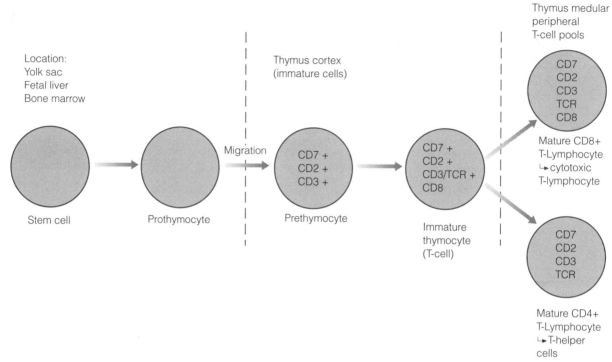

Figure 54-1 T-cell development begins at a primary hematopoietic site such as the bone marrow and ends in the thymus. In the thymus, T-cells undergo T-cell antigen receptor (TCR) rearrangement. The T-cell population is then selected for tolerance to self antigen and for reactivity to self-MHC receptors that will eventually bear foreign antigen. The immature thymocyte expresses TCR as well as CD4 and CD8 concurrently. T-cells are fully mature when they express either CD4 or CD8. CD4+ cells differentiate into T-helper cells that orchestrate the adaptive immune response. CD8+ cells develop into cytotoxic T-lymphocytes that kill infected cells as well as neoplastic and foreign cells.

Cell-Mediated Immunity   Cell-mediated immunity is most easily demonstrated by the process of eliminating viral infection. Viruses have both extracellular and intracellular phases. An antigen-presenting cell (APC) may take up virus in two ways—through **phagocytosis** and through **direct viral infection.** Viruses that are phagocytized are fused with vesicles containing digestive enzymes. Viral peptides are then processed, bound to class II MHC molecules, and presented on the APC cell surface to CD4+ T-lymphocytes. The T-cells recognize the antigen-MHC complex via the TCR, stabilized by the CD4 receptor. A **costimulatory signal** between the APC's **B7 receptor** and the T-helper cell's **CD28 receptor** is required as a "confirmation" signal for T-cell activation. This up-regulates **CD40 ligand** expression in T-helper cells, which serves to drive B-cell **isotype switching,** a key step in antibody **affinity maturation** (see Figure 55-2 in Humoral Immunity section).

T-helper cells differentiate and are activated to secrete signaling peptides, or **cytokines,** depending on the nature of the pathogen to be eliminated. T-helper cells universally secrete **IL-2** upon activation, which stimulates proliferation of many immune cells including B-cells, cytotoxic lymphocytes (CTL), and T-helper cells. T-helper cells differentiate into two types: T$_h$1-cells and T$_h$2-cells. **T$_h$1-cell** differentiation is stimulated by APC-secreted **IL-12. T$_h$1-cells** primarily

promote immunity against small extracellular pathogens such as viruses and bacteria, eliminated through phagocytosis and cell killing. Both CD40L and the cytokine **interferon-γ (IFN-γ)** promote B-cell isotype switching toward IgG production. IFN-γ also superactivates macrophage phagocytosis and antigen presentation by up-regulating their oxidative killing machinery and MHC expression, respectively. T$_h$1-cells also secrete **tumor necrosis factor (TNF),** which activates neutrophil phagocytosis and CTL-mediated elimination of virally infected cells.

T$_h$2-cells are differentiated toward eliminating large extracellular pathogens, such as parasites. T$_h$2-cell differentiation is driven by **IL-4,** secreted by mast cells and basophils after a parasite encounter. T$_h$2-cells in turn secrete more cytokines like IL-4 itself, which promotes B-cell isotype switching to IgE, the primary anti-parasitic antibody. **IL-5** promotes eosinophil function, the primary parasite killer cell. Eosinophils recognize the Fc portion of IgE via **Fcε receptors,** which activate the extracellular release of **major basic protein** and other enzymes that attack the parasite's cell membranes. See Figures 54-2 and 54-3.

To initiate intracellular compartment surveillance, APCs take up virus through direct infection. Viral peptides produced during replication are processed differently than

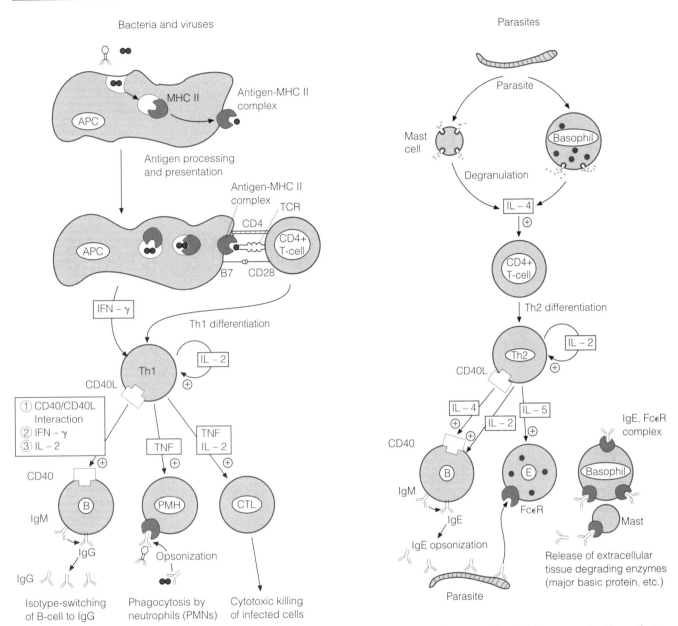

Figure 54-2 Cell-mediated immunity against intracellular pathogens, such as viruses. This pathway uses class I MHC to present antigens that are found in the cytosolic compartment of any cell. CD8+ T-lymphocytes are subsequently activated and mature into cytotoxic T-cells, which kill infected cells. T-helper cells are also involved in augmenting this immune response.

those that are phagocytized; intracellularly replicated viral particles are ultimately associated with class I MHC molecules. **This antigen-MHC I complex specifically activates CD8+ T-lymphocytes, which are then stimulated to differentiate into cytotoxic lymphocytes.** One important molecular interaction includes the up-regulated CD40L/CD40 receptors.

The CD40L-CD40 interaction activates CTLs to produce several cell-killing mediators. **Fas ligand** surface expression is up-regulated, which binds to **Fas** on infected cells and thereby induces cell **apoptosis**. The CD40L-CD40 interaction also promotes the production of **perforin, granzymes,** and

caspases that kill cells by inserting into the plasma membrane of the infected cell, forming a pore that leads to cell lysis. CTLs recognize virus-infected cells by their TCRs binding to class I MHC molecules, presenting the specific viral peptide to which they are sensitized. This activates the cytotoxic machinery described above. Finally, the T-helper cell's CD40L also binds CD40 on B-cells, promoting activation and antibody production.

Immunologic memory to a pathogen is established through the differentiation of a subpopulation of activated T-helper, B-, and CD8+ T-cells into their own respective memory cells. If the body is re-exposed to the antigen, it

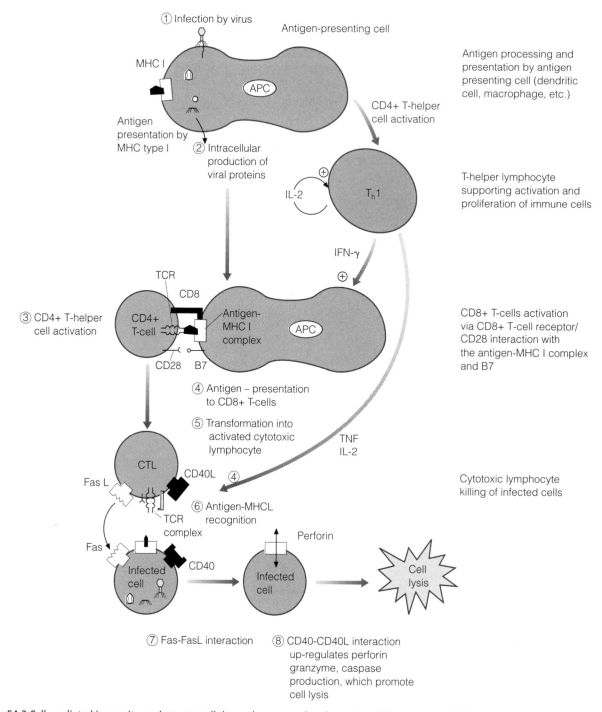

① Infection by virus

Antigen-presenting cell

MHC I

Antigen processing and presentation by antigen presenting cell (dendritic cell, macrophage, etc.)

APC

CD4+ T-helper cell activation

Antigen presentation by MHC type I

② Intracellular production of viral proteins

IL-2 ⊕ T_h1

T-helper lymphocyte supporting activation and proliferation of immune cells

IFN-γ ⊕

TCR

CD8

③ CD4+ T-helper cell activation

CD4+ T-cell

Antigen-MHC I complex

APC

CD8+ T-cells activation via CD8+ T-cell receptor/ CD28 interaction with the antigen-MHC I complex and B7

CD28   B7

④ Antigen – presentation to CD8+ T-cells

⑤ Transformation into activated cytotoxic lymphocyte

TNF IL-2

CTL

Fas L

CD40L ④

Cytotoxic lymphocyte killing of infected cells

⑥ Antigen-MHCL recognition

TCR complex

Perforin

Fas

Infected cell

CD40

Infected cell

Cell lysis

⑦ Fas-FasL interaction

⑧ CD40-CD40L interaction up-regulates perforin granzyme, caspase production, which promote cell lysis

Figure 54-3 Cell-mediated immunity against extracellular pathogens, such as bacteria and fungi. Class II MHC are used to present antigens endocytosed by antigen-presenting cells, such as macrophages to CD4+ cells. These cells are activated and mature into T-helper cells that subsequently promote B-lymphocyte maturation, plasma cell antibody production, and the phagocytic activity of macrophages, neutrophils, and eosinophils in the elimination of bacteria and fungi.

will be able to mount a faster, more effective immune response with more efficient elimination of the pathogen, the process we commonly refer to as "immunity."

Clinical Discussion

Transplant Rejection   There are two types of allograft rejection: humoral (antibody-mediated) and cellular (T-

Table 54-1 Types of rejection and pathogenesis

Rejection Type	Timing	Pathogenesis
Hyperacute rejection	Minutes to < 48 hr	• Classically upon reperfusion of allograft → graft failure • Preformed antibodies to HLA, ABO Ag, and vascular endothelium are in circulation and bind immediately to vasculature, causing complement activation, platelet aggregation, and thrombosis → vasculitis and ischemia
Accelerated rejection	7–10 days	• Humoral: anti-HLA antibodies • Cellular: T-lymphocyte mediated, from prior sensitization • 60% graft loss
Acute rejection	7 days–3 months	• Development of cellular and humoral immunity, often due to inadequate immunosuppression • Signs and symptoms: graft pain, warmth, edema, fever, malaise, fatigue, and signs of specific organ failure
Chronic rejection	Months to years	• Unclear etiology: presumably humoral and cellular • Signs and symptoms of specific organ failure • Diagnosed by biopsy, showing concentric vessel narrowing and ischemic disease of the graft

lymphocyte-mediated). In **humoral rejection,** antibodies are formed by B-cells that recognize foreign antigen on allograft tissue. These antibodies bind allograft tissue and activate complement, which leads to platelet aggregation and thrombosis. Ischemic injury and ultimately transplant rejection ensues.

There are two pathways in **cell-mediated allograft rejection:** the direct and indirect pathways. In the **direct pathway,** recipient CD4+ T-helper cells and CD8+ T-cells recognize foreign class II and class I **human leukocyte antigens** (HLA, the MHC in humans), respectively, on **dendritic cells** (APCs) carried in the donor organ. The T-cells are then activated and cause a local increase in vascular permeability, lymphocyte and macrophage infiltration, and cell lysis of allograft tissue. In the **indirect pathway,** foreign HLA is processed like any foreign antigen and presented by the host's own APCs to T-cells; this eventually leads to transplant rejection.

Therefore, an important clinical issue is **HLA matching** of the donor to the transplant recipient. There are six HLA types to match: HLA-A, HLA-B, and HLA-C (those that contribute to class I HLA) and HLA-DP, HLA-DQ, and HLA-DR (those in class II HLA). Individuals are likely to match with siblings, having a 25% chance of matching. However, the likelihood of matching falls dramatically between unrelated individuals. Matching affords prolonged survival of the graft. With the exception of identical twins, lifelong immunosuppression is necessary to prolong graft survival and is accomplished with such drugs as azathioprine, steroids, cyclosporine, antilymphocyte globulins, and monoclonal anti-T-cell antibodies. Immunosuppression unfortunately also makes the recipient susceptible to opportunistic infections. (See Table 54-1.)

Case Conclusion With the suspicion of acute kidney transplant rejection, our patient is started on prednisone and stabilized hemodynamically with diuretics and ACE inhibitors. His immunosuppressive dosing regimen is increased and his symptoms eventually resolve. At this time, IL continues to have normal functioning of his kidney allograft.

Thumbnail: Cytokines and Their Actions

Cytokine	Cell origin	Cell target	Stimulus for release and subsequent actions
Cytokines Released from Local Insult			
IL-1	Macrophages Infected cells	T- and B-cells Neutrophils Epithelial cells Dendritic cells	Secretion stimulated by infection → • Acts on hypothalamus to induce fever • Stimulates cell growth • T-cell differentiation, IL-2 production
IL-6	Macrophages Neutrophils	Hepatocytes T- and B-cells	Phagocytosis of microbe stimulates → • Production of acute phase proteins (e.g., ESR) • Promotes T- and B-cell growth and differentiation
TNF-α	Macrophages Mast cells/basophils Eosinophils NK cells T- and B-cells	All cells except RBCs	Local tissue damage or infection → • Induces fever, anorexia, shock • Causes capillary leak syndrome • Enhanced cytotoxicity, NK cell function • Acute phase protein synthesis
TNF-β	T- and B-cells	All except RBCs	• Cell cytotoxicity, lymph node, and spleen development
Cytokines of Anti-viral Immunity			
IFN-α/β	Macrophages Infected cells	All cells, especially neighboring cells	Viral infection → induces antiviral state; antitumor activity • Up-regulates MHC class I antigen expression • ↓ Protein synthesis in infected cell • ↑ RNase expression → degrades viral RNA
Cytokines of T-helper Type 1 Cells			
IFN-γ	T_h1 cells NK cells	Macrophage NK cells B-cells Dendritic cells	Bacterial/viral infection → antigen presentation • Promotes T_h1 cell differentiation • Regulates macrophage and NK cell activation • Stimulates B-cell growth and IgG isotype switching
IL-2	T_h1 cells	T-helper cells CD8+ cells B-cells	• Activates all branches of adaptive immunity to proliferate and differentiate (activates cytokine production, effector functions)
IL-12	APC: macrophages, dendritic cells	T-helper cells CD8+ T-cells NK cells	• Promotes T_h1 proliferation • CTL activation • NK cell activation
Cytokines of T-helper Type 2 Cells			
IL-4	T_h2 cells	B-cells T-helper cells	Helminthic infection and allergen exposure → • Stimulates B-cell growth; IgE isotype switching • Recruits eosinophils • Promotes T_h2 cell proliferation • Inhibits macrophages/delayed-type reaction
IL-5	T_h2 cells	B-cells Eosinophils	• Activates eosinophils IgE binding via FcεR • Stimulates B-cell differentiation
IL-10	T_h2 cells	Macrophages	• Inhibits macrophage activation
Cytokines of Mast Cells			
Histamine Serotonin	Mast cells	Vascular endothelium	Helminthic infection and allergen exposure → • Increased vascular permeability → hypotension, edema
Lipid Mediators		Smooth muscle cells	• Bronchiole contraction → bronchospasm • Intestinal hypermotility → diarrhea

Key Points

▶ Cell-mediated immunity is the arm of the immune system specialized in targeting intracellular pathogens (e.g., viruses, mycobacteria, fungi), as well as tumor cells and foreign cells

▶ Specific recognition of pathogens is accomplished by antigen presentation on major histocompatibility complexes of antigen-presenting cells to T-lymphocytes

▶ Activated T-helper cells release cytokines that activate and support all branches of the adaptive immune system

▶ A subset of T-cells and B-cells persists as memory cells that can respond with great efficacy upon re-exposure of the body to the original pathogen

Questions

1. The following is a series of immunological events that occurred during the course of IL's transplant rejection. Which step did *not* occur?

    A. Antigen-presenting cells from the donor and the recipient take up HLA protein from the allograft and present it to recipient T-helper cells on class I and class II HLA receptors

    B. B-cells are activated by T_h2 cells to proliferate and isotype switch to producing IgG, which bind to allograft vascular endothelium and activate complement, causing thrombosis and ischemic injury to the graft

    C. Activated T-helper cells secrete IL-2 and thereby promote proliferation and maturation of B-cells, CD4+ T-cells, CD8+ T-cells, and monocytes into plasma cells, T_h1 cells, cytotoxic T-lymphocytes, and macrophages, respectively

    D. TNF-α is released from activated macrophages, creating symptoms such as fever and malaise, promoting allograft edema by increasing local vascular permeability, and promoting allograft rejection by enhancing NK cell cytotoxicity

    E. The CD40-CD40L interaction between allograft dendritic cells and IL's T-helper cells promote cytotoxic lymphocyte activity by up-regulating *Fas* ligand receptor expression, which binds *Fas* on infected cells and induces apoptosis of that cell

2. There is an immunodeficiency of the interferon-γ receptor that leads to serious infections caused by the BCG vaccine for *Mycobacterium tuberculosis* and nontuberculous mycobacteria. What immune machinery would be defective in this deficiency?

    A. There is a lack of signal to the hypothalamus to induce enough of a febrile reaction to eliminate mycobacterial infection

    B. This deficiency yields a defective mechanism of specific antigen recognition, thereby shielding mycobacterial species from immune recognition

    C. This deficiency prevents the up-regulation of MHC class I and RNase expression, thus preventing intracellular mycobacteria from having their antigen presented to T-helper cells as well as preventing degradation of the pathogen's genomic material

    D. This deficiency prevents the proliferation of subtype 1 T-helper cells and the subsequent activation of oxidative killing by macrophages required to fully eliminate phagocytized mycobacteria

    E. This deficiency prevents the activation of B-cells to isotype switch toward IgE production, preventing the elimination of mycobacteria

HPI: SM is a 25-year-old African-American woman who presents with a **fever, "butterfly" facial rash, oral lesions,** and **joint pain.** She began to experience fatigue and malaise 4 weeks ago. She then developed a persistent low-grade fever and painful oral ulcers. She then noticed discomfort in both her wrists and knees, which has worsened over the past week. After a few days of lying in bed, she decided to step outside "to get some sun" and subsequently developed a rash over her nose and cheeks. In addition, she notes sharp **chest pain upon inspiration.** She was previously healthy, taking no medications. She has two aunts who have "some sort of skin disease."

PE: T 38.5°C HR 86 BP 135/85 RR 20 SaO₂ 98%

On exam, SM is ill appearing, in no acute distress. Her exam is significant for an **erythematous, raised rash over her nose and cheeks.** She has multiple **ulcerated lesions on her labia and gingiva** and cervical lymphadenopathy. She has bilaterally symmetric diminished lung movement with diffuse crackles and a palpable spleen tip. She has grossly normal-appearing **wrists and knees with tenderness** upon palpation and passive flexion. No neurologic deficits.

Labs: WBC 3500/μL Hgb 10.0 Hct 30% Plt 105,000/μL; PT 13 seconds **PTT 42 seconds; Coombs' test +; antinuclear antibody (ANA) +; anti-Sm antibody +; RPR +.**

Thought Questions

- What are the fundamental functions of the adaptive immune system?

- What is humoral immunity and what function does it serve in the defense against invading pathogens? How does humoral immunity eliminate such pathogens?

- How do effectors of humoral immunity develop the ability to distinguish between self and nonself?

- What diseases occur when there are derangements in the ability to distinguish between self and nonself? How are these diseases diagnosed and treated?

Basic Science Review and Discussion

Roughly speaking, there are two compartments in the body that require immune surveillance: the extracellular and intracellular space. Extracellular pathogens include bacteria and toxic particles such as exotoxins; intracellular pathogens include viruses and mycobacteria (although these, too, have an extracellular phase). Because extracellular pathogens float freely outside of the cell, soluble antibodies are required to recognize and attack them. Intracellular pathogens, however, successfully hide from such antibodies. The immune system protects all other cells by sacrificing infected cells in order to eliminate the pathogen within.

Antibodies Antibodies, or **immunoglobulins (Ig),** are products of antigen-activated B-lymphocytes and are the main effectors of humoral immunity. They provide the function of **pathogen recognition** by binding to specific portions of a pathogen's molecular structure, called an **epitope.** Epitopes can include any molecule, such as peptides, carbohydrates, lipids, and nucleic acids. This binding serves to neutralize and tag the particle for final elimination through phagocytosis. Figure 55-1 is a diagram of an IgG antibody.

There are five immunoglobulin isotypes: IgG, IgM, IgE, IgA, and IgD, each with their own functional niche. Upon activa-

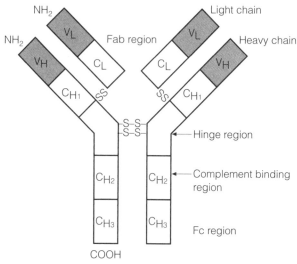

Figure 55-1 Schematic structure of the immunoglobulin G molecule. The basic structure of all antibodies consists of two heavy chains and two light chains covalently linked by disulfide bonds. There is a variable region, which includes both amino termini of the heavy and light chains, and serves to *recognize* antigen through specific epitope binding. The constant regions, of which there are three per heavy chain and one per light chain, *communicate* with and thereby activate the rest of the immune system through various mechanisms. The Fc (constant) region includes portions that bind C1q of the classic complement pathway as well as a portion that binds Fc receptors found on macrophages, natural killer cells, B-cells, neutrophils, and eosinophils.

tion of the humoral immune response, the primary antibody raised against extracellular pathogens is **IgM,** a pentameric molecule that generally has a low **affinity** (single molecular binding force) but high **avidity** (summed binding force from having more points of attachment) to an antigen. This IgM response is followed by the development and proliferation of **IgG,** a monomeric antibody that has high affinity but low avidity (strong binding with fewer points of attachment) to that same antigen. Both IgM and IgG activate the complement cascade and both serve as B-cell surface antigen receptors, which stimulate B-cell proliferation and differentiation into antibody-secreting **plasma cells.**

IgA is the major antibody found in secretions and serves the purpose of protecting mucosal surfaces from invading microorganisms. **IgE** is the major antibody elicited in allergic reactions and antiparasitic humoral immunity. **IgD** is present on mature B-cell surfaces, although its role has not yet been elucidated. Table 55-1 lists some of the basic characteristics of the five antibody classes.

B-Lymphocytes and Antibody Development B-lymphocytes are the primary cell mediators of humoral immunity. Their primary function is to produce antibodies that neutralize pathogens by recognition of specific antigenic epitopes. B-cells arise from pluripotent stem cells that differentiate into lymphoid progenitors in the bone marrow and fetal liver. They recognize the Fc region of IgG as well as opsonizing complement components that facilitate phagocytosis of antigen for subsequent presentation. They also recognize whole, unprocessed extracellular antigen through surface-bound Igs, which serve as B-cell receptors for B-cell activation. In order to allow for recognition of such a vast diversity of possible epitopes, B-cells have developed a mechanism of creating an equally vast and diverse repertoire of antibodies from relatively few genes. This is accomplished through two stages: (1) **antigen-independent rearrangement** of immunoglobulin gene segments and

(2) **antigen-dependent somatic mutation** (point mutation) of these genes. In the first stage, heavy chain genes result from a combinatorial rearrangement of the V, D, J, and C segments. Light chains, which are either of the κ or λ subtype, are generated by the rearrangement of V and J segments. Given 10,500 possible heavy chain segments and 320 possible light chain segments over 3 million possible antibodies can be produced. Somatic mutation of these rearrangements followed by positive selection of B-cells that produce antibodies with progressively higher affinity to antigen, a strongly binding, highly specific antibody is produced in a process termed **affinity maturation.** This process yields a B-cell that produces one antibody type. But within the population of B-cells in an individual, a virtually infinite array of antibodies that recognize almost any molecule can be produced.

Development of Tolerance to Self-Antigen Random rearrangement and somatic mutation of developing B-cells generate self-reactive antibodies that must be changed or eliminated to avoid self-damage. **Central B-cell tolerance** occurs in immature B-cells within the bone marrow where they first develop. Those cells that strongly interact with widely expressed self antigens are **negatively selected** through induction of apoptosis. In addition, self-reacting B-cells also undergo **B-cell receptor editing** by reactivating their Ig gene recombination machinery to modify the receptor specificity. This "pruning" process occurs continually in the B-cell population as it expands and refines it ability to differentiate between benign and nonbenign particles, self and nonself. **Peripheral B-cell tolerance** occurs once mature B-cells are released into circulation. Those B-cells that repeatedly recognize self-antigen becomes anergic, or immunologically inactivated.

Antibody-Mediated Immunity Development of antibody-mediated immunity begins with a new infection by a pathogen, such as a bacterium or parasite. **Pattern-recognized antigens** such as lipopolysaccharide (LPS) on

Table 55-1 Properties of immunoglobulins

Property	IgG	IgA	IgM	IgD	IgE
Structure	Monomer	Monomer/dimer	Monomer/pentamer	Monomer	Monomer
Function	1. Secondary antibody response 2. Complement activation 3. B-cell antigen receptor 4. Placentally transferred Ig	Secretory immunoglobulin preventing microbial attachment to mucous membranes	1. Primary antibody response 2. Complement activation 3. B-cell antigen receptor (monomer)	Mature B-cell marker	1. Allergy 2. Antiparasitic response
Relative % age	80%	10%	9%	0.04%	0.0003%
Binding cells via Fc receptor	1. Macrophages 2. Neutrophils 3. NK cells (LGL)	Lymphocytes	Lymphocytes	None	1. Mast cells 2. Basophils 3. B-cells

gram-negative bacteria or **multivalent (or repeating) antigens** such as polysaccharides induce **T-cell-independent activation** of B-cells. These antigens activate B-cells by binding the **B-cell receptor (BCR) complex,** consisting of surface immunoglobulin IgM or IgD, in a pattern- or dose-dependent fashion. This directly induces B-cell proliferation and differentiation into antibody-producing plasma cells.

Most antigens (especially proteins) are neither multivalent nor pattern recognized like LPS. Such antigens require "help" from T-helper cells to produce an antibody response, which is described as **T-cell-dependent activation.** This is accomplished through **antigen presentation,** a process wherein a pathogen is ingested and processed by an antigen-presenting cell to produce a small peptide fragment, which is then covalently bound to **major histocompatibility complex** (MHC) receptor. An antigen that comes from the extracellular space (like bacteria) is presented on type II MHC to a CD4+ T-helper cell, which "helps" the rest of the immune system to respond effectively to this antigen. Antigen-presenting cells include dendritic cells (or Langerhans cells, if in the skin or mucosal), macrophages, follicular dendritic cells in the spleen, B-lymphocytes, and microglia in the CNS.

Once an antigen is bound to type II MHC, it is presented to T-helper cells via the **T-cell receptor (TCR)** and the **CD4 receptor.** A "confirmatory" second signaling interaction then occurs between the APC surface protein **B7** and the T-cell's **CD28,** which is required for T-helper cell activation. Without this second signal, no activation occurs and the lymphocyte is actually rendered immunologically nonfunctional, or **anergic.** Other interactions include those between the T-helper cell's **CD40 ligand (CD40L)** to **CD40** on B-cells, which stimulates B-cell proliferation and antibody production—effects that are also supported by cytokines secreted by T-helper cells.

Finally, the antibodies produced by plasma cells must be "tailored" for optimal elimination of the specific pathogen. The first step is **isotype switching** (or class switching), a process whereby a B-cell is stimulated to produce antibodies of a particular isotype (e.g., IgG or IgE). IgGs, which opsonize microbes (tagging them for phagocytosis) provide optimal defense against small extracellular pathogens (e.g., bacteria and viruses). IgE antibodies are more suited for parasite elimination, as they bind to Fcε receptors on eosinophils, the cellular mediators of antiparasitic defense. Activated B-cells initially produce IgM, a low-affinity antibody. Once the CD40-CD40L interaction occurs, isotype switching is initiated. Different cytokines direct final antibody isotype production. T-helper cells activated by extracellular bacteria or viruses differentiate into T-helper type 1 cells (T_h1) and those stimulated by parasites differentiate into T-helper type 2 cells (T_h2). **T_h1 cells secrete IFN-γ,** which promotes IgG isotype switching and

phagocytic killing. **T_h2-cells secrete IL-4,** which promotes IgE class switching, as well as **IL-5,** which activates eosinophils for parasitic elimination. Similarly, T-helper cells in the respiratory and gastrointestinal mucosa stimulate IgA class switching. The final step in "tailoring" the humoral immune response is affinity maturation of the antibody, as described above. From this point, most activated B-cells differentiate into antibody-producing **plasma cells.** However, a fraction differentiate into **memory B-cells,** which circulate for months to years, providing immunological memory, ready to respond to a pathogen if it were to re-infect the body. (See Figure 54-1 in Cellular Immunity section.)

Clinical Discussion

Autoimmune disease   Autoimmune disease results from failure of the immune system to maintain tolerance to self antigen, causing immune-mediated destruction of the body's own cells and tissues. This results from the production of antibodies against self antigens or activation of self-reactive T-cells, which may be due to either an intrinsic abnormality in lymphocytes or abnormalities in the display of self antigens. For the most part, autoimmune disease is thought to arise from failures of peripheral tolerance rather than central tolerance. Autoimmune diseases are associated with specific subtypes of **human lymphocyte antigens** (HLA: the name of human MHC), often preceded by infectious prodromes. It is thought that the local innate immune response to tissue infection up-regulates costimulators and cytokines that activate and break anergy of self-reactive T-cells. Alternatively, some microbes may have antigens that are similar to self antigens, a phenomenon termed "molecular mimicry." Antibodies and T-cells from such an infection may later cross-react with self antigen, causing an inflammatory response to one's own tissue. This is thought to be the underlying basis of poststreptococcal rheumatic heart disease, where IgG developed to group A *Streptococcus pyogenes* epitopes cross-react with proteins in cardiac muscle tissue. Finally, tissue injury may release antigen normally sequestered from the immune system, causing autoimmune reaction against intracellular self antigen; this can occur after trauma to immune-protected sites such as the cornea and the testes.

Systemic lupus erythematosus   **Systemic lupus erythematosus (SLE)** is a multisystemic autoimmune disease that arises from the failure to maintain tolerance to self antigen. This results in the presence of a large array of autoantibodies to nuclear and cytoplasmic antigens, particularly **antinuclear antibodies (ANA).** These antibodies can react to red cells, platelets, lymphocytes, and phospholipid-associated plasma proteins. These antibodies can mediate a **type II cytotoxic hypersensitivity** reaction resulting in hemolytic anemia, leukopenia, and thrombocytopenia. Tissue injury also

Table 55-2 Criteria for diagnosis of systemic lupus erythematosis [do not memorize]

Criterion	Description
1. Malar rash	"Butterfly-shaped" rash, flat, erythematous rash of sun-exposed areas
2. Discoid rash	Erythematous raised patches
3. Photosensitivity	Skin rash from sun exposure
4. Oral ulcers	Often painless oral or nasopharyngeal ulceration
5. Arthritis	Nondegenerative arthritis of two or more joints with tenderness, swelling, and effusion
6. Serositis	Pleuritis, pericarditis
7. Renal disorder	Proteinuria, RBC casts
8. Neurologic disorder	Seizures, psychosis
9. Hematologic disorder	Hemolytic anemia, leukopenia, lymphopenia, thrombocytopenia
10. Immunologic disorder	Anti-dsDNA + anti-Sm antibodies; anti-phospholipid Ab (false positive VDRL)
11. Anti-nuclear antibody	Anti-nuclear antibody (in virtually 100% of patients with SLE)

The presence of four out of eleven criteria is diagnostic of SLE; the presence of both anti-double-stranded DNA and anti-Sm antibodies is virtually diagnostic of SLE.

results from **immune complex-mediated disease (type III hypersensitivity)**, which can lead to glomerulonephritis, arthritis, and vasculitides.

SLE is a common disease, occurring predominantly among women of child-bearing age and is more common and severe among African-American women. There is a familial clustering of the disease. SLE presents classically as an acute or chronic, recurrent, and remitting febrile illness with damage to the skin, joints, kidney, and serosal membranes. For formal diagnosis, the American Rheumatology Association developed the criteria as described in Table 55-2. Symptomatic exacerbations are treated with corticosteroids and immunosuppressant drugs.

Case Conclusion   SM is diagnosed with systemic lupus erythematosus. She is treated with the nonsteroidal anti-inflammatory drug (NSAID) naproxen and with a course of prednisone for her exacerbation of symptoms. She is subsequently maintained on low doses of NSAIDs with intermittent steroid tapers. She is currently doing well on this lifelong regimen, monitored regularly by her rheumatologist.

Thumbnail: Autoimmune Diseases

Disease	Pathogenesis	Clinical manifestations
SLE	Antinuclear antibodies and other antibodies cause immune complex disease and hematologic cytotoxicity	Young, female, child-bearing age, African-American; rash, arthritis, serosal damage, glomerulonephritis, pancytopenia, neurologic disorders
Sjögren syndrome	Lymphocytic infiltration and destruction of lacrimal and salivary glands	Women, 35–45 years old; dry eyes, dry mouth (xerostomia), parotid gland enlargement
Scleroderma	Unknown etiology; excessive fibrosis throughout the body (skin, GI tract, kidneys, heart, muscles, lungs, and microvasculature) from abnormal immune activation	Women, 50–60 years old; localized or diffuse skin fibrosis; diffuse visceral fibrosis and organ dysfunction; ischemic tissue injury from microvascular disease; CREST syndrome: Calcinosis, *Raynaud* phenomenon, *Esophageal* dysmotility, *Sclerodactyly, Telangiectasia*
Inflammatory myopathies	Dermatomyositis: immune-mediated inflammation of skin and muscle; ischemia from capillary damage Polymyositis: muscle inflammation from cell-mediated injury Inclusion- body myositis: muscle inflammation; possible CTL injury	Lilac discoloration of upper eyelids, periorbital edema; rash over knees, knuckles, and elbows Symmetric muscle weakness; inflammatory change in heart, lungs, and blood vessels Begins with distal muscle involvement (weakness), especially knee extensors and wrist/finger flexors; asymmetric
Mixed connective tissue disease	High titers of antibodies to RNP	SLE + polymyositis + systemic sclerosis
Vasculitides	Necrotizing inflammation of blood vessel walls	Fever, fatigue, weight loss, occlusion of blood vessels, and ischemia

CTL, cytotoxic lymphocytes; RNP, ribonucleoprotein.

Key Points

▶ Adaptive immunity is a branch of immunity that makes possible specific recognition of pathogens, as well as rapid proliferation of the immune cells that eliminate such pathogens

▶ Humoral immunity is a branch of adaptive immunity that allows specific recognition of soluble pathogens via soluble mediators called immunoglobulin

▶ B-lymphocytes, the cells that produce immunoglobulins, undergo a process of "pruning" whereby cells that recognize self antigen are selected to die or undergo B-cell receptor editing to prevent them from reacting to self antigen

Questions

1. The following is a list of SM's clinical symptoms, with their underlying immunopathology. Which is *least* likely to be correct?

   A. Arthritis: immune complex deposition in synovial membranes

   B. Malar rash: immunoglobulin- and complement-mediated injury at the dermoepidermal junction of the skin

   C. Pleuritic chest pain; chronic pleuritis and chronic interstitial fibrosis

   D. Palpable spleen tip; follicular hyperplasia in spleen with abundance of IgG- and IgM-producing plasma cells

   E. Anemia, leukopenia, and thrombocytopenia; immune complex-mediated injury to hematologic components

2. There is a receptor called CTLA-4 that can be up-regulated and act as an antagonist to costimulatory B7 surface protein. Soluble CTLA-4 protein is in trials for preventing graft-versus-host disease in bone marrow transplant patients. Through what mechanism is this likely to work?

   A. CTLA-4 binds B7, preventing the necessary second signal required to initiate the immune reaction against a certain foreign antigen; it can thus prevent donor bone marrow T-lymphocytes and other immune cells from being immunologically activated against host antigen

   B. CTLA-4 binds B7 and inhibits binding of the host antigen to MHC receptor, thus preventing antigen presentation to donor lymphocytes and subsequently preventing immunologic attack of host tissue

   C. CTLA-4 acts as a general immunosuppressant, preventing activation of T-lymphocytes from the donor, preventing damage to host tissue

   D. CTLA-4 prevents the expression of CD40 in antigen-presenting cells, thus preventing the subsequent sensitization of donor T-lymphocytes to host tissue

   E. CTLA-4 down-regulates the expression of CD28, thereby preventing the needed second signal

HPI: CD is a 4-year-old boy who presents to the ER **lethargic** with a **high fever** and a **diffuse petechial rash.** The child's illness began 3 days ago when he developed a low-grade fever and a sore throat. The next day, he was seen by his pediatrician and was found to be slightly febrile with pharyngitis. His throat was cultured and he was sent home with supportive care. Today he developed a diffuse petechial rash and a fever peaking at 104°F. He complains of a **headache, joint pain, nausea,** and **vomiting** and has become more lethargic.

PMH: An **admission for pneumococcal pneumonia** at the age of 1, which resolved without complication.

PE: T 39.6°C HR 145 BP 80/50 RR 24 SaO$_2$ 95% on room air

He is **toxic appearing, somnolent** but arousable. His exam is significant for **nuchal rigidity** with a positive **Kernig's and Brudzinski's sign,** diffuse **petechial rash,** and bilateral knee inflammation. He has no focal neurological deficits.

Labs: WBC 36,000/μL, Hct 40%, Plt 110,000/μL

He is hemodynamically stabilized; 2 blood cultures are sent and IV ceftriaxone is initiated for presumed **meningitis.** Head CT shows no evidence of a mass lesion. A lumbar puncture is performed, which reveals grossly cloudy CSF with an elevated opening pressure, and increased protein and decreased glucose content. Microscopically, the CSF reveals elevated WBC with a neutrophil predominance and gram-negative intracellular diplococci. The patient is admitted. At day 2, blood and CSF cultures grow **Neisseria meningitidis.** IgM and IgG levels to meningococcus are elevated.

Thought Questions

- What is innate immunity? What are its cellular and humoral components?

- What are the major categories of deficiencies in innate immunity?

- What are the clinical manifestations that occur with these immunodeficiencies?

- How are these immunodeficiencies diagnosed and treated?

Basic Science Review and Discussion

The **innate immune system** is the most primitive division of immunity and represents **the first line of defense** against pathogens such as bacteria, foreign cells such as allografts, and tumor cells. The means of immune protection are less specific than that of adaptive immunity and broadly include protective barriers like skin, mucosal epithelium, and stomach acid as well as pattern recognition proteins that recognize and eliminate broad classes of pathogens by binding to commonly expressed molecular patterns like lipopolysaccharide (LPS) on gram-negative bacteria. **Unlike the adaptive immune system, this branch of immunity does not require prior exposure to a pathogen to be activated and thus is an important line of defense against pathogens to which the body is naïve.** But like adaptive immunity, innate immunity has both a humoral and a cellular component that interacts and works synergistically to eliminate pathogens.

The humoral components of innate immunity consist of **antimicrobial peptides,** soluble **pattern recognition proteins,** and **complement proteins.** The antimicrobial peptides include defensins that bind microbes and create pores within their membranes, causing cell lysis. There are also a number of soluble pattern recognition proteins, called **collectins,** capable of binding carbohydrates unique to microbial membranes. These proteins tag extracellular pathogens for phagocytosis and activate the inflammatory response via the complement cascade.

The **complement system** is an important part of innate immunity consisting of several proteins that mediate three main functions: (1) **opsonization** of extracellular pathogens, (2) **cell lysis** via the formation of the membrane attack complex, and (3) **cell signaling** via by-products of the cascade that activate local inflammation. There are three pathways through which complement is activated: (1) **the alternative pathway,** (2) **the lectin pathway,** and (3) **the classical pathway.** These pathways converge upon the formation of C3b, a central component that activates several arms of the immune response. The alternative and lectin pathways rely on pattern recognition proteins and are important for first-time infections where there are no specific antibodies available for opsonization. In contrast, the classical pathway relies on pre-existing immunoglobulins for its action. Opsonization neutralizes and tags a pathogen for phagocytosis. This subsequently initiates a cascade of proteolysis and activation of complement proteins. The small peptides released from the cascade (e.g., C2a–C5a) serve as cytokines that promote the inflammatory response by recruiting leukocytes and increasing local vascular permeability to facilitate leukocyte transmigration. In addition, cytokines initiate the adaptive immune response by promoting antibody production to the specific antigens involved. Finally, the terminal complement proteins form the **membrane attack complex,** a transmembrane pore that inserts into microbial membranes and thereby promotes leakage of leukocyte-recruiting bacterial proteins, bacterial lysis, and phagocytosis. (See Figure 56-1 and Table 56-1.)

The cellular arm of innate immunity includes **neutrophils, monocytes-macrophages,** and **natural killer (NK) cells.** Once microorganisms are opsonized and cytokines are released, neutrophils and macrophages are recruited to the site of inflammation. These cells use pattern recognition receptors to recognize microbial polysaccharide structures and opsonins that facilitate phagocytosis. These cells also do not require prior exposure to a pathogen in order to be activated. Once phagocytized, microorganisms within phagosomes are partially degraded by the digestive enzymes of lysosomes. However, the most effective killing action comes from the reactive oxygen and nitrogen intermediates of NADPH oxidase and inducible nitric oxide synthase (iNOS), respectively. **NADPH oxidase** products mediate **rapid oxidative killing,** whereas **iNOS products** provide a **slower, more sustained mechanism of killing** of extracellular pathogens. NK cells eliminate intracellular pathogens by attacking cells

infected by virus (as well as tumor cells and transplanted cells) via important differences in surface protein expression. They can detect absent or reduced expression of self-MHC class I receptors on foreign cells and infected cells (as many viruses evade cytotoxic T-cell killing by inhibiting MHC expression). They also kill cells with stress-induced expression of surface proteins MIC-A and MIC-B.

Clinical Discussion: Defects in the Complement System The Thumbnail describes defects of the complement system and their clinical manifestations. The severity of disease reflects the relative importance of each component in their defense against infection.

Diagnosis of complement deficiency

- Consider complement deficiency in anyone with recurrent encapsulated bacterial infections
- Consider MAC deficiency in anyone with recurrent or disseminated *Neisseria* infections

Diagnostic tests

- **Total hemolytic complement activity (CH$_{50}$)** → low or undetectable for most complement deficiencies (C1–C8)
- **Serum C3 and C4:** different profiles suggest different complement deficiencies

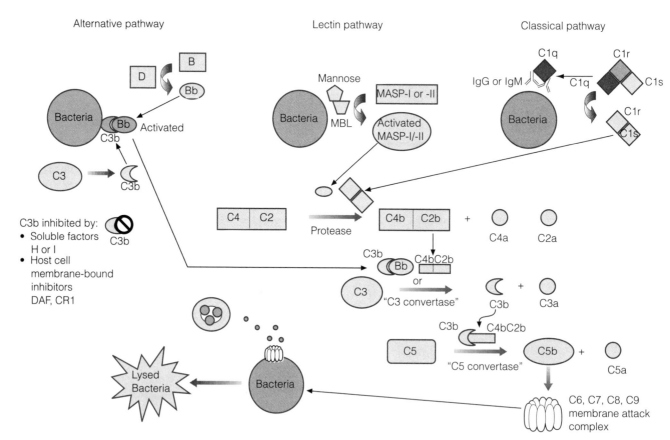

Figure 56-1 The complement cascade. There are three possible pathways that all converge upon the conversion of C3 to C3b. It is a proteolytic cascade that releases small cytokine fragments and eventually leads to the formation of the membrane attack complex.

Table 56-1 Complement components and their actions

Complement component	Action
C3b	**Opsonin** of the alternative pathway; complexes with Bb to produce C3 convertase
MBL	**Opsonin** of the lectin pathway; binds polysaccharides unique to microorganisms
2 IgG or 1 IgM	**Opsonin** of the classic pathway; binds specific antigen and C1q releasing C1r/C1s
DAF, CR1, MCP	**Cell surface-bound protein** *inhibitors of C3b* that protect host cells
Factor H or I	**Soluble** *inhibitors of C3b*; prevents activation of complement cascade
MASP-I or MASP-II	**Lectin pathway** *protease* that cleaves C4/C2 → C4b/C2b + C4a + C2a
C1r/C1s	**Classic pathway** *protease* that cleaves C4/C2 → C4b/C2b + C4a + C2a
C3bBb	**Alternative pathway** *C3 convertase* that cleaves C3 → C3b + C3a
C4b/C2b	**Classic pathway** *C3 convertase* that cleaves C3 → C3b + C3a
C4a	Weak **anaphylatoxin**; evokes *histamine release* from basophils and mast cells
C3b	1. Complexes with C4b/C2b to form "**C5 convertase**": cleaves C5 → C5b + C5a 2. Amplification of alternative pathway loop by producing more C3b to complex with Bb to form C3bBb, the "**C3 convertase complex**" 3. **Opsonin** for neutralization and tagging of particles for phagocytosis 4. Promotes *immune complex binding* to macrophages and neutrophils 5. Promotes *solubilization of immune complexes* 6. C3b bound to particles *promotes antibody production* to particle antigens
C3a	1. **Anaphylatoxin**; evokes histamine release from basophils and mast cells 2. Acts on endothelial cells to *promote vascular permeability*
C5b	Binds covalently to microbial membranes (esp. gram-negative bacteria and enveloped viruses) → **nucleates formation of membrane attack complex** with C6, C7, C8, and C9
C5a	1. **Anaphylatoxin**; evokes histamine release from basophils and mast cells 2. Potent *chemoattractant* for monocytes and neutrophils 3. Acts on endothelial cells to *promote vascular permeability*
C5, C6, C7, C8, C9	**Membrane attack complex**: polymerizes to form a transmembrane pore → weakens membrane integrity and allows leakage of immune mediators that promotes leukocyte recruitment for phagocytosis of microorganism

MBL, mannose-binding lectin; Ig, immunoglobulin; MASP, MBL-associated serine protease; DAF, decay accelerating factor; CR1, complement receptor 1; MCP, membrane cofactor of proteolysis.

- **Quantitation of complement factors** to identify specific complement deficiency

Treatment of complement deficiency and other cellular innate immunodeficiency

- Acute infection: broad-spectrum intravenous **antibiotics**

- Chronic/recurrent infection: prophylactic antibiotics, **vaccination** against pneumococcus, meningococcus, and *H. influenzae*

- **C1 INH concentrate** infusion for hereditary angioedema: aborts acute attacks; prophylaxis for surgical procedures

- **Gene therapy** for complement deficiencies may have a role in the future

Case Conclusion CD's meningococcal meningitis and bacteremia resolved with antibiotic therapy. Given his recurrence of major encapsulated bacteria infection, a complement deficiency was suspected. Subsequent CH_{50} testing revealed no detectable activity. C3 and C4 levels were normal. Quantitative testing of complement factors revealed a C5 deficiency. CD's family was subsequently educated on the significance of this disease, the necessity for vaccination against encapsulated bacteria, and the need for immediate medical attention with any signs of infection. CD is doing well otherwise and shows no signs of neurologic sequelae from the meningitis.

Thumbnail: Complement Deficiencies

Defect	Disease	Possible mechanisms
C1q, C1r, C1s, C2, or C4	**Immune complex syndromes:** SLE, discoid lupus, glomerulonephritis, vasculitis; ↑ risk of septicemia in C2 deficiency	**Classical pathway defect** Impaired processing and clearance of immune complexes
C3, H, or I	**Recurrent, *severe* pyogenic infections** with encapsulated bacteria, e.g., pneumococcus, meningococcus → pneumonia, otitis media, sinusitis	**Alternative pathway defect** Inefficient opsonization by C3b may cause susceptibility to infection; inability to dismantle C3 convertase
C5, C6, C7, or C8 MAC deficiency	**Recurrent, disseminated neisserial infections,** commonly meningococcal meningitis; immune complex diseases	**Defective membrane attack complex:** bacterial cell lysis may be required for effective killing of this pathogen
C1 esterase inhibitor (INH) protein	**Hereditary angioedema:** episodic, localized, nonpitting edema without pruritis on face or limb in response to trauma/stress; painful bowel edema; life-threatening laryngeal edema	**Uncontrolled C1 activity,** with breakdown of C4 and C2 and release of vasoactive peptide, and kinin causes edema

SLE, systemic lupus erythematosus; MAC, membrane attack complex.

Key Points

▶ The innate immune system is the more primitive branch of immunity that uses nonspecific means to exclude or eliminate infection.

▶ It uses physical barriers like skin, as well as pattern recognition of molecular structures unique to microorganisms, to provide protection from and elimination of infection.

▶ The humoral component consists of several antimicrobial peptides, soluble pattern recognition proteins, and the complement cascade, which directly attack or opsonize microbes, and promotes further amplification of the inflammatory response.

▶ The cellular components include neutrophils, macrophages, and NK cells that eliminate pathogens by phagocytosis followed by lytic and oxidative killing or by killing cells infected with intracellular pathogens.

Questions

1. The following is a list of aspects of CD's history and physical exam that would make one suspicious of a complement deficiency. Which is the *least* correct?
   A. Previous history of pneumococcal pneumonia
   B. Current meningococcal pneumonia
   C. Petechial rash
   D. Arthritis
   E. Nuchal rigidity with a positive Kernig's and Brudzinski's sign

2. Five years later, CD experienced another episode of meningococcal infection with a less severe and more indolent course with symptoms limited to low-grade fever, polyarthritis, petechial rash, and hematuria, but no evidence of meningitis. What may be a possible pathophysiologic explanation for this?
   A. CD has developed a faster, more efficient innate immune response to *N. meningitidis* due to his previous exposure to the bacterium
   B. CD's infection is marked by symptoms of immune complex deposition reflecting the availability of IgG to meningococcus that can limit the spread of infection via the classic pathway and other mechanisms of adaptive immunity
   C. CD has been able to compensate for his lack of C5 protein by up-regulating other proteins of the complement cascade and thereby improve the efficiency of this line of defense
   D. CD's natural killer cells, having been previously exposed to meningococcus, can now more efficiently destroy bacteria of this species, thereby limiting spread of infection
   E. The reactive intermediates of NADPH oxidase and iNOS limit the infection by providing a rapid as well as slow and sustained oxidative killing of phagocytized bacteria

HPI: IG is an 8-year-old girl who presents to the ER with **shortness of breath, diffuse urticaria, angioedema,** and **hypotension.** She had been snacking on cashews when, within minutes, she began to "feel a lump in her throat" and hoarseness. She simultaneously developed **facial swelling** and a diffuse, **intensely pruritic rash.** She also had nausea, and vomiting with **crampy abdominal pain.** On the way to the hospital, she developed **chest tightness, wheezing,** and difficulty breathing. She takes no medication nor does she have any drug allergies. She has no known atopic disease but has a **family history of asthma.**

PE: T 37.7°C HR 124 BP 82/53 RR 26 SaO$_2$ 90% on room air
On exam, she is ill appearing and in moderate respiratory distress. Her exam is significant for **facial** and **periorbital non-pitting edema, perioral cyanosis,** and **stridorous breath sounds.** She has supraclavicular retractions and her lungs have **diffuse wheezing** on auscultation. Her cardiac exam is unremarkable. Her abdomen is soft, mildly distended, with **diffuse periumbilical tenderness.** She has diffusely distributed large, irregularly shaped **pruritic, erythematous wheals** on her trunk and extremities.

She is given 100% oxygen by nasal cannula. Intravenous access is established and she is given fluids and subcutaneous epinephrine until she is hemodynamically stabilized. She is given intravenous diphenhydramine, ranitidine, methylprednisolone and albuterol for her anaphylactic reaction and bronchospasm. She is then admitted, with close monitoring over the next 24 hours.

Thought Questions

- What are the four types of hypersensitivity?

- What are the common hypersensitivity conditions and their clinical manifestations?

- How are hypersensitivity conditions diagnosed?

- How are common hypersensitivity reactions treated?

Basic Science Review and Discussion

Hypersensitivity is a pathologically exaggerated immune response to a foreign antigen, or **allergen,** that results in local or systemic inflammation. Such reactions are all preceded by previous exposure to the antigen to which the body develops humoral or cellular immunity. Allergic reactions tend to localize at sites exposed to the environment such as skin, eyes, and the respiratory and gastrointestinal tract. Allergens may consist of a foreign peptide, which can induce an inflammatory reaction once the body is re-exposed. Alternatively, an allergen may be a nonpeptide (also known as a **hapten**), like a drug, that binds to a host antigen and thereby forms a hapten-peptide complex. This complex becomes a novel antigen that the body sees as foreign. An antibody may be formed to this antigen that may be able to recognize self antigen as well. This can result in autoimmune disease, as in hemolytic anemias where red blood cells are destroyed due to IgG binding, with or even without the presence of the original hapten.

There are four types of hypersensitivity reactions. **Type I, immediate hypersensitivity,** involves the activation of mast cells upon binding of an allergen to cell-associated IgE. This occurs in atopic diseases like asthma, eczema, and allergic rhinitis, all of which have a strong familial association. Type I reactions also occur in more systemic diseases like anaphylaxis, urticaria, and angioedema, which can occur in both atopic and nonatopic individuals. **Type II, cytotoxic hypersensitivity,** is mediated by preexisting IgGs that bind **cell-associated antigen,** thereby causing immune-mediated destruction of that cell; this occurs in autoimmune hemolytic anemias and thrombocytopenias. **Type III, immune complex hypersensitivity,** results from the development of IgGs to a **soluble antigen** that forms immune complexes, which subsequently deposit in tissue and initiate a local inflammatory response. This is found in diseases like rheumatoid arthritis and systemic lupus erythematosus. Lastly, **Type IV, delayed-type hypersensitivity,** is a **cell-mediated** immune reaction where a previously sensitized T-lymphocyte mediates a local inflammatory response upon re-exposure to an antigen. This activates CD4-positive T-helper cells and/or CD8-positive cytotoxic activity and is often delayed, as it takes time to activate and recruit T-lymphocytes. Figure 57-1 shows the four hypersensitivity reactions and Table 57-1 describes their pathogenesis.

Clinical Discussion: Hypersensitivity Each type of hypersensitivity reaction is accompanied by its own set of pathophysiologic consequences and subsequent clinical manifestations. (See Thumbnail) As they represent distinct immunologic phenomena with their own sets of participating signaling proteins and receptors, the means of diagnosis and treatment are distinct for each disease.

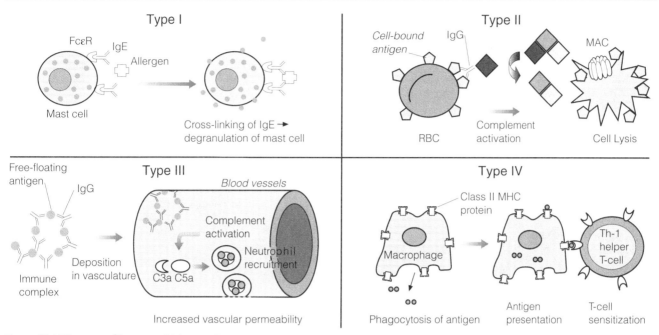

Figure 57-1 Diagrams of hypersensitivity reactions.

Table 57-1 **The pathogenesis of hypersensitivity reactions**

Type	Hypersensitivity reaction	Pathophysiologic consequences
I: Immediate anaphylactic IgE-mediated mast cells	1. Allergen exposure (drugs, food, insect venom) leads to IgE development 2. **Sensitization:** IgE binds mast cells → proliferate → take up residence in cutaneous and mucosal tissue 3. Upon re-exposure, mast cells recognize allergen, which bind and cross-links cell-bound IgE (also found in basophils) 4. This elicits immediate release of histamine, serotonin, chemokines, prostaglandins, leukotrienes, proteases, heparin, and PAF 5. Late-phase reaction 6–12 hrs later with infiltration of granulocytes and monocytes	• **Histamine, leukotrienes, prostaglandins, and serotonin** promote vasodilation, local vascular permeability (which allows influx of plasma proteins like complement and immunoglobulins) and bronchoconstriction • **Leukotrienes** also mediate leukocyte-endothelial cell adhesion and chemotaxis • **Cytokines** mediate eosinophil recruitment, which produces histaminase and arylsulfatase that degrade histamine and leukotrienes, respectively, thereby reducing inflammation • **Thromboxane/PAF:** platelet aggregation
II: Cytotoxic IgG-mediated	1. **Hapten** (e.g., drug) attaches to cell surface protein → IgG forms to self antigen 2. Infection can also induce formation of self antigen cross-reacting IgG → complement activation 3. Membrane attack complex and leukocytes mediate direct cell lysis	• **Hemolytic anemias:** IgG to RBC surface antigen→ direct RBC lysis • **Autoimmune thrombocytopenic purpura:** IgG coat platelets → platelets destroyed in the spleen by macrophages • **Rheumatic fever:** IgG to GAS cross-reacts with cardiac cell antigen → carditis
III: Immune complex Complexes of antigen, IgG antibody, and/or complement	**Arthus reaction:** *localized* immune complex formation → complement activation, local inflammation, neutrophil infiltration, and thrombosis **Serum sickness:** *systemic* inflammatory reaction to diffuse immune complex deposition from high levels of antigen in the serum; causes widespread complement activation (e.g., drug reaction)	• **Glomerulonephritis:** poststreptococcal (esp. after skin infections); antibody to GAS forms IC that deposits in glomerulus, promoting complement activation, PMN recruitment, and local inflammation • **Arthritis:** IC deposition on synovial membranes of joints • **Vasculitis:** IC deposition in vessels
IV: Delayed Cell-mediated: cytotoxic T-cell and T-helper cells	1. Allergen is phagocytized by an antigen presenting cell (e.g., macrophage) 2. Antigen is presented on class II MHC receptors to T-helper cells, which are then sensitized to allergen 3. Upon re-exposure, T-lymphocytes are re-activated and mount an immune response that requires hours to days to fully manifest clinically; thus it is termed "delayed-type hypersensitivity"	• **Contact hypersensitivity:** direct skin contact with allergen, like poison oak, binds surface protein of skin cells; cell-mediated immunity is directed against this foreign-host peptide antigen; repeat exposure leads to direct cytotoxic killing of such cells • **Tuberculin skin test:** previous exposure to *M. tuberculosis* establishes cell-mediated immunity; PPD injection causes an erythematous wheal within 48–72 hours

PAF, plate activating factor; GAS, group A β-hemolytic *Streptococcus pyogenes;* IC, immune complex.

Thumbnail: Common hypersensitivity syndromes

Disease	Etiology/Pathophysiology	Clinical Manifestations	Diagnosis & Treatment
Type I: Immediate Hypersensitivity			
Allergic Rhinitis	Animal and plant proteins (mold, pollen), insect debris IgE-mediated atopic disease	Nasal congestion, sneezing Itchy nose, ears, eyes Eosinophilia, ↑ IgE	Dx: Skin testing, RAST Tx: Antihistamines Cromolyn Corticosteroids Pseudoephedrine
Allergic Dermatitis/Eczema	Atopic disease of unknown etiology	Pruritic, exudative, or lichenified rash on face, neck, upper trunk, wrists, flexor or extensor surface of arms and legs	Dx: Clinical, ↑ IgE Tx: Skin moisturizers Topical corticosteroids Antihistamine for pruritis
Anaphylaxis, Urticaria & Angioedema	Massive mast cell degranulation leads to systemic vasodilation → hypotension ↑ vascular permeability → cutaneous (angioedema) and visceral (bowel) edema Smooth muscle contraction→ bronchospasm	Diffuse pruritis Urticaria: red wheals Facial/periorbital edema Stridor and wheezing Respiratory distress Hypotension N, V, Abdominal pain/cramps Eosinophilia	Dx: Clinical Tx: Subcutaneous epinephrine IV fluids Oxygen/possible endotracheal intubation IV Antihistamine Bronchodilator—IV β2 agonist or methyxanthines (aminophylline) steroids
Drug Allergy	Mast cell surface IgE recognize drug/self antigen epitope whenever a person is exposed to drug → causes Type I response	Pruritic erythematous urticarial, maculopapular rash; onset 7–21 days after drug exposure May develop angioedema	*Acute desensitization*—slowed administration to prevent massive anaphylaxis *Chronic desensitization* administered over weeks to form IgG to IgE
Type II: Cytotoxic Hypersensitivity			
ABO/Rh Hemolytic Anemia	IgG from host serum or Rh-negative pregnant woman bind RBC surface antigen: 1. Surface antigens A or B in transfusion reactions 2. Rh in Rh-positive fetuses of Rh-negative mothers	Rapid onset anemia—tachycardia, hypotension, fever, CHF symptoms, jaundice, splenomegaly *Erythroblastosis Fetalis:* neonatal jaundice, anemia kernicterus, hydrops	Dx: Direct/indirect Coombs test +, ↑ BUN/Cr Prevention: Rho(D) Ig to Rh-negative post-partum women and newborns Tx: stop transfusion, oxygen, epinephrine, corticosteroids
Drug-induced and other Autoimmune Hemolytic Anemia	Drug acts as a hapten when bound to cell-surface protein → IgG is formed to RBC antigen → RBC lysis or spherocyte formation → splenic sequestration	Rapid onset anemia as above ↓ Hct, reticulocytosis, indirect hyperbilirubinemia	Dx: Direct Coombs' test + Tx: Stop drug, prednisone immmunosuppressant drugs Splenectomy IV immune globulin
Idiopathic Thrombocytopenic Purpura	Hapten phenomenon leads to IgG formation against platelets → phagocytized by splenic macrophages	Platelet count 5000–75,000 Bleeding diathesis; petechial hemorrhages; purpura, easy bruising	Dx: ↑ bleeding time Normal PT/PTT Tx: Platelet transfusion Splenectomy
Rheumatic fever	After upper respiratory GAS infection, IgG formed cross-reacts with cardiac muscle cells and other tissue	Fever, abdominal pain Migratory polyarthritis Erythema nodosum Carditis, chorea Subcutaneous nodules	Dx: Streptozyme, ASO titer Tx: Penicillin for GAS Prednisone for carditis Aspirin (anti-inflammatory) Haloperidol for chorea

Common hypersensitivity syndromes

Disease	Etiology/Pathophysiology	Clinical Manifestations	Diagnosis & Treatment
Type III: Immune-Complex Hypersensitivity			
Glomerulonephritis	IgG formed to GAS forms immune complex that is deposited in glomerulus → complement activation, inflammation	After GAS skin infection Abrupt onset hematuria, oligouria, hypertension, edema, proteinuria, hypocomplementemia	Dx: Streptozyme, ASO titer Tx: Control hypertension hyperkalemia, edema, and acidosis; penicillin for GAS
Rheumatoid Arthritis	Rheumatoid Factor binds Fc region of IgG and forms immune complexes with complement → deposit on synovial membrane → arthritis; associated with HLA-DR4	Fever, malaise, weight loss, morning stiffness → arthralgia, arthritis, joint deformities (esp. PIP, MCP joints, wrists, knees, ankles, toes), subcutaneous nodules, pleural effusion, vasculitis	Dx: Rheumatoid Factor Tx: Aspirin or other NSAID COX-2 inhibitors Prednisone (if severe) Other anti-inflammatories Methotrexate Cyclosporine
Type IV: Delayed-Type Hypersensitivity			
Contact Dermatitis	Chemical irritant or protein allergen induce T-cell recruitment and activation → skin inflammation	Erythematous, pruritic, edematous rash → vesicular/bullous transformation → weepy, crusted, infected rash	Dx: Clinical Tx: Topical or systemic corticosteroids; topical antibiotics for infected skin

Dx = diagnosis; Tx = treatment; RAST = Radioallergosorbent test (ELISA or antibody test against common allergens); CHF = congestive heart failure; PIP = proximal interphalangeal joint; MCP = metacarpal phalangeal joint; PT = prothrombin time; PTT = (activated) partial thromboplastin time; ASO = anti-streptolysin; Fc region = constant fragment of immunoglobulin; HLA-DR4 = human leukocyte antigen DR4; NSAID = non-steroidal anti-inflammatory drug; COX-2 = cyclooxygenase-2.

Case Conclusion   Twelve hours later, IG develops a repeat of her symptoms: facial swelling, respiratory distress, and hypotension. She is again resuscitated. She is monitored for another 24 hours and is discharged.

Key Points

- ▶ There are four types of hypersensitivity reactions:
  - ▶ Type I: immediate; mast cell-bound IgE-mediated → mast cell degranulation
  - ▶ Type II: cytotoxic; IgG bind cell surface antigen, which activates complement and promotes cell lysis
  - ▶ Type III: immune complex-mediated; IgG bind soluble antigen, forming immune complexes that deposit in vessels and tissue causing inflammation and tissue damage
  - ▶ Type IV: delayed-type; T-cell-mediated immunity against antigen
- ▶ Type I reactions cause disease that includes pruritis, vasodilation, increased vascular permeability, and smooth muscle contraction and happen with rapid onset, causing such diseases as atopic disease and anaphylaxis

- ▶ Type II reactions include disease of hematologic cytotoxicity from the development of IgG to surface antigen of blood cells; for example, drug-induced hemolytic anemia
- ▶ Type III reactions cause inflammation at sites in the vasculature where immune complexes can deposit, such as glomeruli, synovial membrane, small vessels, and at vessel bifurcations
- ▶ Type IV reactions result from recognition of hapten self antigen complexes or chemically modified self antigen by T-lymphocytes, which may result in cytotoxicity to host tissue

Questions

1. The following is a list of events in the pathogenesis of IG's hypersensitivity reaction. Which is *least* likely to have occurred?

   A. Cashew proteins were recognized by mast cell-associated IgE causing degranulation

   B. Massive degranulation of mast cells caused large systemic release of histamine, serotonin, prostaglandins, leukotrienes, and cytokines

   C. IgE bind soluble cashew protein, thus forming immune complexes that activate complement and promote vascular permeability resulting in angioedema and laryngeal edema

   D. Inflammatory cytokines released at the gastrointestinal tract caused local vasodilation and an increase in vascular permeability causing bowel edema manifesting as nausea, vomiting, and abdominal pain

   E. The recrudescence of her symptoms 12 hours later resulted from the late-onset infiltration of neutrophils, eosinophils, basophils, and monocytes to sites of mast cell degranulation

2. CD is a 25-year-old medical student who presents with a pruritic, erythematous maculopapular rash on her trunk. She had used a new detergent to wash her clothes and subsequently went for a run in the woods. The next day, she developed this rash. She did have one episode of pruritis after trying a new soap last year and has probably been exposed to poison oak before. She asks, "could this be due to an allergic reaction to the detergent or could I have run by some poison oak? If so, would this rash go away with diphenhydramine (Benadryl)?" What is the *most* accurate assessment of her dermatitis and what is the treatment?

   A. Her rash is consistent with a type I hypersensitivity reaction to poison oak and would be relieved by antihistamines

   B. Her rash is consistent with a type IV hypersensitivity reaction to poison oak and would not be relieved by antihistamines but can be treated with topical steroids

   C. Her rash is consistent with a type I hypersensitivity reaction to a substance in her detergent and can be relieved by antihistamines

   D. Her rash is consistent with a type IV hypersensitivity reaction to a substance in her detergent and can be relieved by topical steroid, not antihistamine

   E. Her rash is consistent with direct irritation of the skin by the detergent and can only be relieved by washing off the area and waiting for the inflammation to subside

> **HPI:** BD is a 12-month-old boy who presents with 1 day of **fever, cough,** and **dyspnea.** The mother recorded a fever of **102.3°F** and notes increased **irritability, rhinorrhea,** frequent **ear pulling, diarrhea,** and **vomiting.** The cough began yesterday and has progressed to rapid breathing. This is his **sixth respiratory tract infection in the last 5 months,** which includes one episode of bronchitis, three episodes of otitis media, and one episode of pneumonia requiring hospitalization.
>
> **PE:** T 39.4°C BP 97/52 HR 135 RR 49 SaO_2 95% on room air
> On exam, he is in **mild respiratory distress.** His weight is 10% less than that of the last recorded weight, which was in the fifth percentile. His exam is significant for **erythematous and purulent tympanic membranes, thick green sputum in the nasopharynx,** chest retractions, diffuse ronchi, and diminished capillary refill. His **chest X-ray** showed **diffuse infiltrates.**
>
> He was immediately given oxygen, nebulized albuterol, and antibiotics. He was admitted for pneumonia and the immunologist was consulted to investigate the possibility of a primary immunodeficiency.

Thought Questions

- What are the common forms of primary immunodeficiency?

- What are the underlying defects of such immunodeficiencies?

- What are the clinical manifestations of these diseases?

Basic Science Discussion and Review

There are many primary immunodeficiencies affecting many divisions of the immune system. These immunodeficiencies highlight the importance of each component of immunity.

Immunodeficiencies caused by defects in phagocytic function prevent the immune system from carrying out the final steps in microbial killing. (See Table 58-1.) This leads to persistent microbial infection, which clinically manifests as chronic abscess formation and abnormal wound healing. Immunodeficiencies caused by defects in leukocyte recruitment to sites of infection or injury cause patterns of poor wound healing and inadequate pus formation (the clinical manifestation of adequate neutrophil infiltration).

Most immunodeficiencies of humoral immunity manifest themselves between 6 months and 2 years of life, after protective maternal antibodies clear from circulation in infants. These generally predispose the child to infections by organisms requiring opsonization and phagocytosis for final elimination. These include small extracellular pathogens such as encapsulated bacteria. Individuals with deficiencies in specific isotypes are susceptible to infections at the sites usually protected by those immunoglobulin isotypes (e.g., IgA deficiencies predispose people to infections of mucosal surfaces, like gastritis). See Table 58-2.

Those with deficiencies in cell-mediated immunity from T-lymphocyte abnormalities exhibit poor immune defense against organisms that have a significant intracellular phase requiring antigen presentation by macrophages. These immunodeficiencies are marked by increased susceptibility to viruses, mycobacteria, and fungi. See Table 58-3.

Table 58-1 Phagocyte defects

Immunodeficiency	Pathogenesis	Clinical manifestations
Chronic granulomatous disease	**Deficiency in NADPH oxidase** causing impaired production of reactive oxygen intermediate production → impaired cell killing results in granulomas, which represent an attempt by phagocytes to contain the spread of infection	Commonly X-linked; *defective clearing of a few microbial species;* staphylococcal infections in first months of life; later, groin, cervical, or axillary abscesses, osteomyelitis, lung/liver abscess, colitis; *Serratia* and *Nocardia* infections
Leukocyte adhesion deficiency	**Defect in tight adhesion of neutrophils** to endothelium preventing normal migration to site of infection	*Abnormal wound healing,* progressive neonatal periumbilical necrosis; recurrent surface infections; neutrophilia without adequate pus formation
Chédiak-Higashi syndrome	**Mutation of lysosomal trafficking gene** impairs normal trafficking and release of vesicle contents preventing chemokine release, PMN chemotaxis, and T-cell stimulation; abnormal pigment handling	*Progressive local infections without pus formation;* partial oculocutaneous albinism; late-onset lymphoproliferative disease

There are also a number of immunodeficiencies that arise from defects in both B- and T-lymphocytes. These diseases cause marked susceptibility to all types of infection (viral, bacterial, and fungal) from dysfunctional antibody-mediated *and* cell-mediated immunity leading to high rates of morbidity and mortality, often at earlier ages. In addition, affected individuals may have other disease manifestations specific to the underlying genetic defect that caused the immunodeficiency syndrome. See Table 58-4.

Table 58-2 Deficiencies of humoral immunity (B-cell defects)

Immunodeficiency	Pathogenesis	Clinical manifestations
Bruton's X-linked γ-globulinemia	**Failure of precursor B-cells to differentiate into mature B-cells** due to mutations in *Bruton tyrosine kinase; no light chains*; X-linked → **immunoglobulin deficiency** causes defect in clearing of organisms requiring phagocytosis; absent or few B-cells and plasma cells • All immunoglobulin levels depressed • Underdeveloped lymphoid germinal centers	• Males; after 6 months • *Recurrent bacterial infections* of the respiratory tract: pharyngitis, sinusitis, otitis media, bronchitis, pneumonia • Common bacteria: *H. influenzae, S. pneumoniae, S. aureus* • Common viruses: enteroviruses → gastritis → encephalitis • *Giardia lamblia:* ↓ IgA; gastritis • *Mycoplasma* infection causes arthritis • Treatment: IV immunoglobulin replacement
Common variable immunodeficiency	**Deficient production of all different antibody classes** due to immature circulating B-cells that can recognize antigen, respond, but fail to fully mature to plasma cells → nodular B-cell hyperplasia	• Can present during adulthood • *Chronic pulmonary infections,* chronic giardiasis, intestinal malabsorption, atrophic gastritis with pernicious anemia • S/Sx of lymphoid hyperplasia: fever, weight loss, anemia, splenomegaly, lymphadenopathy, thrombocytopenia, lymphocytosis Treatment: IV immunoglobulin replacement
Isolated IgA deficiency	**Inability to produce IgA antibodies;** associated with congenital intra-uterine infection (toxoplasmosis, rubella, CMV) or following treatment with phenytoin or other medications in genetically susceptible individuals → halted B-cell differentiation	• Caucasian, familial • Asymptomatic or recurrent respiratory infections, chronic diarrheal disease • Associated with atopic disease, arthritis, SLE

Table 58-3 Deficiencies of cellular immunity (T-cell defects)

Immunodeficiency	Pathogenesis	Clinical manifestation
DiGeorge syndrome	Failed development of the 3rd and 4th pharyngeal pouches causing congenitally absent thymus and parathyroids → **loss of T-cell-mediated immunity** and parathyroid function; deletion in chromosome 22q11	• ↓ Circulating T-cells → poor defense against fungal and viral infections • Congenital heart defects • Facial abnormalities • Hypocalcemic tetany
Hyper-IgM syndrome	A mutation causes abnormal **CD40/CD40L interaction** preventing: 1. Activation of CTLs and macrophages → poor cell-mediated immunity 2. B-cells from isotype switching from IgM to IgA, IgG, or IgE → poor opsonization (also a humoral immunodeficiency)	• Male: X-linked inheritance • Recurrent pyogenic infections (because IgG levels are low) • *Pneumocystis carinii* pneumonia • Autoimmune hemolytic anemia, thrombocytopenia, neutropenia (from IgM antibody reaction)

Case Conclusion The immunology consultant performs an evaluation on BD and discovers that he has a history of poison ivy contact dermatitis and no prior episodes of thrush. His family history is significant for a granduncle who died of pneumonia as a child. On exam, he has no lymphadenopathy. His CBC with a differential smear reveals lymphopenia with a marked decrease in mature B-cells as determined by immunohistochemistry. Serum immunoglobulin levels shows marked decreases in all five classes of immunoglobulin. BD is subsequently diagnosed with Bruton's X-linked γ-globulinemia and is treated with immunoglobulin replacement.

Table 58-4 Combined B- and T-cell defects

Immunodeficiency	Pathogenesis	Clinical manifestations
Severe combined immunodeficiency syndrome (SCID)	**Impaired humoral and cell-mediated immunity** caused by multiple defects in T-, B-, and NK-cell development, e.g., adenosine deaminase deficiency • RAG-1 and -2 gene mutations impair V(D)J rearrangement • JAK3 protein kinase deficiency	• X-linked or autosomal recessive • Severe fungal, bacterial, and viral infection • Affected infants rarely survive beyond 1 year without treatment • Treated with pluripotent hematopoietic stem cell transplant
Wiskott-Aldrich syndrome	**Progressive T-lymphocyte depletion** in circulation and in paracortical (thymus-dependent) areas of lymph nodes → loss of cellular immunity, poor antibody development to polysaccharide and protein antigens; poor IgM levels	• X-linked disease • Recurrent fungal, bacterial, and viral infection • Thrombocytopenia • Eczema • Early death
Ataxia telangiectasia	Mutant ATM gene causes **defect in monitoring of DNA repair** and coordination of DNA synthesis in cell division; maldevelopment of the thymus	• Respiratory tract infections • Cerebellar ataxia: truncal *ataxia* • Oculocutaneous *telangiectasia* • Lymphomas and carcinomas
Hyper-IgE syndrome	Mechanism and gene defect unknown → **very high IgE levels,** abnormal neutrophil chemotaxis, diminished antibody responses to immunizations	• *Recurrent skin and lung abscesses* • Staphylococcal infections and other pyogenic infections • Recurrent bone fractures, scoliosis

Thumbnail: Immunodeficiency

- Defects in phagocytic function prevent final digestion and elimination of many infections with many consequences, including abscess formation
- Defects in humoral immunity lead to infections by small organisms requiring opsonization and phagocytosis for final elimination (extracellular infections)

- Defects in cellular immunity cause susceptibility to infections by mycobacteria, fungi, and viral infection (intracellular infections)

Key Points

▶ The specific profiles of susceptibility to different infections illustrate the specific function of the defective immune component of an immunodeficiency

▶ Complement deficiencies are marked by susceptibility to infections by bacteria that require the opsonizing activity of complement, particularly encapsulated organisms such as *Neisseria meningitidis*

▶ B-lymphocyte immunodeficiencies are marked by susceptibility to organisms that require opsonization by antibodies, especially in the gastrointestinal mucosa where IgA serves as an important defense

▶ T-lymphocyte immunodeficiencies are marked by susceptibility to mycobacterial and fungal infection, both of which require a robust, cell-mediated immunity to suppress

Questions

1. What is the significance of BD's prior history of poison ivy contact dermatitis without history of thrush?

   A. It suggests an abnormal delayed-type hypersensitivity reaction that is associated with his immunodeficiency syndrome

   B. The contact dermatitis suggests atopic disease, which makes him susceptible to respiratory tract infection and inflammation

   C. This suggests an autoimmune skin disease activated by recognition of poison ivy antigen acting as a hapten by binding dermal cells, eliciting cell-mediated immunity against BD's cell surface antigen

   D. Having no prior history of thrush makes the diagnosis of immunodeficiency in the protection of the upper respiratory tract mucous membranes questionable

   E. This past medical history suggests normal cell-mediated immune function

2. LE is a 10-year-old boy who presents to an immunology clinic after his sixth hospitalization for diarrhea. His immunoglobulin panel reveals an absence of IgA. What is the immunopathology underlying this immunodeficiency?

   A. The absence of IgA, the first immunoglobulin raised against pathogens, prevents proper neutralization of bacteria, making LE more susceptible to gastritis

   B. The absence of IgA prevents intravascular clearing of bacteria, making LE susceptible to recurrent gastritis, causing diarrhea

   C. The absence of IgA prevents the opsonization of intraluminal parasites of the gastrointestinal tract, making LE susceptible to chronic amebiasis

   D. The absence of IgA prevents the opsonization of pathogens within the gastrointestinal tract, thus making LE more susceptible to gastrointestinal bacteria infection, gastritis, and subsequent diarrhea

   E. The absence of IgA prevents complement fixation, which is essential for initiating the inflammatory reaction, and opsonizing and eliminating bacteria, thus making LE susceptible to recurrent gastritis

Case 54

1. B
2. D

Case 55

1. E
2. A

Case 56

1. E
2. B

Case 57

1. C
2. D

Case 58

1. E
2. D

Answers

Case 1

1. B Vancomycin and linezolid will cover methicillin-sensitive staphylococci, but should be reserved for methicillin-resistant organisms. Penicillin and ampicillin are increasingly ineffective against *S. aureus,* as the introduction of penicillin in the early 1940s selected for penicillinase-producing strains. Approximately 85% to 90% of *S. aureus* strains in both the hospital and the community are now resistant to penicillin/ampicillin. The first-generation cephalosporins (e.g., cefazolin) will cover methicillin-sensitive strains of *S. aureus*. Of note, cefazolin has poor penetration into the CNS, and nafcillin should be used instead of the former in the case of staphylococcal meningitis.

2. C; 3. C Methicillin-resistant *S. aureus* (MRSA) has carriage rates as high as 25% to 50%. Groups at higher risk for MRSA include injection drug users, persons with insulin-dependent diabetes, patients with dermatologic conditions, patients with long-term in-dwelling intravascular catheters, and health care workers.

4. D *S. epidermidis* species tend to be much more antibiotic resistant than *S. aureus* species, with a methicillin resistance rate of approximately 80%.

Case 2

1. D Streptolysin O and streptolysin S both contribute to β-hemolysis. As streptolysin O is inactivated by oxidation (oxygen-labile), it cases β-hemolysis only when the colonies grow under the surface of a blood agar plate. Because streptolysin S is oxygen stable, it is responsible for β-hemolysis when colonies grow on the surface of a blood agar plate.

2. C Group A streptococcus is the only streptococcal species that is bacitracin susceptible, needs M-protein for virulence, and has the species name of *S. pyogenes*. Group A streptococci are the most likely infectious agents to trigger poststreptococcal nonsuppurative infections, albeit such immunologic complications have rarely been seen following group C or group G infections. All streptococcal species are catalase negative, which distinguishes them from the catalase-positive staphylococcal species.

Case 3

1. B Nutritionally variant streptococci (NVS) require pyridoxal or thiol group supplementation for growth. A streak of *S. aureus* on a sheep blood agar plate can provide these factors to the surrounding media so that the nutritionally variant *Streptococcus* species will grow as satellite colonies around the *S. aureus* streak. Alternatively, 0.001% pyridoxal or 0.01% L-cysteine can be added to the agar media to promote growth of these *Streptococcus* species. Unsupplemented tryptic soy broth will not support the growth of NVS, and *S. pneumoniae* cannot provide these factors to the surrounding media to allow satellite growth of NVS

colonies. Charcoal yeast extract agar plates are designed to allow culture of *Legionella* species.

2. D In the setting of infective endocarditis, emboli from the vegetative valvular lesion can lodge in the distal vasculature and immune complexes can form, leading to "stigmata" of endocarditis, such as

Stigmata	Mechanism	Description
Roth's spots	Immunologic	Retinal hemorrhage with a central area of clearing
Osler's nodes	Immunologic	Erythematous painful nodes at the tips of digits
Janeway lesions	Vascular	Erythematous painless macules on the palms and soles
Splinter hemorrhages	Vascular	Petechiae underneath the nail bed

Case 4

1. D The following are CDC guidelines for the prevention of VRE:

Situations in which the use of vancomycin is appropriate:

1. Treatment of serious infections due to β-lactam-resistant gram-positive organisms

2. Treatment of serious infections due to gram-positive organisms in patients with serious β-lactam allergies

3. Treatment of antibiotic-associated colitis (AAC) when treatment with metronidazole has failed or if the AAC is potentially life threatening

4. Prophylaxis for endocarditis for certain procedures based on American Heart Association recommendations

5. Prophylaxis for certain surgical procedures involving implantation of prosthetic materials in hospitals with a high rate of MRSA or MRSE.

Situations in which the use of vancomycin should be discouraged:

1. Routine surgical prophylaxis, unless the patient has a severe allergy to β-lactam antibiotics

2. Empiric treatment for febrile neutropenic patients, unless a gram-positive infection is suspected and the institution has a high rate of MRSA

3. Treatment of one positive blood culture for coagulase-negative *Staphylococcus* if other blood cultures drawn at the same time are negative (i.e., likely contamination)

4. Continued empiric use in patients whose cultures are negative for β-lactam-resistant gram-positive organisms

5. Prophylaxis for infection or colonization of in-dwelling central or peripheral intravascular catheters

6. Selective decontamination of the gastrointestinal tract

7. Eradication of MRSA colonization

8. Primary treatment of antibiotic-associated colitis

9. Routine prophylaxis for infants with very low birth weight

10. Routine prophylaxis for patients on continuous ambulatory peritoneal dialysis or hemodialysis

11. Treatment of infection due to β-lactam-sensitive gram-positive microorganisms in patients with renal failure (for ease of dosing schedule)

12. Use of vancomycin solution for topical application or irrigation.

2. A VanA exhibits high-level resistance (MIC > 128 μg/mL) to vancomyin and is resistant to teicoplanin (an investigational glycopeptide antibiotic). VanB exhibits moderate-level resistance (MIC 16–64 μg/mL) to vancomycin and is sensitive to teicoplanin. VanC, VanD, and VanE exhibit low-level resistance to vancomycin (MIC 8–16 μg/mL) and are sensitive to teicoplanin.

Case 5

1. B The most common location for diagnosed actinomycosis is the angle of the jaw.

2. A *Listeria monocytogenes* is a nonfilamentous gram-positive rod that forms strongly catalase-positive, β-hemolytic colonies with a distinctive tumbling motility at 25°C in semisolid medium. This agent causes sepsis and meningitis in neonates and in immuno-suppressed adults. The infection is acquired usually from unpasteurized milk or vegetables contaminated with animal feces. The treatment for *Listeria* infections is ampicillin plus or minus aminoglycosides. Trimethoprim-sulfamethoxazole (TMP-SMZ) can be used for penicillin-allergic patients.

Case 6

1. C *B. anthracis* has natural resistance to sulfa drugs, trimetho-prim, aztreonam, and third-generation cephalosporins (such as ceftriaxone and ceftazidime). Antimicrobial agents that should be considered in addition to ciprofloxacin or doxycycline in the treat-ment of inhalational anthrax include penicillin or ampicillin, vancomycin, rifampin, chloramphenicol, clindamycin, imipenem, and clarithromycin.

2. D Given that the incubation period for inhalational anthrax is between 2 and 43 days, antimicrobial prophylaxis should be con-tinued for 60 days to prevent germination of the spores and subsequent disease.

Case 7

1. C Because this patient does not know the date of his last tetanus shot, he should be considered nonimmune. With this dirty wound, he should receive both tetanus toxoid and tetanus immune globulin for immediate protection.

2. B *C. tetani* is an anaerobic, motile, gram-positive spore-forming rod. The spores are resistant to both heat and many detergents.

3. D Tetanospasmin, produced by *C. tetani,* is the cause of the clinical syndrome of tetanus. *C. botulinum* produces botulinum toxin in its pathogenesis. *E. coli* O157:H7 produces a shiga-like toxin that causes diarrhea. The major pathogenic factor of *V. cholerae* is a potent exotoxin. The causative organisms of malaria, of which *Plasmodium falciparum* is one, do not produce toxins.

Case 8

1. B Botulinum toxin is the most potent bacterial toxin known—one microgram of purified toxin is able to kill 200,000 mice. The toxin is released only upon the death and autolysis of the organ-ism, and is thus classified as an exotoxin. Its activity is limited to the peripheral nervous system, where it is internalized into the presynaptic membrane at the neuromuscular junction and blocks the release of acetylcholine. Antibiotics have no direct effect on the toxin. The currently used antitoxin is of equine origin and is usually given as polyvalent A, B, and E antitoxin. Injection of botu-linum toxin is used in medical settings to treat strabismus and blepharospasm and has gained popularity recently as a cosmetic approach to lessen wrinkles (Botox).

2. A Infant botulism, the most common form of the disease in the U.S., arises from germination of ingested spores with subsequent toxin production within the intestine. Honey has been identified as a source of contaminated spores and is thus not recommended to be given to infants less than 12 months of age. There are no recommendations for prophylactic antibiotics. The disease is acquired through ingestion of spores, so respiratory precautions are not appropriate. There is no vaccine for botulinum toxin. Breast-feeding has no effect on botulism.

Case 9

1. C Antibiotics that kill off normal flora but allow *C. difficile* to survive create ecological conditions for *C. difficile* overgrowth. Because metronidazole kills *C. difficile,* it is less likely to give rise to the infection than other antibiotics. Clindamycin (A) and cephalosporins (B, D, and E) kill a broad spectrum of bacteria but do not harm *C. difficile;* these antibiotics are associated with some of the highest rates of pseudomembranous colitis.

2. B Toxic megacolon can be a lethal complication; this is why anti-motility drugs are relatively contraindicated for *C. difficile* colitis. Gas gangrene (A) is due to *C. perfringens. C. difficile* does not cause the other listed conditions.

Case 10

1. C Rifampin will turn all of an individual's secretions, such as urine, sweat, tears, and stool, an orange color. Contact lenses can be permanently stained with this orange discoloration. This side effect is a source of great consternation to individuals who are not warned of its possibility.

2. E *Moraxella catarrhalis,* formerly called *Branhamella catarrhalis,* is a gram-negative cocci that causes upper respiratory infections, including sinusitis, otitis media, and, occasionally, pneumonia.

Case 11

1. B *Bacillus cereus* strains can produce two different toxins: a heat-stable toxin that can lead to an illness after 2 to 7 hours and a heat-labile toxin that causes disease manifestations 8 to 14 hours after ingestion. The syndrome of *Clostridium perfringens* diarrhea usually occurs 8 to 14 hours after ingestion of the preformed toxin.

2. C *Campylobacter jejuni* is a gram-negative rod that is S shaped or comma shaped on Gram stain.

Case 12

1. B The combination of an appropriate β-lactam antibiotic and an aminoglycoside is the most effective combination against *P. aeruginosa.* Penicillin does not have activity against *P. aeruginosa.* Both (C) and (E) are incorrect answers because combinations of two β-lactam antibiotics, even if they both have activity against *P. aeruginosa,* are antagonistic. Cefuroxime in (D) is a second-generation cephalosporin without activity against the organism.

2. C Neutropenia in cancer patients is a risk factor for necrotizing enterocolitis. The syndrome can also occur in young infants and is often fatal.

Case 13

1. C *Streptococcus sanguis,* one of the *Viridans* streptococci, is a common cause of endocarditis; however, it is gram positive and usually grows more quickly than 6 days. *Pseudomonas* accounts for about 10% of endocarditis in intravenous drug users. It is a long, thin gram-negative rod and usually grows more quickly than 6 days. The morphology of short, gram-negative rods in this case argues for a *Haemophilus* species. *H. parainfluenza* and *H. aphrophilus* are members of the HACEK (*Haemophilus, Actinobacterium, Cardiobacterium, Eikenella,* and *Kingella*) group of organisms, which are fastidious, slow growing, and require incubation with CO_2. They cause about 5% of infective endocarditis and are becoming more frequently isolated with improved culture techniques. *H. influenza* is also a potential cause of endocarditis, but growth is usually faster than 6 days. Speciation of *Haemophilus* isolates depends heavily upon nutritional growth requirements, particularly V-factor (NAD: nicotinamide adenine dinucleotide) and X-factor (hemin). *H. influenza* requires both V- and X-factors. *H. aphrophilus* requires X-factor but not V-factor. *H. parainfluenza* requires V-factor but not X-factor (the *para* prefix among *Haemophilus* species is used to indicate they do NOT require X-factor).

2. A Disease caused by *H. influenza* is rare before the age of 3 months, presumably due to the protective effect of maternal anti-bodies. This illustrates the importance of humoral, rather than cellular, immunity in protection against disease. The primary determinant of immunity is high titers of anti-capsular antibody. There are no known nonhuman reservoirs of Hib. The respiratory tract is the most common portal of entry for infection, and Hib generally invades by passing between, rather than through, respiratory epithelial cells.

Case 14

1. E This patient has chancroid. Culture for chancroid is very insensitive. RPR testing may be negative during primary syphilis, as it may take 2 to 3 weeks to turn positive after infection. Repeated RPR testing over this time period is necessary to eliminate syphilis. Additionally, the chancre of primary syphilis is usually nontender. Lymphogranuloma venereum (LGV) is caused by *Chlamydia trachomatis* serovars L1, L2, and L3; chlamydia serology should be positive if this were the diagnosis. Donovanosis, or granuloma inguinale, is caused by *Calymmatobacterium granulomatis* and would not be associated with lymphadenopathy.

2. B Erythromycin is the best treatment for chancroid. Other options include azithromycin, ceftriaxone, ciprofloxacin, and possibly TMP-SMZ.

Case 15

1. D Overall, *E. coli* is the most common cause of UTIs, and the resistance pattern of local *E. coli* strains will influence community prescribing habits for these infections. *E. coli* is also the only gram-negative rod listed. *Enterococcus faecalis* (E) is a gram-positive coccus that frequently causes UTIs. When *S. aureus* (A) is found in the urine, it often is a secondary result of bacteremia rather than a primary infection. *S. saprophyticus* (B) is a coagulase-negative staphylococcus that can cause urinary tract infections in young women. Corynebacteria (C) are gram-positive rod skin flora. Their presence in a urine culture indicates contamination through improper collection.

2. B Uncomplicated cystitis causes dysuria, frequency, and urgency. The presence of systemic symptoms, such as rigors (A) or vomiting (D) and pain at the costovertebral angle, where the kidneys lie (C), all point to pyelonephritis. While gross hematuria (E) can be caused by infection alone, it is more often due to trauma, tumor, or kidney stones, and a work-up is mandated.

3. C Nitrofurantoin is a useful antibiotic because it works selectively in the bladder, after being concentrated in the urine. Because of this selective action, it is not appropriate for patients with pyelonephritis, as it will not kill bacteria in the bloodstream or kidneys. The drug will also not work in patients with renal failure, whose kidneys do not concentrate the drug. Whereas quinolones such as ciprofloxacin or levofloxacin are often used for UTIs, trovafloxacin would not be used because it can cause serious liver toxicity. Imipenem (A) is a parenteral, extremely broad-spectrum antibiotic that would never be used in the outpatient setting. Azithromycin (B) is rarely used for UTIs because its spectrum and achievable drug levels do not match well with urinary tract pathogens. It is more often used for respiratory and ENT infections. Metronidazole (E) is used to treat vaginal infections (bacterial vaginosis or trichomonas), but UTIs are usually due to aerobic bacteria not killed by this drug.

Case 16

1. D Cholera toxin results in a secretory diarrhea only; the patient's symptoms suggest dysentery. *E. coli, Salmonella,* and *Shigella* can all present with either secretory or bloody diarrhea, depending on the strain. Bloody diarrhea is caused by organisms that directly invade the intestinal epithelial cells or produce a cytotoxic toxin. *Vibrio parahaemolyticus,* although microbiologically related to *Vibrio cholerae,* produces diarrhea through direct invasion, causing dysentery.

2. E Oral rehydration therapy, because of its simplicity and low cost, has reduced cholera mortality by 10-fold. Preventing cholera is crucial, and involves improving water supplies and reminding travelers to take precautions. Boiled water, in a soup, should be safe, however. The cholera toxin is not a strong antigen, and no good cholera vaccine is available. Finally, there is little role for antibiotics in cholera. Ciprofloxacin is useful in traveler's diarrhea with *Shigella* or *E. coli* (although it is contraindicated for *E. coli* O157:H7 because of an increased incidence of hemolytic-uremic syndrome). Gut decontamination is sometimes performed before surgery, or in an attempt to treat refractory hepatic encephalopathy.

Case 17

1. E Gastric non-Hodgkin's lymphoma (MALToma) is associated with *H. pylori* infection. Treatment of the *H. pylori* is associated with tumor regression. Hepatitis B virus is associated with hepatocellular carcinoma. EBV is associated with Burkitt's lymphoma, CNS lymphoma, and body cavity lymphomas. The other organisms listed are not associated with malignancies.

2. B The urease breath test depends on living organisms hydrolyzing ^{13}C- or ^{14}C-urea into ammonia and $^{13}CO_2$ or $^{14}CO_2$, which is detected in a breath sample. Thus, a positive test indicates active infection. Serology is sensitive and specific in diagnosing infection, but remains positive after successful eradiation of infection. Culture is the least sensitive of the diagnostic tests for *H. pylori* and requires endoscopy to obtain tissue samples. Stool PCR and the CAMP test do not test for *H. pylori.*

3. A This patient has nonulcer dyspepsia. Her positive serology indicates past or current infection with *H. pylori;* however, a link between nonulcer dyspepsia and *H. pylori* infection has not been established. Thus, the patient does not require *H. pylori* treatment in this case. If a duodenal ulcer had been seen on endoscopy, treatment of *H. pylori* would be indicated and the regimen in (B) would have the highest rate of eradication. An H_2 blocker such as ranitidine may help relieve her symptoms of dyspepsia.

Case 18

1. A Although gastrointestinal tularemia can be acquired by ingestion of *F. tularensis* organisms, *Brucella melitensis* is commonly acquired through the ingestion of unpasteurized goat's milk cheese (often imported from Mexico).

2. B Splenectomized patients are at high risk for disseminated infection with this organism and often present with DIC and sepsis after a dog bite.

Case 19

1. A Enteric pathogens, such as *Salmonella* and *Shigella,* are often distinguished from normal fecal flora by using plates such as MacConkey agar or Hektoen agar, which allow easy selection of lactose nonfermenters. The enterobacteriaceae and *Salmonella* are glucose fermenters, oxidase negative, and nitrate reducing (B–D). *Salmonella* does produce hydrogen sulfide, which distinguishes it from *Shigella* and most enterobacteriaceae.

2. E *Salmonella typhimurium* is a nontyphoidal strain of *Salmonella* that causes gastroenteritis. Typhoid fever (D) is caused by *Salmonella typhi* and *S. paratyphi.* Typhus (A–C) is a group of unrelated rickettsial diseases.

Case 20

1. B Only patients with active pulmonary or laryngeal tuberculosis are infectious. Patients with positive smears and cavitary disease have a higher organism load and are more infectious than patients who have positive cultures but no organisms found on direct sputum smears. Infections at other anatomic sites (A and E) do not make a patient infectious unless there is concomitant pulmonary TB. Positive skin tests (C) are a marker for past exposure, but do not necessarily indicate active disease; indeed, patients with overwhelming TB infection can have negative PPDs.

2. B Pyrazinimide is one of the four first-line TB drugs. The other listed drugs are second line because of decreased or less proven efficacy, the necessity for parenteral administration (streptomycin), serious side effects (PAS and cycloserine), or cost and reservation for other uses (levofloxacin).

3. C All the first-line drugs can cause hepatotoxicity, the major toxicity of TB therapy. INH can cause neuropathy (which can be prevented by co-administration of vitamin B_6), ethambutol can cause optic neuritis, rifampin can cause serious drug-drug interactions (particularly with HIV protease inhibitors), and pyrazinimide causes hyperuricemia (although this is usually asymptomatic).

4. C Active tuberculosis at any site (the presence of culturable organisms or evidence of progressive disease) mandates multidrug therapy. For patients with latent tuberculosis infection (A), treatment with a single drug will suffice to kill the small number of organisms. The calcified granulomas in patient B are a sign of old disease; he does not need new treatment unless he becomes symptomatic. The patients (D) and (E) have had low-risk exposures and would not be treated unless there was evidence of a change in skin tests.

Case 21

1. E As with tuberculosis therapy, treatment of rapidly growing mycobacterial infections is usually very prolonged. Most skin and soft tissue infections require a combination of debridement and long courses of therapy; pulmonary infections may require even more than 6 months of appropriate chemotherapy for cure.

2. B The various prophylactic regimens for MAC in HIV infection (usually initiated at CD4 counts ≤ 50 cells/μL) include azithromycin 1200 mg orally every week, clarithromycin 500 mg orally twice a day, and rifabutin 300 mg orally every day.

Case 22

1. D *Listeria* can be cultured through routine techniques. The other organisms on this list, all intracellular pathogens, are usually diagnosed through serology.

2. E Rocky Mountain spotted fever is transmitted by ticks. Lyme disease is also spread by ticks, but the causative agent is a spirochete. Scrub typhus and rickettsial pox are spread by mites. There is no insect vector for Q fever.

Case 23

1. C Reactivation of *Coxiella burnetii* infection occurs in female mammals during pregnancy, with high concentrations of organisms found in the placenta; the risk of *C. burnetii* transmission to humans at animal births is high.

2. D Pulmonary anthrax is known as "woolsorter's disease," as this condition often occurred in farm workers around massive amounts of sheep wool containing *B. anthracis* spores. *Brucella melitensis* can cause disease (brucellosis) in humans after exposure to goats or sheep. *B. ovis* primarily causes genital diseases in rams. *Francisella tularensis* is the agent of tularemia and usually follows exposure to rabbits, deer, and rodents.

Case 24

1. E β-lactams (penicillins and cephalosporins) are often used to treat community-acquired pneumonia because they cover the most common causes (pneumococcus and gram-negative organisms such as *Moraxella* or *Haemophilus influenzae*). These drugs do not cover atypical agents, and are usually given in combination with one of the other classes listed for atypical coverage, unless a firm etiologic diagnosis has been made. Ketolides are a new class of antibiotic that cover atypical organisms and have stronger pneumococcal coverage than the macrolides.

2. D *Legionella* is not known to be a colonizer; if it is found on culture, it should be treated. While *Mycoplasma* and *Chlamydia* cultures are rarely sent, these organisms can be found in asymptomatic subjects, so their mere presence does not require treatment. *Moraxella, Haemophilus,* and *Pneumococcus* can also be colonizers in asymptomatic patients. However, they should be treated in a patient with clinical signs of pneumonia and one of these organisms predominating in a sputum Gram stain and culture.

3. B Mycoplasma are tiny free-living organisms that lack a cell wall. Because they have no cell wall, β-lactam antibiotics are ineffective against them. Bacteria (*Klebsiella, Moraxella,* and *Pneumococcus*) as well as yeast have cell walls. Because human cells do not have cell walls, the biosynthetic pathways for cell wall generation are important antibiotic targets.

4. B Mycoplasma are extracellular parasites. The other agents all act intracellularly in human cells. Although the elementary bodies of *Chlamydia* are extracellular, they are equivalent to spores; the reticular bodies, which are intracellular, are the form that carry out metabolism and reproduction.

Case 25

1. D This patient has PID, most likely complicated with a perihepatitis known as Fitzhugh-Curtis syndrome. She has no particular evidence of either TOA or TOC, though this cannot be ruled out without an ultrasound. Cervicitis is an infection of just the cervix; patients have no adnexal tenderness and can be managed as outpatients.

2. C Patients with PID should be treated presumptively for GC and *C. trachomatis.* Treatment of GC can include a second- or third-generation cephalosporin or high-dose azithromycin, as resistance to penicillins and spectinomycin has been demonstrated. *C. trachomatis* can be treated with macrolides such as erythromycin and azithromycin as well as tetracyclines. However, tetracyclines are not used in pregnant patients because of effects on fetal teeth.

Case 26

1. C *Borrelia burgdorferi* and *Babesia microti* are transmitted by the same species of tick (*Ixodes dammini*) in the same endemic areas (northeast U.S.). Up to 50% of patients diagnosed with babesiosis have serologic evidence of past infection with *Borrelia.* The other choices are not causes of arthritis in this scenario.

2. E Colorado tick fever is caused by an arbovirus transmitted by the wood tick (*Dermacentor andersoni*). (Note: the only other viral infection spread by ticks in the U.S. is Powassan encephalitis.) Lyme disease is caused by the bacteria *Borrelia burgdorferi,* spread by the *Ixodes dammini* tick. Rocky Mountain spotted fever is caused by the bacterium *Rickettsia rickettsiae,* spread by the *Dermacentor andersoni* or *Dermacentor variabilis* tick. Tulareamia is caused by the bacterium *Francisella tularensis,* spread by the *Dermacentor* ticks or *Amblyomma americanum.* Babesiosis is caused by the parasite *Babesia microti,* spread by the *Ixodes dammini* tick.

Case 27

1. A Leptospirosis is a zoonotic disease of humans, acquired most frequently from contact with urine of infected animals. The contact often occurs in contaminated water sources such as sewers or stagnant bodies of fresh water. Leptospira are not documented to be spread from person to person, nor do they form spores. Trichinosis develops after ingestion of infected pork, not leptospirosis.

2. A This is a classic Jarisch-Herxheimer reaction, similar to that seen in treatment of syphilis and other spirochetal diseases. Although the pathophysiology is not completely understood, the reaction is thought to be due to the killing of organisms with release of toxins or from a release of chemokines (i.e., tumor necrosis factor, IL-6, or IL-8) by phagocytic cells in response to treatment. Penicillin is the antibiotic of choice, and no resistance has been described. The organism is present in blood, urine, and CSF and can be cultured from all of these sites prior to treatment. Co-infection would be exceedingly unlikely.

Case 28

1. C All the treponemes cause skin disease, and most affect other organ systems as well. Pinta (which means "painted") affects only the skin (although the skin manifestations alone can be devastating and stigmatizing). Yaws and bejel can affect skin and bones. Syphilis affects skin and bones, but its dreaded manifestations are the cardiovascular, CNS, and ocular symptoms of tertiary syphilis.

2. D Classic manifestations of tertiary syphilis include cardiovascular disease (aortic aneurysms), CNS disease (tabes dorsalis or general paresis), ocular disease, and the formation of lesions called gummas. Most skin manifestations are found at earlier stages; the chancre is the hallmark of primary syphilis, and the maculopapular rash and condylomata lata are found during the secondary stage.

3. D Syphilis is one of the very few pathogens where drug resistance has not become a clinical problem. It is still exquisitely sensitive to penicillin. The only reason not to use penicillin is if the patient has a severe allergy to the drug. Primary syphilis is a systemic infection and topical treatment is not possible. Neurosyphilis is still treated with penicillin, although the antibiotic is given via continuous IV to achieve higher CNS levels. Penicillin is the only drug approved for use in pregnant patients.

Case 29

1. A Two diseases are transmitted to humans by the same deer tick vector, *Ixodes:* human granulocytic ehrlichiosis (HGE), which is caused by the *Ehrlichia phagocytophila* group and babesiosis, caused by *Babesia microti.* Human monocytic ehrlichiosis is caused by *Ehrlichia chaffeensis* and spread by *Amblyomma,* the Lone Star tick; Rocky Mountain spotted fever is caused by *Rickettsia rickettsii* and spread by *Dermacentor variabilis,* the dog tick; West Nile

virus is spread by the *Culex* mosquito; Colorado tick fever is also spread by the dog tick.

2. B Ninety percent of Lyme disease is found in the following ten states: Connecticut, Rhode Island, New Jersey, New York, Delaware, Pennsylvania, Massachusetts, Maryland, Minnesota, and Wisconsin.

Case 30

1. E Resistance varies by the host and by the prior exposure of that host to antivirals. Approximate proportions of resistance in the U.S. population are as follows:

- 3% in normal hosts
- 5% to 7% in immunocompromised patients (such as organ transplant recipients and recipients of chronic corticosteroids)
- 15% in bone marrow transplant patients and advanced HIV (due to extensive prior acyclovir exposure)

2. B Asymptomatic viral shedding occurs 4.3% of the days tested in a year, accounting for 10% risk per year of transmission to an uninfected partner.

Case 31

1. B Foscarnet (and cidofovir) are second-line drugs against CMV, used to treat ganciclovir-resistant virus. Acyclovir, valacyclovir, and famciclovir are all active against HSV-1 and HSV-2, but not CMV, which lacks the viral thymidine kinase required for their activation. Lamivudine is a reverse transcriptase inhibitor, used to treat HIV and HBV.

2. D HIV patients are only at risk of CMV infection once they have reached a CD4 count below 50. These patients receive regular eye exams to detect retinitis (the most common site of infection) before vision is affected and irreversibly lost. CMV can also cause colitis in HIV patients, but they would be symptomatic with diarrhea; diagnosis requires endoscopic biopsy of the colon. Neutropenia (an absolute neutrophil count < 500) is actually a contraindication to digital rectal exam, because of the risk of bacteremia and subsequent sepsis. CMV can also cause CNS infection and rarely pneumonitis in HIV patients (pneumonitis is much more common in transplant patients), but asymptomatic patients are not screened.

Case 32

1. B Although there is some evidence of initiating antiretroviral therapy in the face of acute infection and such studies are currently in progress, most clinicians support acute HIV infection with symptomatic therapy alone at this point.

2. A Retroviruses contain single-stranded, linear, positive-polarity RNA and a viral reverse transcriptase protein that "transcribes" the RNA genome into DNA upon viral entry into the host cell.

Case 33

1. A Mosquito repellant is thought to be the only effective measure against WNV infection. There is no evidence that handling dead infected birds or other infected animals can lead to WNV infection.

2. D Convincing epidemiologic evidence, especially from the 1999 New York outbreak, shows that older age is a risk factor for death from WNV infection and an increased incidence of chronic neurologic sequelae.

Case 34

1. E This patient has acute hepatitis, and the most likely cause is hepatitis A. Although sexual transmission is possible, the most likely source is food. Hepatitis B could potentially be transmitted from a sexual partner, a needlestick exposure from work (he should be vaccinated), or vertically (although vertical transmission would result in chronic hepatitis rather than acute disease in an adult). Ticks are not vectors for agents of acute viral hepatitis.

2. C For nonimmune patients with potential future exposures to hepatitis A, preventive therapy is indicated. Rural Mexico would be a high prevalence area for hepatitis A, so she is at risk for acute infection. Vaccination is indicated in all travelers to endemic areas. Because it takes 2 to 4 weeks to develop protective antibodies from vaccination, immune globulin is indicated for patients in whom the potential exposure will occur in less than 1 month. Rimantadine is not effective against hepatitis A.

Case 35

1. B Anti-HBs shows protective immunity against the hepatitis virus. Production of this antibody is stimulated by past exposure to the virus, or by administration of the recombinant HBV vaccine. Anti-HBc is a marker of past exposure to the virus, but in some cases current infection is still possible. HBeAg is a marker for high viral loads, and therefore high infectivity. Anti-HBe Ab indicates relatively low infectivity (although this test is rarely used in clinical practice). Finally, HBsAg is a marker for current infection.

2. D Lamivudine is active against both HBV and HIV, as is tenofovir. Adefovir is also active against both viruses, but nephrotoxicity prevents adefovir from being used at the higher HIV dose. These drugs have activity against HBV because HBV replication includes a reverse transcriptase step. Other HIV drugs, including the rest of the nucleoside analogues like AZT and ddI, are not active against HBV.

Case 36

1. C Ribavirin disrupts replication of many RNA viruses by interfering with replication. Hepatitis B is a DNA virus that can be treated with another set of drugs interfering with the reverse transcrip-

tion step in its replication cycle. There are no antiviral drugs for the other viral hepatitides.

2. B The Sin Nombre virus is a Hantavirus that causes a pulmonary edema syndrome. This virus is found in the western U.S., and is thought to be transmitted through aerosolized mouse urine. The other listed viruses cause hemorrhagic fever, but not pulmonary edema. Lassa and Ebola are found in Africa, and Junin and Machupo are found in South America, although cases have occurred in other countries due to travel or importation of infected animals.

Case 37

1. E Influenza can be distinguished from a generic upper respiratory infection (such as B) by the severe constitutional symptoms it causes. Despite the commonly used phrase "stomach flu," gastrointestinal disturbances are minimal or absent in influenza. Patient A's diarrhea is likely due to another viral cause, or to bacteria or parasites. Patient C appears to have acute hepatitis, which could be caused by hepatitis A or B. The symptoms of patient D are worrisome for measles; he may not have been immunized against this disease.

2. D Zanamivir and oseltamivir are both neuraminidase inhibitors. Hemagglutinin (B) is the other major surface protein of influenza virus, used for binding to target cells. No drugs currently target it. Protease and reverse transcriptase (C and A, respectively) are drug targets in HIV. Dihydrofolate reductase (E) is inhibited by sulfa drugs, and is a target in bacteria and parasites.

3. D Allergy to eggs is a contraindication to the vaccine because eggs are used to grow the virus for vaccine production. Because influenza virus is a killed virus, it is safe for AIDS patients (A) and pregnant women (C) to receive. Patients with severe pulmonary or cardiac disease (E) benefit the most from vaccination because they are the most likely to die from influenza, and vaccination programs should target them. Whereas the pneumovax should not be repeated more than every 5 to 7 years (D), the influenza vaccination needs to be given every year to maximize protection against currently circulating virus.

4. C Oseltamivir (and zanamivir) are neuraminidase inhibitors active against both influenza A and B. Amantadine (A) and rimantadine (E) are both only active against influenza A. Stavudine (B) is a nucleoside reverse transcriptase inhibitor active against HIV. Nelfinavir (D) is a protease inhibitor active against HIV.

Case 38

1. D Hepatitis B is a DNA virus. The rest of these viruses contain RNA.

2. C It is possible that the mother may not acquire infection, and thus there may be no risk to the fetus. If she does acquire rubella during the first trimester, there is a 90% chance that the fetus will be affected to some degree. Infection is diagnosed by rubella-specific antibody titer rises on paired serum samples. Despite the fact that no fetal abnormalities have been observed in cases of inadvertent administration of vaccine to pregnant women, live-attenuated rubella vaccine is contraindicated during pregnancy. IVIg has shown no benefit in protecting the fetus. Ribavirin is not effective against rubella virus and is significantly teratogenic.

3. D The rubella vaccine is a live, attenuated virus. Viral shedding in respiratory secretions of vaccinees may persist for up to 4 weeks after immunization. Thus, vaccine should not be given to individuals who may be at risk of passing the infection on to those at greatest risk of complications—pregnant women. The husband in D should not be offered the vaccine until after his wife has delivered, and then the couple should both be vaccinated. The nurse in C should be required to be immune *prior* to starting a job that puts him in close contact with pregnant women; thus, he needs to be vaccinated. The woman in B should be vaccinated 1 month prior to conception. Unlike other immunosuppressive diseases and/or medications, mild or asymptomatic HIV is not a contraindication to vaccination in children or adults.

Case 39

1. A This student has the "common cold," which is most likely caused by a rhinovirus. RSV may cause a similar picture in adults but is more likely to cause pneumonia and bronchitis in young children and the elderly. Enteroviruses more typically cause a nonspecific acute febrile illness or aseptic meningitis—respiratory tract infections occur uncommonly. This would be the right season for influenza infection; however, her lack of fever and myalgias argue strongly against influenza and she shouldn't be given antiflu therapy. *S. pneumoniae* would be more likely to cause pneumonia, sinusitis, meningitis, or endocarditis, which she does not have.

2. D Acute hemorrhagic cystitis is a unique infection of the urinary tract due to adenovirus; serotypes 11 and 21 are the most commonly implicated. The disease typically affects young men and resolves in 5 to 6 days. A kidney stone should have shown up on the CT scan, particularly with ongoing symptoms, and the pain of kidney stones is more typically located in the flank with radiation to the groin. The lack of pyuria and negative culture argue against bacterial UTI. Gonorrhea would present with urethritis, not cystitis. The lack of hypertension, normal renal function, and nondysmorphic RBCs differentiate cystitis from glomerulonephritis.

Case 40

1. C OPV is a live, attenuated virus ingested orally. It replicates in the gastrointestinal tract and is secreted in the feces. Thus, secondary infections may occur, which is helpful in immunizing nonvaccinated contacts but may lead to acute disease in immunocompromised hosts. Additionally, mucosal immunity may be induced by OPV as it replicates in the gastrointestinal tract. IPV is a subcutaneous injection of nonreplication competent virus and is safe in immunocompromised hosts. It does not induce mucosal immunity. Both IPV and OPV contain all three serotypes of virus,

and booster shots are required to maintain immunity for both IPV and OPV.

2. D This patient has classic symptoms and findings of myocarditis, and Coxsackie B virus is a common cause. Prolonged, or even permanent impairment of cardiac function may be seen after viral myocarditis. Pneumococcal pneumonia would present with cough, fever, and a lobar infiltrate on x-ray. Pericarditis may present with similar symptoms (chest pain, arrhythmias, and shortness of breath), although tuberculous pericarditis is uncommon. Chlamydial infections have been associated with atherosclerosis; however, the causal link is not established. Herpes zoster may be a cause of chest pain when the dermatomal distribution of the outbreak corresponds to the left anterior chest wall. The findings of congestive heart failure are not consistent with zoster.

Case 41

1. B Amphotericin B can lead to renal injury, ranging from mild renal tubular acidosis to severe renal toxicity with nephrocalcinosis. Hypokalemia and hypomagnesemia are frequent side effects from this medication, as well as the more rare hepatotoxicity and bone marrow suppression.

2. D *Mucor* and *Rhizopus* form nonseptate, true hyphae with broad irregular walls and branches that form at right angles (90°).

Case 42

1. E Flucytosine, which is given orally, is converted to 5-fluorouracil, which is an antimetabolite that may result in bone marrow suppression. Drug levels of flucytosine may be monitored, as higher levels correlate with toxicity. The other answers are all potential side effects of amphotericin.

2. C *Cryptococcus* does not secrete any toxins, but rather relies on its capsule to evade host defenses through inhibition of phagocytosis and antibody production. Additionally, phenoloxidase uses the mycotoxic host catecholamines epinephrine in the process of melanogenesis, thus protecting the yeast.

Case 43

1. E Blood cultures growing yeast could theoretically be contaminants, but the physician is obligated to treat them. Yeast can colonize the other listed sites without causing disease, although yeast skin and UTIs are often diagnosed and treated. True yeast pneumonias are exceedingly rare; usually yeast in the sputum is a colonizer of the oropharynx.

2. A Amphotericin B has both infusion-related toxicity (fever and chills) as well as cumulative nephrotoxicity, but doctors still frequently use the drug because they have the most clinical experience with it. Expensive lipid-based formulations have been developed to try and reduce these side effects. Topical antifungals

(B, C, and D) all have minimal side effects. The new antifungal, caspofungin (E), also has minimal reported side effects.

3. E Caspofungin, an echinocandin, blocks β-glycan synthesis required to make yeast cell walls. This is analogous to the *antibacterial* antibiotic penicillin (B). Polyenes, such as amphotericin and nystatin (A and D), and azoles, such as fluconazole (C), target ergosterol, a component of the yeast cell *membrane*.

Case 44

1. E In an immunocompetent patient, *Coccidioides* causes an acute pneumonia, which is self-limited and most experts do not recommend treatment. A majority of people living in *Coccidioides* endemic areas show skin test evidence of prior infection with the fungus. Of the listed drugs, levofloxacin is an antibacterial antibiotic, and terbinafine is usually reserved for onychomycosis; only fluconazole and amphotericin are routinely used for serious fungal infections.

2. B Spherules filled with endospores are pathognomic for *Coccidioides*. Special medium can be used to induce *Coccidioides* grown in the lab to form spherules to confirm identification. A report of round encapsulated yeast would most often imply *Cryptococcus*. Acutely branching hyphae would suggest molds such as *Aspergillus* or *Pseudallescheria boydii*. (Although dimorphic fungi take the form of molds at room temperature, they usually appear as yeast in pathological specimens from tissues at body temperature.) Do not confuse bacterial cocci, such as *Staphylococcus*, with *Coccidioides*. Finally, a morula is the hallmark of ehrlichiosis.

3. C The most likely dimorphic fungus to be acquired in Arizona would be *Coccidioides*. *Histoplasma* is found in the midwest, *Blastomyces* in the southeast. *Penicillium marneffei* is another endemic dimorphic fungus that infects HIV patients in Southeast Asia. It is not found in the U.S., except in patients who have traveled to that region in the past. *Spororthrix schenkii* is yet another dimorphic fungus, but is not restricted to a specific endemic area. It lives in the dirt and classically infects gardeners, particularly those stuck by rose thorns.

Case 45

1. C Glucose-6-phosphate dehydrogenase (G6PD) deficiency is the most common enzyme deficiency in humans, with an estimated 400 million people worldwide harboring this defect. Various drugs can trigger hemolytic anemia in a G6PD-deficient state, including primaquine. Hence, G6PD levels should always be checked prior to initiating primaquine therapy for the eradication of the intrahepatic stage of *P. vivax* and *P. ovale*.

2. E Approximately 5% of native and imported malaria cases are the result of coinfection with *P. falciparum* and another *Plasmodium* species (i.e., *ovale, vivax,* or *malariae*), as the *Anopheles* mosquito can carry multiple malarial species concomitantly. It may be difficult to distinguish the different species on the patient's blood smear, however. Hence, the treatment of presumed *P. falci-*

parum almost always involves concomitant treatment for the intrahepatic stage of *P. vivax* and *P. ovale* (as seen in PF's case by the use of pyrimethamine in addition to the quinine).

Case 46

1. E Both trophozoites and cysts of *Giardia lamblia* can be identified in stool and are diagnostic of infection; however, false negatives are common. The newer stool assays for *Giardia* antigens are more sensitive than microscopic stool examination for making the diagnosis. Culture of *Giardia* is not routinely done, and serology is not helpful in making the diagnosis in acute infection.

2. C Cysts are the infectious form of *Giardia lamblia*. The other statements are true about the trophozoite stage.

Case 47

1. A The recommendations in choice (B) reflect 2001 U.S. Public Health Service guidelines. PCP occurs primarily at CD4 counts less than 200 cells/μL, but may occur at higher counts. *Pneumocystis* disseminates in only 1% to 3% of AIDS patients, but may be found in the liver, spleen, bone marrow, skin, or thyroid gland. PCP is felt to result most commonly from reactivation of latent infection, and thus isolation is not needed. However, if tuberculosis is suspected, respiratory isolation is mandatory to prevent transmission of this highly contagious pathogen.

2. C Patients with deficiencies in cell-mediated immunity are at risk of PCP. Chronic high-dose corticosteroids, CD4 cell depletion in HIV, and malnourishment in premature newborns are risk factors. CGD is an X-linked autosomal recessive that presents with recurrent infections with catalase-positive bacteria (*S. aureus, S. marsescens,* and *B. cepacia*) and fungi (*Nocardia* and *Aspergillus*) with granuloma formation.

Case 48

1. B Microscopic examination of genital secretions is a quick and efficient method of diagnosing trichomoniasis. In women, the sample is best collected from the vaginal canal during a speculum exam. In men, the organism infects the urethra and prostate, so prostate massage can increase the yield. Midstream urine culture is used to diagnosis bacterial urinary tract infection; culture of an early morning, first-voided urine sediment in men may be effective for diagnosing *Trichomonas*. Clue cells are seen in bacterial vaginosis, not trichomoniasis. Serology and ultrasound are not effective in diagnosing trichomoniasis.

2. D This patient has vulvovaginal candidiasis. It is most commonly a result of overgrowth of *Candida* spp. colonizing the genital or gastrointestinal tract. It is only rarely transmitted by sexual partners. Antibiotic use may alter the microbiological environment of the genital tract, killing bacteria and encouraging the overgrowth of yeast. PID and infertility may be sequelae of untreated chlamydia or gonorrhea, not commonly from yeast infections. RPR testing is positive in syphilis, and although evaluation for STDs may be indicated, a positive RPR is not specifically due to *Candida*. Infection with human papilloma virus, not yeast, is associated with cervical cancer.

Case 49

1. B Both *Toxoplasma* and *Plasmodia* (the agents of malaria) are blood and tissue sporozoa, obligate intracellular parasites with no organelles of locomotion. The other primary human infection with this class of organisms is *Pneumocystis carinii* pneumonia (PCP). Intestinal sporozoa include *Isospora belli* and *Cryptosporidium parvum*. *Trypanosoma cruzi*, the causative agent of Chagas disease, is a flagellated trypanosome. *Giardia* is an intestinal flagellate. *Naegleria fowleri* is a free-living amoeba that causes a rapidly progressive, usually fatal disease called primary amebic meningoencephalitis (PAM) when the organism invades directly through the nasal mucosa and cribriform plate while diving or swimming in infected fresh water. *Trichomonas* is a common motile urogenital protozoan.

2. B *Toxoplasma* is often transmitted by cat feces and undercooked lamb, beef, or pork. It is not found in fish or ticks. *Bartonella* may be transmitted from cat scratches.

Case 50

1. E All of the answers here are cestodes and may cause intestinal infection. *Diphyllobothrium latum* is acquired by eating raw freshwater fish from Scandinavia, Central Africa, or Chile. Adult tapeworms, the longest of the tapeworms causing human disease, may reach 25 m, consist of 3000–4000 proglottids, and produce over 1 million eggs per day. Patients are usually asymptomatic, although the tapeworm absorbs large quantities of vitamin B$_{12}$ and may cause megaloblastic anemia. Proglottids usually disintegrate in the intestine before being expelled, leaving only eggs in the stool. The eggs described here and epidemiological evidence presented are characteristic of *D. latum*.

2. C Echinococcal infections in humans produce cystic lesions in affected organs, most often the liver and lungs. *E. granulosis* produces unilocular cysts, whereas *E. multilocularis* produces multiloculated liver cysts. *Taenia saginata* (the beef tapeworm) and *Hymenolepis nana* (the dwarf tapeworm) are both cestodes that cause intestinal infection. *Schistosoma mansoni* is a liver fluke, a trematode that may produce liver fibrosis, but not cysts. *Onchocerca volvulus*, a nematode, is the cause of river blindness.

Case 51

1. C River blindness (onchocerca volvulus) is spread by the Simulium blackfly. The fly's preferred habitat is near fast-flowing streams, which explains the name of this illness. Ascaris, pinworm, and Guinea worm are all spread by ingestion. Hookworm may be ingested, but it can also be contracted through the skin.

2. C Trichinosis is most often contracted by eating undercooked pork, but can also be transmitted by eating undercooked walrus, bear, boar, cougar, or horse meat. Sushi lovers should beware of anisakiasis, transmitted by raw fish. Pinworm is usually transmitted by ingesting worms from another human host. Although it is an intestinal nematode, *Strongyloides* is usually transmitted through the skin, not by ingestion. Elephantiasis is spread through insect vectors.

Case 52

1. C *Paragonimus westermani* is the lung fluke. Adult worms cause nodules in the lung and occasionally brain. *Clonorchis* and *Opisthorchis* are biliary flukes. *Fasciolopsis buski* and *Schistosoma mansoni* affect the intestine and the mesenteric veins, respectively.

2. B Praziquantel opens parasite calcium channels, allowing calcium into muscle cells and causing contraction. Levamisole and pyrantel pamoate are nicotinic agonists that act at the neuromuscular junction. Other antiparasitic drugs use the other mechanisms listed. Mebendazole and albendazole affect microtubules and block transport processes. Pyrimethamine, used for malaria and toxoplasmosis, inhibits dihydrofolate reductase, an enzyme required for folate synthesis. Metronidazole kills anaerobic bacteria and certain protozoans because their anaerobic electron transport pathway metabolizes it into a toxic free radical compound.

Case 53

1. A Cardiomyopathy. Chagas disease commonly causes intestinal motility problems in the esophagus or colon by impairing smooth muscle function, but it does not cause malabsorption.

2. D *Trypanosoma brucei* is an exclusively extracellular protozoan parasite, which unlike *Trypanosoma cruzi* does not have an intracellular form. *Plasmodium* species (the agents of malaria), *Babesia*, and *Leishmania* all act intracellularly. *Pneumocystis carinii* also acts extracellularly, but is classified as a fungal rather than as a protozoan species on the basis of DNA sequence similarities.

Case 54

1. B Transplant rejection is largely a T$_h$1 division cell-mediated immunity phenomenon promoting IgG production and cytotoxic activity. In acute rejection, there are presumably no preformed antibodies or prior T-lymphocyte sensitization. Therefore, the whole process of antigen presentation, T-helper cell activation, and subsequent activation of different cells starts from the time of the transplant. Recognition of "foreignness" by T-helper cells occurs through the direct and indirect pathways of sensitization, either by recognition of foreign HLA with foreign antigen on dendritic cells carried over by transplantation or by antigen processing and presentation by endogenous antigen presenting cells of the recipient. These antigens (especially the allograft's surface MHC) activate T$_h$1-cells to release IL-2 and other cytokines that promote immune cell proliferation, B-cell IgG isotype switching, as well as

CTL and macrophage activation toward cell killing and phagocytosis. CD40L is then up-regulated in T-helper cells, which bind CD40 on B-cells, CTLs, and even dendritic cells to activate them further. TNF-α released from the site of inflammation promotes local edema by increasing vascular permeability and promoting cytotoxicity. Thus (A), (C), (D), and (E) are incorrect.

2. D Mycobacteria are eliminated by opsonization by IgG, phagocytosis, and oxidative degradation by macrophages. Without IFN-γ receptors, the IFN-γ cytokine cannot signal the activation of NADPH oxidase and inducible nitric oxide synthase (iNOS) to produce superoxide intermediates, crucial for the final elimination of phagocytized mycobacteria. IL-1 and TNF-α are responsible for acting on the hypothalamus to induce fever; thus (A) is incorrect. TCR and BCR are the receptors responsible for specific antigen recognition; thus (B) is incorrect. IFN-α and IFN-β are responsible for inducing "the antiviral state" among cells, which includes up-regulation of class I MHC to promote antigen presentation of intracellular pathogens, down-regulation of overall protein synthesis to prevent virus assembly, and increase of RNase synthesis to help degrade viral RNA. *Mycobacteria* become intracellular when phagocytized but remain outside of the cytosolic compartment and thus are not presented by class I MHC; genomic nucleic acids also consist of DNA not RNA. Thus mycobacteria are not treated like viruses during the elimination process; (C) is incorrect. Finally, IL 4 is responsible for B-cell isotype switching to IgE, which is not involved in elimination of mycobacteria; (E) is incorrect.

Case 55

1. E The hematologic abnormalities found in SLE are caused by type II cytotoxic hypersensitivity reaction against red blood cells, white blood cells, and platelets, not by immune complex deposition. Immune complex-mediated tissue injury generally results from deposition of immune complexes in tissue causing arthritis, glomerulonephritis, and vasculitis; (A) is incorrect. Antibodies against antigen at the dermo-epidermal region cause direct damage to the region resulting in the erythematous and bullous lesions of the malar rash and discoid lupus; (B) is incorrect. Chronic lung interstitial inflammation may result in diffuse crackles of pulmonary fibrosis; (C) is incorrect. SLE is associated with immune injury due to a diffuse array of antibodies, and thus the spleen may become enlarged from follicular hyperplasia and increased plasma cell activity; thus (D) is incorrect.

2. A CTLA-4 antagonizes B7 on APCs preventing the appropriate binding to CD28 on T-helper cells, thus blocking the needed second signal to allow proper activation of the immune response. This will theoretically prevent sensitization of donor T-lymphocytes against the "foreign" antigen of host tissue, thus suppressing graft-versus-host disease among bone marrow transplant recipients. All of the others are incorrect mechanisms.

Case 56

1. E Nuchal rigidity as evidenced by the Kernig's and Brudzinski's sign is the least specific of all those listed. A positive Kernig's sign

is neck pain elicited by passive knee extension with hips flexed at 90°. A positive Brudzinski's sign is neck pain elicited by passive neck flexion. Both are signs of meningeal irritation from any cause of meningitis, and do not necessarily reflect the presence of a complement deficiency. Answers (A) and (B) are incorrect, as people with complement deficiencies do have increased risk of pneumococcal and meningococcal infection. Those with terminal complement deficiencies are more likely to present with recurrent disseminated neisserial infection including meningococcal and gonococcal septicemia and meningitis. Answers (C) and (D) are incorrect as complement deficiency can present with arthritis and petechial rash, reflecting the presence of immune complex disease.

2. B People with C5 deficiencies, as well as other terminal component (MAC) complement deficiencies, are subject to recurrent neisserial infections as well as immune complex disease. However, after the first infection, the subsequent infections are often marked by less severe disease with milder symptoms such as low-grade fever, arthritis, rash, at times nephritis (associated with hematuria). This reflects the development of adaptive immunity to *Neisseria* spp. and the availability of plasma cells producing specific IgG binding extracellular bacteria forming immune complexes. Overwhelming infection and immune complex formation could surpass the body's ability to clear immune complexes leading to their deposition in joints, vessels, and glomeruli. For those with MAC deficiencies, whereas the infection is better contained, there is still a defect in the final elimination of bacteria resulting in a more indolent course due to persistent infection. Answers (A) and (D) are incorrect as both the complement cascade and natural killer cells represent parts of the innate immune system that are independent of prior exposure to pathogens. Answer (C) is incorrect as it is unknown whether this mechanism exists. Answer (E) is incorrect as these oxidative killing mechanisms exist in phagocytes and are unaffected by complement deficiencies.

Case 57

1. C This answer describes a type III immune complex-mediated hypersensitivity reaction. IG's condition is most consistent with an anaphylactic reaction, or type I immediate hypersensitivity reaction to a cashew allergen. This is mediated by mast cell-bound IgE followed by mast cell degranulation and release of several mediators rather than an immune complex disease. In this reaction, previous exposure to cashew proteins have established IgE-bound mast cells that recognize this allergen and reside in skin, respiratory, and gastrointestinal mucosal. The presence of this allergen systemically probably set off massive mast cell (and basophil) degranulation, releasing several mediators involved in immediate hypersensitivity. The presence of the allergen in the gastrointestinal tract caused local inflammation and mucosal edema resulting in nausea, vomiting, and abdominal pain. These initial symptoms are usually followed by a late-phase reaction where there is a recrudescence of symptoms due to later-onset infiltration by neutrophils, basophils, eosinophils, and monocytes recruited by the release of chemokines in this reaction. Thus (A), (B), (D), and (E) are incorrect.

2. D The fact that the rash presented the day following her exposure to the allergen suggests a type IV or delayed-type hypersensitivity reaction. This type of reaction could have occurred with either poison oak or laundry detergent. With poison oak, direct contact causes plant oils to bind some cell surface protein. This is then seen as a foreign antigen and the body will mount a cell-mediated cytotoxic immune response to this antigen. This requires hours to days to manifest itself clinically. Simple chemicals, as might be found in her laundry detergent, can also be leached into her skin, especially where she has been sweating. These can bind cell surface proteins, which are then seen as foreign to the body. Thus a cell-mediated immune response can similarly be mounted against this antigen. To decide which of these potential allergens was the culprit, one must pay attention to the distribution of the rash, which corresponds to the area covered by her clothing rather than the area that would be brushed by low-lying poison oak leaves. Therefore her laundry detergent should be the culprit. Finally, type IV hypersensitivity reactions are not histamine related as are type I hypersensitivity reactions. Thus, her rash is not likely to be alleviated by antihistamines (except for the pruritis) and instead should be treated with a general anti-inflammatory agent such as topical corticosteroids, which are effective in this type of reaction. Thus (A), (B), (C), and (E) are incorrect.

Case 58

1. E BD's past medical history suggests an intact cell-mediated immune system responsible for the delayed-type hypersensitivity reaction of poison ivy contact dermatitis and the defense against fungal infections by *Candida albicans,* the main pathogen of thrush. This, in fact, does not necessarily represent the presence of immunodeficiency, as such a history suggests a *normal physiologic* response by T-lymphocytes to poison ivy antigen and is the very immune mechanism that fights off fungal infections; (A) is incorrect. BD's disease is unrelated to mast cell- and IgE-mediated immediate hypersensitivity as suggested by (B). BD's disease is not an autoimmune disease, which represents *hyper*function of the immune system; it is, in fact, *hypo*function of the immune system; (C) is incorrect. Finally, as recurrent infection to mucosal membranes such as the respiratory tract may suggest poor defense against common mucosal pathogens, the lack of prior thrush suggests a more specific immunodeficiency in antibody production important in elimination of encapsulated bacteria like *H. influenzae.*

2. D IgA is the main immunoglobulin of secretions and serves to protect all mucosal surfaces from infection and penetration by the many microbes that pass through the lumen. The congenital absence of IgA would make one susceptible to infections at these sites, which include the gastrointestinal and respiratory tracts. Such an infection would manifest as a recurrent gastritis and diarrhea. Unfortunately, this immunodeficiency cannot be treated with intravenous immunoglobulin replacement as can IgG deficiencies.

Index